Female and Male Contraception

Female and Male Contraception

Editor: Justin McCarthy

AMERICAN
MEDICAL PUBLISHERS
www.americanmedicalpublishers.com

AMERICAN
MEDICAL PUBLISHERS
www.americanmedicalpublishers.com

Cataloging-in-Publication Data

Female and male contraception / edited by Justin McCarthy.
p. cm.
Includes bibliographical references and index.
ISBN 979-8-88740-123-2
1. Contraception. 2. Male contraception. 3. Conception. 4. Human reproduction.
5. Fertility, Human. I. McCarthy, Justin.
RG136 .F46 2023
613.94--dc23

American Medical Publishers,
41 Flatbush Avenue,
1st Floor, New York,
NY 11217, USA

ISBN 979-8-88740-123-2 (Hardback)

Contents

Preface

This book was inspired by the evolution of our times; to answer the curiosity of inquisitive minds. Many developments have occurred across the globe in the recent past which has transformed the progress in the field.

Contraception is a method of preventing pregnancy. It generally prevents the egg and sperm from fusing together, which results in pregnancy. Vaginal rings, female and male sterilization, oral contraceptive pills, intra uterine devices (IUDs), injectables, lactational amenorrhea techniques, and implants are the most common forms of contraception. These techniques work through various mechanisms and are successful in preventing and unwanted pregnancy. Condoms are the only contraceptive method that can stop a pregnancy, as well as the spread of sexually transmitted infections such as HIV. Females have a number of choices for birth control, which range from intrauterine devices and patches to pills, while males have only two effective birth control methods, namely, vasectomy and condoms. This book explores all the important aspects of female and male contraception. It consists of contributions made by international experts. This book will prove to be immensely beneficial to students and researchers in this field.

This book was developed from a mere concept to drafts to chapters and finally compiled together as a complete text to benefit the readers across all nations. To ensure the quality of the content we instilled two significant steps in our procedure. The first was to appoint an editorial team that would verify the data and statistics provided in the book and also select the most appropriate and valuable contributions from the plentiful contributions we received from authors worldwide. The next step was to appoint an expert of the topic as the Editor-in-Chief, who would head the project and finally make the necessary amendments and modifications to make the text reader-friendly. I was then commissioned to examine all the material to present the topics in the most comprehensible and productive format.

I would like to take this opportunity to thank all the contributing authors who were supportive enough to contribute their time and knowledge to this project. I also wish to convey my regards to my family who have been extremely supportive during the entire project.

Editor

1

Determinants of modern contraceptive use among sexually active men in Ethiopia: Using EDHS 2016 national survey

Tamrat Shaweno[1*] and Zerihun Kura[2]

Abstract

Background: Recently, the focus of family planning programs has changed from female oriented to men oriented, or both partner oriented to have effective outcomes. Although, contraceptive use among sexually active women was exhaustively researched; there is still a huge gap on modern contraceptive use and its determinants among sexually active men in Ethiopia.

Objectives: We assessed the determinants of contraceptive use among sexually active men in Ethiopia using national survey data.

Method: The data source for this study was the 2016's Ethiopian Demographic and Health Survey of men aged above 15–59 years. We analyzed data of 12, 688 sexually active men in the past 12 months prior to the survey using STATA version 14.1. Bivariate and multivariable multinomial logistic regression analysis was conducted and statistical significance was set at p value < 0.05.

Result: From a total of 12, 688 sexually active men in Ethiopia, 9378 (73.9%) didn't use any modern contraception or use traditional methods, 2394 (18.9%) use partner methods for those who reported using a method through their partner (such as pill, IUD, injections, female sterilization and Norplant) and the rest 916 (7.2%) used male methods for those who reported using male only methods (such as condoms and male sterilization). In the adjusted multinomial logistic regression model, men's age categories 25–34 years (AOR:2.0; 95%CI = 1.5–2.5), 35–44 (AOR: 2.8; 95%CI = (2.0–3.8), and 45$^+$ years (AOR: 1.5; 95%CI = 1.0–2.6), being rural resident (AOR: 1.60; (95%CI = 1.3–2.2), married and living with partner (AOR: 0.03; (95%CI = 0.01–0.06), who attended secondary (AOR:1.2; (95%CI = 0.8–1.9) and higher (AOR: 1.4; (95%CI = 1.2–2.5) education, whose partner was working (AOR: 1.6; (95%CI = 1.3–2.2), having three and above children (AOR: 0.5; (95%CI = 0.3–0.8), reading newspaper/ magazines at least once a week or less than once a week, listening to radio at least once a week, watching television at least once a week and watching television less than once a week were significantly associated with use of male method than traditional/no method as compared to their respective references.

Conclusion: Modern contraceptive use among sexually active men in Ethiopia is low and multiple factors determined it. Close monitoring and supporting of sexually active men with age above 25 years, rural background, higher educational level, whose partner was working, having three and more children and little exposure to media may increase men's use of modern contraceptives.

Keywords: Modern contraceptive, Male method, EDHS 2016, Ethiopia

* Correspondence: babiynos@gmail.com
[1]Department of Epidemiology, Faculty of Public Health, Jimma University, Jimma, Ethiopia

Introduction

The importance of modern contraceptive use is now well recognized, not only to improve women and child health, but also to contribute to related issues such as gender equality, better child health, an improved response to HIV, greater education outcomes and poverty reduction [1]. To reaffirm the promise of universal access to reproductive health and family planning, the international community is giving special attention to regions and countries lagging behind [1–3]. Huge gaps exist in demand for family planning satisfied with modern contraceptives in countries where overall contraceptive use is low or where many sexually active groups rely on traditional methods of contraception [2, 3]. At the end of 2015, less than half of total demand for contraceptives was being met with modern methods in 54 countries (of which more than 60% are in Africa) [4]. Between 2015 and 2030, the time period of the 2030 Agenda for Sustainable Development, contraceptive use is projected to increase particularly in countries where less than half of reproductive age groups currently use contraception [4]. In line with this vision, Ethiopia has committed to increase the modern contraceptive prevalence rate from 35% to 55% amongst married women by 2020 and reducing the total fertility rate from 4.6 to 3.0 [5]. Family planning programs have traditionally focused primarily on women; men being over looked and given lesser attention [6]. Although, some studies have highlighted the influence of men on reproductive decisions such as contraceptive use, still information is scarce with regard to contraceptive use among sexually active men [6, 7]. Men, particularly in male-controlled contexts, play a great role in influencing fertility choices [8]. However, male involvement in family planning remains limited [9, 10]. In addition, research examining determinants of couples' modern contraceptive use has ignored men's crucial role [11, 12], which has eventually resulted in underlining the idea of contraceptive use as women's concern, leaving little or no role for men [13–15]. It was observed [16] that men, particularly in low socio economic settings, prefer large numbers of children both as a source of labor and profitable gain, and as a source of respect. Men's role as central decision makers, are believed to determine men's and couples' use of contraceptives [17, 18]. A men's agreement of the use of contraception is a key for effective family planning programs [19, 20]. A study illustrated that men had complete decision making supremacy and the ability to result in compliance or submission from their partners [16].

Even though, different family planning programs excluded the participation of men [20, 21], in recent years, efforts are ongoing to extend men's participation in reproductive health and use of contraceptives [22]. Findings indicated that discussion of family planning with a health worker, region, education, wealth index, number of surviving children and fertility preference were most significantly associated with modern contraceptive use among men [23, 24]. Studies from different parts of Ethiopia indicated that, over 90% of men supported and approved of using family planning; however, 36% of men didn't know about male contraceptive methods [25, 26]. But, to advocate including men in contraceptive programs, information is still scarce on determinants of modern contraceptive use among men in Ethiopia [23, 24]. Moreover, the variations of modern contraceptive use among sexually active men in Ethiopia by different variables including socio-economic characteristics, interaction with health system and access to media, and behavioral and attitudinal factors remains limited. We hypothesized that, socio-demographic factors, interaction with health system, access to media and behavioral/attitudinal factors influence modern contraceptive use among sexually active men in Ethiopia. A better understanding of determinants of modern contraceptive use among sexually active men in Ethiopia could be helpful to develop intervention strategies relevant to Ethiopia. Therefore, this study aimed to explore determinant factors that influence modern contraceptive use among sexually active men in Ethiopia using 2016 EDHS national survey data.

Methods

Study design and data set

The data set used for this study was obtained from 2016 Ethiopian Demographic Health Surveys conducted from January 18, 2016 to June 27, 2016, across the country. The survey was a population-based cross-sectional study and it is available from the MEASURE DHS database at https://dhsprogram.com/data/available-datasets.cfm. For the surveys, there were two stages. In the first stage, the total of 645 clusters (202 in urban and 443 in rural) were randomly selected proportional to the household size from the sampling strata and in the second stage, 28 households per cluster were selected using systematic random sampling. The sample allocations were derived with information obtained from the 2011 EDHS. From a total of 16, 533 men, 14, 176 were eligible for an interview. A total of 12,688 eligible men were interviewed yielding a response rate of 89.5% [27]. Data were weighted to adjust for differences in probability of selection and to adjust for non-response. Our analysis was restricted to the 12, 688 (weighted) men who reported being sexually active in the 12 months prior to the survey and we excluded men who reported that either them or their partners were infecund.

Study variables

The outcome variable for this study was modern contraceptive use. We categorized modern contraceptive use into three outcome categories. These included:

'traditional/no method' for those who reported current use of traditional or natural methods (like periodic abstinence, lactational amenorrhea and use of withdrawal method) or not using modern contraceptive methods which are ineffective in pregnancy prevention; 'partner method' for those who reported use of a method by their partner (like injections, pills, IUD, norplant, female sterilization and); and 'male method', for those who reported using male only methods (like male sterilization and condom use). The explanatory variables were grouped into five categories to see their influence on modern contraceptive use. These included socio-demographic variables (age, residence, number of children and marital status), socio-economic factors (wealth index, education and current working status of the partner), interaction with health system (discussed family planning with health worker), access to media (frequency of reading newspaper/magazine, frequency of listening to radio, frequency of watching TV) and behavioral/attitudinal factors (belief that women who use contraceptive become promiscuous and belief that contraception is a women's business).

Statistical analysis

Bivariate analyses were done to assess the association between predictor variables and outcome variable of the study using X^2 tests. We selected multinomial logistic regression because it is the most suitable for the study of the outcome with three categories. Four multinomial regression models were fitted in this study. In model I we included socio demographic and partners' working status while controlling for other covariates. Model II included socio-demographic variables, partners' working status and total children ever born while controlling for the wealth index variables and variables related to media. Model III included socio demographic variables, partners' working status, total number of children ever born and wealth index while controlling for access to media. In the final model all explanatory variables were included into the model. All analyses were weighted to account for differences in sampling probabilities. Those predictor variables significantly associated with outcome variable were included in the multivariable logistic regression model in which the odds ratio with 95% confidence intervals was estimated to identify the predictors of modern contraceptive use (male method) in Ethiopia. A *p*-value less than 0.05 were employed to declare the statistical significance.

Result

Characteristics of the study participants

From a total of 12, 688 sexually active men in Ethiopia, 9378 (73.9%) didn't use any contraception or use traditional methods, 2394 (18.9%) use partner methods and the rest 916 (7.2%) did use male methods. Approximately, more than one third (35%) of the sexually active men were in the age group 15–24 years and more than two third (69.5%) were from the rural community. Wirth regard to marital status, more than half (56.8%) of men were married and living in marital union. Only few 1607 (12.7%) of the respondents achieved higher education whereas, majority of the respondents attended primary education. Slightly, four men out of five (83.5%) were currently working and majority have no child at the time of the survey (46.3%). With regard to interaction with the health system, exactly three fourth of the respondents didn't discuss about contraception with the health care provider. Only, about 33.9% were categorized as richest in economic class whereas, the rest 15.2, 13.7, 14.3 and 22.9% were richer, middle, poorer and poorest, respectively. With regard to behavioral factors, more than four-fifth disagree that women who use contraceptive become promiscuous and contraception is a women's business [Table 1].

Prevalence of modern contraceptive use among sexually active men

The prevalence of modern contraceptive use in relation to selected socio-demographic characteristics, behavioral factors and access to media was illustrated in Table 2. Concerning the socio-economic characteristics, a significant positive association was observed between age and use of contraceptive partner method. Sexually active men aged between 25 and 34 years (COR:1.6; 95%CI = 1.4–1.9), $P < 0.001$)), 35–44 years (COR:0.7; 95%CI = (0.6–0.9), $P < 0.001$)), and aged above 45 years (COR:0.3; 95%CI = (0.2–0.4), $p < 0.001$)), were more likely to use a partner method compared to none /traditional method users, respectively. On the contrary, men above 35 years (COR:5.9; 95%CI = 5.1–6.8), $P < 0.001$)), were less likely to use a male method than traditional or no method, compared to those men in the age group 15–24 years. Men with urban residence were more likely to use both a partner method (COR:1.5; 95%CI = (1.3–1.6), $P = 0.007$)), and male method (COR:7.5; 95%CI = (6.4–8.7), $P < 0.001$)) compared to those men with rural residence. Married men either living (COR:7.8; 95%CI = (6.- 9.0), $P < 0.001$)) or not living with the partner (COR:7.8; 95%CI = (5.9–10.3), $P < 0.001$)) were more than seven times to report use of a partner method and married men living with the partner (COR:0.1; 95%CI = (0.08–0.12), $P < 0.001$)) were less likely to use a male method compared to traditional method users or non-users. Men with primary (COR:3.8; 95%CI = (2.8–5.3), $P < 0.001$)), secondary (COR:11.7; 95%CI = (8.5–16.2), $P < 0.001$)), and; higher and above (COR: 23.2; 95%CI = (16.8–32.0), $P < 0.001$)) educational status were more likely to use male method than traditional method or non-use of any method compared to those with no

Table 1 Sample characteristics of sexually active men 15–59 years in Ethiopia (2016 EDHS) (weighted)

Characteristics	Number (N)	Percent (%)
Contraceptive use		
None/Traditional methods	9378	73.9
vPartner methods	2394	18.9
Male methods	916	7.2
Socio-demographic factors		
Age		
45^+	1979	15.6%
35–44	2592	20.4%
25–34	3615	28.5%
15–24	4502	35.5%
Residence		
Urban	3866	30.5%
Rural	8822	69.5%
Marital status		
Ever married but not together	375	3.0%
Married and living with partner	7208	56.8%
Never union	5105	40.2%
Education level of respondents		
Higher	1607	12.7%
Secondary	2233	17.6%
Primary	5331	42.0%
no education	3517	27.7%
Current working		
Yes	10,595	83.5%
No	2093	16.5%
Total children over born		
3 and above	4689	37.0%
1-2 children	2126	16.8%
no child	5873	46.3%
Socio-economics factors		
Wealth index		
Poorest	2908	22.9%
Poorer	1810	14.3%
Middle	1739	13.7%
Richer	1925	15.2%
Richest	4306	33.9%
Interaction with health system		
Discussed FP with health worker		
Yes	3159	24.9%
No	9529	75.1%
Access to media		
Frequency of reading newspaper/magazine		
At least once a week	1350	10.6%
less than once a week	2466	19.4%
not at all	8872	69.9%
Frequency of listening to radio		
At least once a week	3793	29.9%
less than once a week	3046	24.0%
not at all	5849	46.1%
Frequency of watching TV		
At least once a week	3433	27.1%
less than once a week	3040	24.0%
not at all	6215	49.0%
Behavioral/attitudinal factors		
Women who use contraceptive become promiscuous		
Don't know	796	6.3%
Agree	1262	9.9%
Disagree	10,630	83.8%
Number of wives/partners		
Two and more wives	472	3.7%
one wife	6736	53.1%
No wife	5480	43.2%
Contraception is a women's business		
Don't know	690	5.4%
Agree	1145	9.0%
Disagree	10,853	85.5%

*TV Television

registered educational status. Similarly, men with the same educational status were more likely to use partner method too, but the odds of use of male method are significantly higher compared to partner method. Men having one or two child (COR:6.6; 95%CI = (5.8–7.5), $P < 0.001$)); and three or more children (COR:3.5; 95%CI = (3.1–3.9), $P < 0.001$)) were more likely to use partner method but less likely to use a male method compared to those men with no children. Men from economic classes of richer (COR: 0.2; 95%CI = (16.8–32.0), $P < 0.001$)), middle (COR: 0.1; 95%CI = (0.1–0.2), $P < 0.001$), poorer (COR: 0.1; 95%CI = (0.1–0.2), $P < 0.001$), and poorest (COR: 0.1; 95%CI = (0.1–0.2), $P < 0.001$) were less likely to use male method as compared richest men. Men who discussed FP (family planning) with health worker (COR: 2.4; 95%CI = (2.2–2.7), $P < 0.001$) were more than two times to use a partner method compared to use traditional methods/no methods. Conversely, these men were less likely to use a male method than traditional or no use of any method compared to those who didn't discuss about FP with health worker (COR: 0.8; 95%CI = (0.7–1.0), $P < 0.001$). Men who agreed that, women who use contraceptive becomes

Table 2 Bivariate association between modern contraceptive use and various background characteristics, EDHS 2016, Ethiopia (weighted)

Characteristics	Partner method vs. none/traditional method			Male method vs. none/traditional method		
Age respondents	COR	*P*-value	%CI	COR	*P*-value	%CI
45+	3.7	0.001	3.2–4.4	0.3	0.001	0.2–0.4
35–44	5.9	0.001	5.1–6.8	0.7	0.001	0.6–0.9
25–34	5.3	0.001	4.6-, 6.1	1.6	0.001	1.4–1.9
15–24	0[b]			0[b]		
Residence						
Urban	1.5	0.077	1.3–1.6	7.5	0.001	6.4–8.7
Rural	0[b]			0[b]		
Marital status						
Ever married but not together	7.8	0.001	5.9–10.3	1.7	0.001	1.3–2.3
Married and living with partner	7.8	0.001	6.7–8.9	0.1	0.001	0.1–0.2
Never union	0[b]			0[b]		
Education of respondents						
Higher and above	2.0	0.001	1.7–2.3	23.2	0.001	6.9–32.0
Secondary	1.0	0.639	0.9–1.2	11.7	0.001	8.5–16.2
Primary	1.0	0.824	0.9–1.1	3.8	0.001	2.8–5.3
None	0[b]			0[b]		
Current working						
Yes	6.0	0.001	4.8–7.4	1.3	0.007	1.1–1.5
No	0[b]			0[b]		
Total children over born						
3 and above	3.5	0.001	3.1–3.9	0.1	0.099	0.1, 0.2
1–2 children	6.6	0.001	5.8–7.5	0.5	0.595	0.4–0.5
No child	0[b]			0[b]		
Socio-economics factors						
Wealth index						
Poorest	0.3	0.001	0.2–0.6	0.1	0.001	0.1–0.2
Poorer	0.7	0.001	0.6, 0.8	0.1	0.001	0.1–0.2
Middle	0.9	0.164	0.8–1.0	0.1	0.001	0.1–0.2
Richer	1.0	0.687	0.9–1.1	0.2	0.001	0.2–0.3
Richest	0[b]			0[b]		
Interaction with health system						
Discussed FP with health worker						
Yes	2.4	0.001	2.2–2.7	0.8	0.031	0.7–1.0
No	0[b]			0[b]		
Access to media						
Frequency of reading newspaper/magazine						
At least once a week	2.0	0.001	1.7–2.3	5.1	0.001	4.3–6.2
Less than once a week	1.634	0.001	1.5–1.8	3.7	0.001	3.2–4.4
Not at all	0[b]			0[b]		
Frequency of listening to radio						
At least once a week	2.0	0.001	1.8–2.3	4.7	0.001	4.0–5.6
Less than once a week	1.323	0.001	1.2–1.5	2.5	0.001	2.1–3.1

Table 2 Bivariate association between modern contraceptive use and various background characteristics, EDHS 2016, Ethiopia (weighted) *(Continued)*

Characteristics	Partner method vs. none/traditional method			Male method vs. none/traditional method		
Age respondents	COR	*P*-value	%CI	COR	*P*-value	%CI
Not at all	0^b			0^b		
Frequency of watching TV						
At least once a week	2.2	0.001	2.0–2.5	9.7	0.001	2.5–11.8
Less than once a week	1.9	0.001	1.7–2.1	3.6	0.001	2.1, 4.6
Not at all	0^b			0^b		
Behavioral/attitudinal factors						
Women who use contraceptive become promiscuous						
Don't know	0.2	0.001	0.1–0.3	0.1	0.001	0.1–0.2
Agree	0.8	0.002	0.7–0.9	0.7	0.016	0.6–0.9
Disagree	0^b			0^b		
Number of wives/partners						
Two and more wives	3.2	0.001	2.5–4.1	0.2	0.001	0.01–0.13
One wife	6.0	0.001	5.3–6.8	0.1	0.001	0.1–0.2
No wife	0^b			0^b		
Contraception is a women's business						
Don't know	0.1	0.001	0.1–0.2	0.2	0.001	0.1–0.3
Agree	0.8	0.010	0.7–1.0	0.5	0.001	0.4–0.7
Disagree	0^b			0^b		

**COR* adjusted odds ratio, *CI* confidence interval, 0^b reference category, *FP* family planning *TV* television

promiscuous were less likely to use a partner method (COR: 0.8; 95%CI = (0.7–0.9)), $P < 0.002$) or a male method (COR: 0.7; 95%CI = (0.6–0.9), $P < 0.016$) than use of traditional method /no method as compared to men who disagreed to the thought that, women who use contraceptive become promiscuous. (For details see Table 2).

Determinants of modern contraceptive use among sexually active men

In the adjusted multinomial logistic regression model, age of men, residence, marital status, partners working, number of ever born children, access to media, frequency of listening to radio and frequency of watching TV were significantly associated with use of male method than partner method compared to use of traditional method / no method. Men aged above 25 years were less likely to report use of partner method than use of traditional /no method compared to men whose age 15–24 years. Contrariwise, these men were less likely to use partner method than use of traditional/no method compared to men aged 15–24 years. Men aged 25–34 years (AOR: 2.0; 95%CI = (1.5–2.5), 35–44 years (AOR: 2.8; 95%CI = (2.0–3.8)), and 45^+ years (AOR: 1.5; 95%CI = (1.0–2.6)) were approximately, 2.0 ($p = 0.004$), 3.0 ($p < 0.01$) and 1.5 times ($p < 0.01$) more likely to use male methods than traditional /no method respectively, compared to men aged 15–24 years. Men with urban residence were nearly two times more likely to use male method than traditional/no methods compared to men from rural residence (AOR: 1.60; (95%CI = 1.3–2.2), ($p <$ 0.001)). Men who were ever married and living with the partner were 0.03 times, ($p < 0.001$) less likely to use male method than traditional/no method compared to men not in marital union (AOR: 0.03; (95%CI = 0.01–0.06)), ($p < 0.001$)). Men whose educational status was secondary (AOR: 1.2; (95%CI = 0.8–1.9), ($p < 0.024$)) and higher (AOR: 1.4; (95%CI = 1.2–2.5), ($p < 0.001$)) were significantly associated with use of male method than traditional /no method compared to men who didn't attend formal education. There were no significant associations observed among partner method users of similar educational category. Men whose partners' work was significantly associated with use of male method (AOR: 1.6; (95%CI = 1.3–2.2), ($p < 0.001$)) than traditional /no method as compared to men whose partners were not working. Having one or two child was not significantly associated with use male method (AOR: 1.2; (95%CI = 0.8–1.8), ($p > 0.050$)) than traditional/no method as compared to men having no children. Men having more than three and above children were 0.5 times less likely to use male method than traditional/ no method as compared to men having no children (AOR: 0.5; (95%CI = 0.3–0.8), ($p < 0.001$)).

With regard to access to media, men reading newspaper /magazine at least once a week (AOR: 1.4; (95%CI = 1.1–1.7), ($p < 0.001$)) and below once a week (AOR: 1.5; (95%CI = 1.2–1.8), ($p < 0.001$)) were more than 1.5 times more likely to use male method than traditional methods as compared to men not reading newspaper /magazine at all. Similarly, men listening to radio at least once a week were more likely to use male method (AOR: 1.5; (95%CI = 1.2–1.9), ($p < 0.002$)) than traditional /no method as compared to men not listening to radio at all. Men watching TV at least once a week (AOR: 1.9; (95%CI = 1.5–2.4), ($p < 0.001$)) and below once a week (AOR: 1.5; (95%CI = 1.1–1.9), ($p < 0.003$)) were approximately two times more likely to use male method than traditional /no method as compared to men not watching TV at all [Table 3].

Discussion

Currently, provision of safe, effective and affordable modern contraceptive methods is emphasized to achieve high levels of demand satisfied for family planning through addressing both women's and men's sexual and reproductive health needs [28]. This study illustrated determinants of modern contraceptive use among sexually active men in Ethiopia using EDHS 2016 national survey. In the final model a total of eight variables showed significant association with modern contraceptive use among sexually active men. In this study, age categories of 25–34 and 35–44 were more likely to use male method or partner method than traditional/no method as compared to men in the age categories of 15–24 years' age. Compared to studies from Kenya [29] and Tanzania [30] this finding is not consistent in which men aged 25 years and above were less likely to report use of a partner method than use of a traditional/no method compared to those under 25 years. Part of explanation for this variation could be the increased awareness of youth reproductive health in Ethiopia might have increased the uptake of male method too. With regard to residence; men residing in the urban part of the country were more likely to use male method than traditional/ no method as compared to men residing in rural part of Ethiopia. Compared to studies from Kenya [29], and Nigeria [31], this finding was consistent in which men from rural community were less likely to use male method than traditional /no method as compared to men from urban. But, it was inconsistent to a study [32] in which residents of rural community were more likely to use modern contraceptives. In this study, men married and living with their partner were less likely to use male method than traditional /no method as compared to men not in marital union at all. Although, we didn't find related literature on this part, our explanation for this could be men living with their partner might have full confidence and trust with their partner so that they can be negligible in use of male method. Concerning to educational status, men who attended secondary and higher education were more likely to use male method than traditional /no method as compared to men who didn't attend any education. Compared to studies from Uganda [23, 32], this finding is consistent in that men with secondary and above level of education were more likely to use modern contraceptives.

Men, whose partners were currently working, were more likely to use partner method or male method than traditional/no method as compared to men whose partners were not currently working. Compared to studies from other settings, this finding was consistent with the study from Nigeria [33] and in which men whose partners were currently working were more likely to utilize modern contraceptives.

In this study, men with number of ever born children equals three or more were less likely to use male method than traditional/no method compared to men without children. Compared to other studies [33], this finding was not consistent in that men with increasing number of children were more likely to use modern contraceptives. The difference can be explained from, men with large family size in Ethiopia may fear to have additional number of children due to economic and social problems, thus they might prefer to use contraceptives.

With respect to access to media, the frequency of reading newspapers/magazines, frequency of listening to radio and frequency of watching TV showed significant association with use of modern contraceptive. Men who read newspapers/magazines at least once or below once a week were more likely to use male method than traditional/no method as compared to men who didn't read newspapers/magazines at all. Similarly, men who listen to radio at least once a week were more likely to use male method than traditional/no method compared to men who didn't listen to radio at all. In the same fashion, men who watch TV at least once or less than once a week were more likely to use partner method or male method than traditional/no method as compared to men who didn't listen to radio or watch TV at all. As we compare to other findings [29, 30], these findings were consistent.

Unlike other studies done so far, wealth index [23, 31, 32], were not independently associated with modern contraceptive use in this study. The explanation can be from differences in study setting, sample size, study design and definitions.

Conclusions

In this study, we considered multiple factors that contributed to modern contraceptive use among sexually active men in Ethiopia. Men with advanced age and urban

Table 3 Multivariate association between modern contraceptive use and various background characteristics, EDHS 2016, Ethiopia (weighted)

Characteristics	Model I		Model II		Model III		Model IV	
Age respondents	aOR	%CI	aOR	%CI	aOR	%CI	aOR	%CI
45+	1.9	1.3–3.0	1.7	1.2–2.9	1.6	1.1–2.8	1.5	1.0–2.6
35–44	3.2	2.3–4.3	3.1	2.2–4.2	3.0	2.2–4.1	2.8	2.0–3.8
25–34	2.3	1.9–2.7	2.2	1.8–2.7	2.1	1.7–2.6	2.0	1.5–2.5
15–24	0^b		0^b		0^b		0^b	
Residence								
Urban	2.0	1.6–2.5	1.9	1.5–2.4	1.8	1.4–2.3	1.6	1.3–2.2
Rural	0^b		0^b					
Marital status								
Ever married but not together	1.2	0.8–1.9	1.1	0.7–1.7	1.0	0.7–1.8	0.9	0.6–1.4
Married and living with partner	0.1	0.06–0.1	0.1	0.05–0.09	0.04	0.03–0.08	0.03	0.01–0.06
Never union	0b		0b		0^b		0^b	
Education level								
Higher	2.1	1.5–3.1	1.8	1.4–3.0	1.6	1.3–2.8	1.4	1.2–2.5
Secondary	1.5	1.1–2.2	1.4	1.1–2.1	1.3	1.0–2.0	1.2	0.8–1.9
Primary	1.3	0.9–1.8	0.9	0.8–1.7	0.8	0.7–1.6	0.6	0.6–1.4
No education	0^b		0^b		0^b		0^b	
Partners working status								
Yes	2.0	1.6–2.5	1.8	1.5–2.4	1.7	1.4–2.3	1.6	1.3–2.2
No	0b							
Total children ever born								
3 and above			0.3	0.1–0.6	0.4	0.2–0.7	0.5	0.3–0.8
1–2 children			0.9	0.6–1.5	1.1	0.7–1.7	1.2	0.8–1.8
No child			0^b		0^b		0^b	
Wealth index								
Rich					1.2	0.8–1.6	1.3	0.9–1.7
Medium					0.6	0.4–1.1	0.8	0.5–1.2
Poor					–		–	
Discussed **FP with health worker**								
Yes							0.7	0.6–0.8
No							0^b	
Access to media								
Frequency of reading newspaper /magazine								
At least once a week							1.4	1.1–1.7
Less than once a week							1.5	1.2–1.8
Not at all							0^b	
Frequency of listening Radio								
At least once a week							1.5	1.2–1.9
Less than once a week							1.3	0.9–1.6
Not at all							0^b	
Frequency of watching TV								
At least once a week							1.9	1.5–2.4
Less than once a week							1.5	1.1–1.9
Not at all							0^b	

******aOR* adjusted odds ratio, *CI* confidence interval, 0^b reference category, *TV* television

residence were more likely to use modern contraceptives. In addition, men who were married and living with their spouse and men with educational level of secondary or higher were more likely to use modern contraceptives. The increasing number of ever born children was also positively associated with modern contraceptive use among sexually active men. Lastly, an exposure to sensitizing medias including newspaper, radio and TV increased the likelihood of modern contraceptive use among sexually active men in Ethiopia.

Thus, close monitoring and follow up of sexually active men with the above identified risk factors is highly recommended. Moreover, reproductive health programs aiming to increase uptake of modern contraceptives in this population of sexually active men in Ethiopia should consider the importance of men education and ensure access to media particularly, newspapers, radio and television.

Abbreviations

CI: Confidence Interval; EDHS: Ethiopian Demographic Health Survey; AOR: Adjusted Odds Ratio; MEASURE DHS: Monitoring and Evaluation to Assess and Use Results Demographic and Health Surveys

Acknowledgements

The authors would like to acknowledge that the Ethiopian Demographic and Health Survey 2016 data used in this study were obtained from the DHS office; they have given permission to access the data, after we have prepared the proposal on the title.

Authors' contributions

TS: Conceived the study ideas, design, and analyzed data and wrote the draft manuscript; TS and ZK participated in the study design, edited the manuscript and contributed to the final analysis. Both authors read and approved the final manuscript.

Author details

[1]Department of Epidemiology, Faculty of Public Health, Jimma University, Jimma, Ethiopia. [2]Biostatistics Unit, Department of Epidemiology, Faculty of Public Health, Jimma University, Jimma, Ethiopia.

References

1. UNFPA. 2016. Universal Access to Reproductive Health. *PROGRESS AND CHALLENGES*, 2016. United Nations Population Fund 605 Third Avenue New York, NY 10158 www.unfpa.org.
2. Agyemang J, et al. Contraceptive use and associated factors among sexually active female adolescents in Atwima Kwanwoma District, Ashanti region-Ghana. Pan Afr Med J. 2019;32:182. https://doi.org/10.11604/pamj.2019.32.182.15344.
3. Prata N, Fraser A, Huchko MJ, Gipson JD, Withers M, Lewis S, et al. Womens empowerment and family planninig: a review of the literature. J Biosoc Sci. 2017:1–31. https://doi.org/10.1017/s0021932016000663 PubMed PMID: 28069078; PubMed Central PMCID: PMCEmpowerment. Epub 2017/01/11.
4. United Nations, Department of Economic and Social Affairs, Population Division (2015). Trends in Contraceptive Use Worldwide 2015(ST/ESA/SER.A/349).
5. FMOH. (Ethiopia). Costed implementation plan for family planning in Ethiopia, 2015/16–2020. Addis Ababa; 2016.
6. Ochako R, Mbondo M, Aloo S, Kaimenyi S, Thompson R, Temmerman M, Kays M. Barriers to modern contraceptive methods uptake among young women in Kenya: a qualitative study. BMC Public Health. 2015;15:118.
7. Gordon C. Women's Education and Modern Contraceptive Use in Ethiopia. Int J Educ ISSN 1948–5476. 2011;3(1):E9.
8. Kofi J. Modern contraceptive use among women in the Asuogyaman District of Ghana: is reliability more important than health concerns? Afr J Reprod Health La Revue Africaine de la Santé Reproductive. 2013;17(2):58–71.
9. Seyife A,Fisseha G,Yebyo H,Gidey G, Gerensea H (2019) Utilization of modern contraceptives and predictors among women in Shimelba refugee camp, northern Ethiopia. PLoS One 14(3):e0212262.dpi: https://doi.org/10.1371/ journal.pone.
10. Yemaneh Y, Birie B. Assessment of knowledge, attitude and utilization of long acting family planning method among women of reproductive age Groupe in Mizan-Aman Twon, bench-Majizone, south West Ethiopia, 2016. Integr J Glob Health. 2017;1:2.
11. Ditekemena J, Koole O, EngmannC MR, Tshefu A, Ryder R, Colebunders R. Determinants of male involvement in maternal and child health services in sub-Saharan Africa: a review. Reprod Health. 2012;9(1):32.
12. David J. Piller. A. Ethiopia: an emerging family planning success story. Stud Fam Plan. 2013;44(4):445–59.
13. USAID. Trends and Determinants of Contraceptive Use among Young Married Women (Age 15–24) Based on the 2000, 2005, and 2011 Ethiopian Demographic and Health Surveys: A Multivariate Decomposition Analysis. 2014. 103; Rockville.
14. Osuafor GN, Maputle SM, Ayiga N. Factors related to married or cohabiting women's decision to use modern contraceptive methods in Mahikeng, South Africa. Afr J Prm Health Care Med. 2018;10(1):a1431. https://doi.org/10.4102/ phcfm.v10i1.1431.
15. Laune F, Alex C. Decision-making patterns and contraceptive use: evidence from Uganda. Popul Res Policy Rev. 2010;29(3):423–39 https://www.jstor.org/stable/40608408.
16. Solanke, et al. Maternal grand multiparity and intention to use modern contraceptives in Nigeria. BMC Public Health. 2018;18:1207. https://doi.org/10.1186/s12889-018-6130-1.
17. Eshete A, Adissu Y. Women's Joint Decision on Contraceptive Use in Gedeo Zone, Southern Ethiopia: A Community Based Comparative Cross-Sectional Study. Int J Fam Med. 2017, Article ID 9389072,9 pages. https://doi.org/10.1155/2017/9389072.
18. de Vargas Nunes Coll C, Ewerling F, Hellwig F, et al. Contraception in adolescence: the influence of parity and marital status on contraceptive use in 73 low-and middle-income countries. Reprod Health. 2019;16:21–33.
19. Mussie A, Tefera B, Tizta T: Factors associated with utilization of long acting and permanent contraceptive methods among married women of reproductive age in Mekelle town, Tigray Ethiopia. BMC Pregnancy Childbirth; 2012.
20. Eshete A, Adissu Y. Women's Joint Decision on Contraceptive Use in Gedeo Zone, Southern Ethiopia: A Community Based Comparative Cross-Sectional Study. Int J Fam Med. 2017;2017, Article ID 9389072:9. https://doi.org/10.1155/2017/9389072.
21. Adelekan A, Omoregie P, Edoni E. Male Involvement in Family Planning: Challenges and Way Forward. Int J Popul Res. 2014;2014(416457):9. https://doi.org/10.1155/ 2014/416457.
22. Geleta D, Birhanu Z, Kaufman M, Temesgen B. Gender norms and family planning decision-making among married men and women, rural Ethiopia: a qualitative study. Sci J Public Health. 2015;3(2):242–50 Retrieved from http://www.sciencepublishinggroup.com/journal/paperinfo.aspx?journalid=251&doi=10.11648/j.sjph.20150302.23.
23. Kabagenyi A, Jennings L, Reid A, Nalwadda G, Ntozi J, Atuyambe L. Barriers to male involvement in contraceptive uptake and reproductive health services: a qualitative study of men and women's perceptions in two rural districts in Uganda. Reprod Health. 2014;11:21.
24. Kabagenyi A, Ndugga P, Wandera Stephen O, Kwagala B. Modern contraceptive use among sexually active men in Uganda: does discussionwith a health worker matter? BMC Public Health. 2014;14:286.
25. Alemayehu B. Assessment of male involvement in family planning use among men in south eastern zone of Tigray, Ethiopia. Scholarly J Med. 2012;2(2):1–10.
26. Kassa M, Abajobir Alemu A, Gedefaw M. Level of male involvement and associated factors in family planning services utilization among married men in Debre Markos town, Northwest Ethiopia. BMC Int Health Hum Rights. 2014;14:33.
27. Central Statistical Agency (CSA) [Ethiopia] and ICF. Ethiopia Demographic and Health Survey 2016. Addis Ababa: CSA and ICF; 2016.

28. USAID/MEASURE EVALUATION. Male Engagement in Family Planning Gaps in Monitoring and Evaluation September 2017; North Carolina, USA.
29. Ochako, et al. Determinants of modern contraceptive use among sexually active men in Kenya. Reprod Health. 2017;14:56. https://doi.org/10.1186/s12978-017-0316-3.
30. Nsanya MK, Atchison CJ, Bottomley C, et al. Modern contraceptive use among sexually active women aged 15–19 years in North-Western Tanzania: results from the Adolescent 360 (A360) baseline survey. BMJ Open. 2019;9:e030485. https://doi.org/10.1136/ bmjopen-2019-030485.
31. Fagbamigbe AF, et al. Demand and unmet needs of contraception among sexually active in-union women in Nigeria: distribution, associated characteristics, barriers, and program implications. SAGE Open. 2018:1–11. https://doi.org/10.1177/2158244017754023 journals.sagepub.com/home/sgo.
32. Hounton S, et al. Patterns and trends of contraceptive use among sexually active adolescents in Burkina Faso, Ethiopia, and Nigeria: evidence from cross-sectional studies. Glob Health Action. 2015;8:29737. https://doi.org/10.3402/gha.v8.29737.
33. Oginni AB, Ahonsi BA, Adebajo S. Trend and Determinants of Unmet Need for Family Planning Services among Currently Married Women and Sexually Active Unmarried Women Aged 15–49 in Nigeria (2003—2013). Afr Popul Stud. 2015;29(1) http://aps.journals.ac.za.

2

Assessment of emergency contraceptives utilization and associated factors among female college students at Debre Tabor town

Tadesse Wuletaw Demissie[1*], Araya Mesfin Nigatu[2] and Getnet Mihretie Beyene[2,3]

Abstract

Background: Unwanted pregnancy is a significant public health problem worldwide. In higher education, students are exposed to the risk of unintended pregnancy, abortion, and its related negative consequences.

Objective: The objective of this study was to assess the magnitude of emergency contraceptives and factors associated with its utilization among college female students at Debre Tabor Town, Northwest Ethiopia.

Methods: A cross-sectional, institutional-based study was conducted from June to October 2017. A multi-stage stratified sampling technique was applied to select the study participants. Data were cleaned, coded, and entered into Epi info 7 and exported to SPSS version 20 for analysis. Bivariable and multivariable logistic regression was used to identify the association between the use of emergency contraception and the predictor variables. The *P*-value less than 0.05 at 95% CI was taken as statistical significance.

Results: A total of 821 respondents participated with a response rate of 97.6%. The finding showed that 33.3% of them have used emergency contraceptives following unprotected sex. Female students' knowledge about emergency contraceptive [AOR: 2.3; 95% CI 1.20, 4.25], age with 20–24 years category [AOR: 2.3; 95% CI 1.21, 4.49] and married [AOR: 2.8; 95% CI 1.22, 6.21] and divorced [AOR: 4.9; 95% CI 1.12, 21.08] students were found to be significant predictors of EC utilization.

Conclusions: This study revealed that the level of emergency contraceptive utilization was low. Students' level of knowledge about an emergency contraceptive, age at present, and marital status were found to be the major predictor for emergency contraceptive utilization. Therefore, responsible bodies should develop strategies that enhance the knowledge level of students at the college level on the effective utilization of emergency contraceptive methods.

Keywords: EC utilization, Ethiopia

* Correspondence: twuletaw@yahoo.com
[1]Department of Nursing, Debre Tabor Health Science College, Debra Tabor, Ethiopia

Plain English summary

Unwanted pregnancy is a significant public health problem worldwide, particularly in developing countries. In higher education, students are exposed to the risk of unintended pregnancy, abortion, and its related negative consequences.

Students were asked to use an interview-based questionnaire for their exposure and utilization of emergency contraceptives and their associated factors.

A total of 821 respondents participated with a response rate of 97.6%. The finding showed that 33.3% of them have used emergency contraceptives following unprotected sex. Female students' knowledge about an emergency contraceptive, age with 20–24 years category, and married and divorced students were found to be significant predictors of EC utilization.

Article summary

Strength

College students were asked using an interview-based questionnaire for their exposure and utilization of emergency contraceptives and their associated factors.

Responsible bodies particularly college higher officials', policymakers, and health professionals were informed to develop strategies that enhance the knowledge level of students on the effective utilization of emergency contraceptive methods; this could enhance female student's knowledge and use of emergency contraceptives.

Limitation

As the study was a cross-sectional egg -chicken dilemma may happen and as the reproductive issues are sensitive, students may feel shame to explain their emergency contraceptive utilization and other reproductive issues fully.

Background

Emergency contraception also called: "post-coital contraception", or "second chance" is a type of modern and traditional contraception that is used after unprotected sexual intercourse, following sexual abuse, misuse of regular contraception, or non-use of contraception [1].

Every year, more than 120 million couples have an unmet need for contraception and 80 million women have unintended pregnancies from which 45 million of them end up with abortion; this mainly results from unsafe sex which is the second most important risk factor for disability and death in the world's poorest communities [2].

As it is difficult to determine the infertile time of the cycle with certainty; emergency contraceptive methods should be provided for any woman concerned about her risk of pregnancy regardless of the cycle and day of exposure; there are two types of emergency contraceptive methods: the emergency contraceptive pill (the "morning after" pill) and the intrauterine device (IUD) [3]. Hormonal emergency contraceptive pills are taken within 72 h of unprotected sexual intercourse and then 12 h late. Whereas progesterone-only pills one pill should be taken as the first dose as soon as convenient, but not later than 3 days (72 h) after unprotected intercourse to be followed by another one pill 12 h later;Levonelle has to be taken within 72 h(3 days) of un protected sex to prevent pregnancy and ellaOne(containing ulipristal acetate) has to be taken within 120 h(5 days) of sex to prevent pregnancy and the copper bearing IUCD be inserted within 5 days of un protected sex when used as an emergency contraceptive method; it is more effective than the contraceptive pill in preventing pregnancy; less than 1% of women get pregnant. The sooner the methods are used, the more effective after the act of an intended intercourse [4].

Even though, users report some side effects of emergency contraceptives like irregular bleeding, headache, nausea, weight, and mood changes [1]. If used correctly, all types of EC pills can decrease the risk of unintended pregnancy by 75% which in turn helps to reduce unplanned pregnancy and unsafe abortion [5].

A systematic review of causes of maternal mortality estimated that abortion accounted for 49% of deaths and millions more have complications; half of the deaths occur in Africa where one in four unsafe abortions is done with teenagers [6].

Despite the technological advancements in modern contraceptive methods, unintended pregnancy is still a big health problem but can be minimized by the proper utilization of emergency contraceptives. However different findings in middle and low-income countries revealed that EC utilization proportion was 29% in China, 21.2% in South Africa, 13.3% in Nigeria, 39.9% in Ghana, and 2.7% in Ethiopia [7–11].

Emergency contraceptives utilization can play an important role in reducing un planned pregnancies and thereby reducing the risk of un planned pregnancy, its associated health risks, social problem and furthermore prevents economic problems, but there were limited studies in the study area. Therefore, the objective of this study was to assess the magnitude of emergency contraceptive utilization and its associated factors among female college students at Debre Tabor Town.

Methods

Study design, setting, and participants

An institutional-based cross-sectional study was conducted to assess the prevalence of emergency contraceptive utilization and associated factors among female college students learning at Debre Tabor Town, Amhara Regional State, and Northwest Ethiopia. The study was conducted among three governmental and two private colleges (namely; Debre Tabor Health Science College, Debre Tabor Poly Technique College, Begemdir Teachers College,

Fekede Egzi College, and Guna Tabor Business and Health Science College) found in Debre Tabor Town from June to October 2017. There were a total of 800 female students attending their education. The town is located 667 km from Addis Ababa (the capital city of Ethiopia) in the Northwest direction of the country and 97 km away from Bahir Dar city (the capital city of the region) toward the east direction.

It has also 4 kebeles (the smallest local administrative units), three public health centers, one general hospital, three medium private clinics, one primary clinic, three drug stores, and two pharmacies with an area of 3187.07 ha. It has 81, 644 estimated total population, and from which 40,985 were women. Of the 40,985 females, 19,252 were within the reproductive age at the time of the study. The estimated annual delivery number within this period was 2751 births [12].

Sample size and sampling techniques

The sample size was determined using a single population proportion formula with the assumption of a 95% confidence interval and a margin of error of 5%. From those who had sexual experience, the proportion of students who practiced emergency contraceptive methods was assumed to be 46.3%(p) taken from the study conducted in southwest Ethiopia Mizan Tapi university brought larger sample size after considering others to have the required sample size [13]. Then, by adding a non-response rate of 10% and multiplying by a design effect of 2, a sample of 840 was determined.

A two-stage sampling technique was used; in the first case departments were selected using the lottery method and then, the sample size was allocated to each department proportional to the number of female students in each department. Finally, participant students were selected from each department proportional to their year of study using a simple random sampling technique.

Data collection procedures

Data were collected using a self-administered Amharic version and a pretested questionnaire facilitated by two diploma nurses and one BSc nurse supervisor. It includes variables like socio-demographic characteristics, sexual and reproductive health history, knowledge, attitude, practice about EC and determinants of emergency contraceptive methods were asked.

Data processing and analysis

Data were entered, edited, and cleaned using Epi-info version 7 and exported to SPSS version 20 for further statistical analysis. The descriptive analysis such as proportions, percentages, frequency distribution, and measure of central tendency was carried out.

Next to this, the bivariate analysis was done to identify whether there was an association between the dependent and independent variables to select the candidate variable for the multivariable analysis. Accordingly, variables found to have an association with the dependent variable less than 0.2 *p*-values were entered into multivariable binary logistic regression using the enter method for controlling the possible effects of confounders. Finally, the variables which had a significant association with p-value < 0.05 were identified as significant variables based on the odds ratio (OR), with 95% CI. The goodness of fit test was also checked.

Operational definitions of terms

Emergency contraceptive utilization

Refers to methods that a woman can use to prevent pregnancy after unprotected sexual intercourse, method failure, or incorrect use.

Data quality control measures

The quality of data was assured by giving pre-test, training for data collectors, and supervisor on the objective of the study and making frequent supervision. The completeness of the questionnaire was checked every other day by the supervisors and principal investigators.

Ethical considerations

Ethical clearance was obtained from the Amhara Public Health Institution. Informed consent was also obtained from each study participant. Individual participant records were coded on each respective questionnaire and accessed only by the research team members to keep confidentiality.

Results

Socio-demographic characteristics of students

In this study, a total of 821 female college students participated in the study yielding a response rate of 97.6%. The mean age of the respondents was 19.9 (SD ±2.28) years. The youngest being 15 and the oldest 35 years old. More than one third (47.5%) of the respondents were between the age of 15–19 years. Above three fourth of (97%), the respondents were Orthodox Christianity by religion. Concerning marital status, 678 (83.7%) of the respondents were single (Table 1).

Reproductive health characteristics

The mean age at first sexual intercourse and first pregnancies were 18.8 (SD ± 2.24) years and 19.9 (SD ± 2.6) years respectively. Eighty-nine (33.8%) of sexually active female students had had a pregnancy and 50(56.2%) of them were below the age of 20 years. Sixty-seven (75.3%) of pregnant respondents reported that their pregnancy was unplanned. Among those who reported unplanned pregnancy, 30(44.8%) failed to prevent pregnancy because of forgetting to take contraceptive methods namely oral contraceptives, and 9(13.4%) having infrequent sex. Similarly, those of untended pregnancies, 55(82.1%) of them end up with induced abortion mainly from governmental health facilities 33(60%). The major reasons for them to terminate

Table 1 Socio-demographic characteristics of female college students Debre Tabor Town northwest Ethiopia, October 2017 ($n = 821$)

Variables	Frequency	Percent
Age (in years)		
15–19	3390	47.5
20–24	386	47.0
> =25	45	5.5
Mean ± SD	19.9 ± 2.3	
Marital status		
Single	678	83.7
Married	98	11.9
Widowed	5	0.6
Divorced	27	3.3
Separated	4	0.5
Religion		
Orthodox	796	97.0
Muslim	20	2.4
Catholic	4	0.5
Protestant	1	0.1
Year of Study		
1st year	562	68.5
2nd year	149	18.1
3rd year and above	110	13.4
Field of study		
Health Science	302	36.8
Non-health Science	519	63.2
Program		
Regular	678	82.6
Extension	143	17.4

their pregnancy were fear of discontinuing from school (50.9%) followed by fear of parents (36.4%) (Table 2).

Among the total participants, 456(55.5%) of them said that they heard information about emergency contraceptives. From these, 228 (50%) of them mentioned friends as their first source of information followed by mass media 105(23.04%) (Table 2).

Knowledge of emergency contraceptive utilization

Among college female students who have heard about EC 456(55.5%), only 254 (55.7%) correctly identified the time of utilization of the method, 246(53.9%) knew the recommended doses, and 169 (37.1%) recognize the recommended time interval between the doses. The index knowledge summary about EC also showed that 207(45.4%) of the respondents had good knowledge of EC (Table 3). Among 263 respondents who had a history

Table 2 Pregnancy and related characteristics among sexually active female college students Debre Tabor Town northwest Ethiopia, October 2017

Variables	Frequency	Percent
Ever had sex (n = 821)		
yes	263	32.0
No	558	68.0
Age at first sex (n = 263)		
15–19	175	66.5
20–24	80	30.4
> =25	8	3.1
Mean (±SD)	18.8 ± 2.2	
Ever been pregnant (n = 263)		
Yes	89	33.8
No	174	66.2
Ever heard about EC (n = 821)		
Yes	456	55.5
No	365	44.5
What is your source of information		
From friends	228	50.0
From health institutions	47	10.3
From mass media	105	23.0
From boyfriends	15	3.3
From parents	17	3.7
From college teachers	44	9.6
Age at first pregnancy (n = 89)		
15–19	50	56.2
20–24	35	39.3
> =25	4	4.5
Unintended pregnancy (n = 89)		
Yes	67	75.3
No	22	24.7
Induced abortion (n = 67)		
Yes	55	82.1
No	12	17.9
Place of abortion (n = 55)		
Untrained abortionist	5	9.1
Private clinic	11	20.0
Government health institution	33	60.0
Self-infliction	6	10.9
Reason for induced abortion (n = 55)		
Fear of discontinuing school	28	50.9
Fear of parents	20	36.4
Economic problem	11	20.0
Since unintended	10	18.2
Stigma	7	12.7

Table 3 knowledge about emergency contraceptive utilization among female college students in Debre Tabor Town northwest Ethiopia, October 2017 ($n = 456$)

Variables	Frequency	Percent
Methods reported as EC		
Oral contraceptive pills	88	19.3
IUCD	15	3.3
Injectable	25	5.5
Condoms	52	11.4
Norplant	9	2.0
Withdrawal	24	5.3
Calendar/rhythm	11	2.4
All mentioned above	147	32.2
I don't know	88	18.6
Mechanism of action of pills as ECs		
Prevent ovulation	76	16.7
Prevent fertilization	73	16.0
Prevent implantation	28	6.1
Induced abortion	19	4.2
All mentioned above	82	18.0
I don't know	178	39.0
Can Ec cause early abortion?		
Yes	169	37.1
No	287	62.9
When taken early, can EC prevent STI?		
Yes	175	38.4
No	281	61.6
Where EC can be obtained?		
Pharmacy	47	10.3
Governmental health institution	70	15.4
Private clinics	22	4.8
All mentioned above	237	52.0
I don't know	80	17.5
Recommended time to take EC pills?		
At any time	111	24.3
Within 72 h	195	42.8
Within 5 days after sex	59	12.9
I don't know	91	20.0
The recommended dose of pills & IUCD respectively?	155	34.0
One dose	91	20.0
Two and above dose	18	3.9
I don't remember	192	42.1
I don't know	169	37.1
Recommended between doses of pills		
12 h apart	27	5.9

Table 3 knowledge about emergency contraceptive utilization among female college students in Debre Tabor Town northwest Ethiopia, October 2017 ($n = 456$) *(Continued)*

Variables	Frequency	Percent
48 h apart	89	19.5
72 h apart	171	37.5
I don't know		
Recommended time for IUCD as EC		
Within 24 h after sex	54	11.8
Within 48 h after sex	11	2.4
Within 72 h after sex	39	8.6
Within 5 days after sex	65	14.3
I don't know	287	62.9
Effectiveness of EC pills		
Very effective (99%)	145	31.8
Effective (75%)	41	9.0
Moderate (50%)	18	3.9
Less effective (30%)	20	4.4
I don't know	232	50.9
Situation(s) that EC should be taken		
When forced to have sex	52	11.4
If condom raptured during sex	27	5.9
When there are missed pills	11	2.4
When there is sex without a contraceptive	30	6.6
All mentioned above	185	40.6
I don't know	151	33.1
Knowledge of EC (summary index)		
Good knowledge	207	45.4
Poor knowledge	249	54.6

of sexual intercourse, 74(28.1%) of them used EC as contraception (Fig. 1).

Attitude

Three hundred sixty-four (44.3%) of the respondents had a good attitude towards EC. Four hundred ninety-one (59.8%) of the respondents replayed that EC will not cause loss of confidence between regular partners; so that 276(33.6%) of the respondents strongly agreed that EC is useful for all at risk females. On the other hand, 230 (28%) of the respondents agreed that will increase the risk of STI including HIV/AIDS (Table 4).

Practice

Among students who had ever been sexually active 28.1% of them used EC and from respondents who had unprotected sexual acts, 33.3% of them used EC. Oral contraceptive pills were the most common method used followed by condoms accounting for 70.3 and 18.9% respectively. However, only 48.6 and 16.2% of them correctly identified the

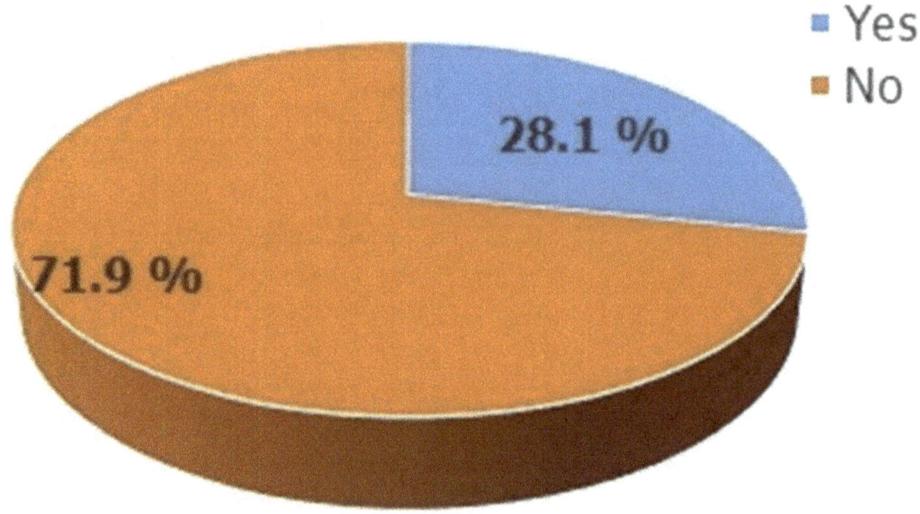

Fig. 1 Prevalence of EC users among college female students who had a history of sexual intercourse, Debre Tabor Town, Northwest Ethiopia October 2017

recommended time limit (that means within 72 h. for pills and within 120 h for IUCD) respectively (Table 5). Twenty-three (62.2%) of the respondents were advised to use emergency contraceptive methods after unprotected sex by their female friends or peers (Fig. 2).

Determinants of emergency contraceptive utilization

The multivariable logistics regression analysis showed that college female students whose age category between 20 and 24 years (AOR = 2.3, 95% CI: 1.21, 4.49) were two times more likely to use EC as a contraception method. Married students (AOR = 2.8, 95% CI: 1.22, 6.21) and divorced once (AOR = 4.9, 95% CI: 1.12, 21.08) were two and five times more likely to use EC as compared to unmarried students respectively. On the other hand, students who had good knowledge (AOR = 2.3, 95% CI: 1.20, 4.25) were two times more likely to use EC as a contraception option (Table 6).

Table 4 Attitude on emergency contraceptive utilization among female college students in Debre Tabor Town northwest Ethiopia, October 2017 (n = 821)

Variables	Response			
	Strongly disagree (%)	Disagree (%)	Agree (%)	Strongly agree (%)
EC causes loose of confidence between regular partners	189(20.6)	491(59.8)	148(18.0)	13(1.6)
EC is good for all females who are at risk	210(25.6)	142(17.3)	193(23.5	276(33.6)
EC increases the risk of STI including HIV/AIDS	183(22.3)	191(23.3)	230(28.0)	217(26.4)
EC is good after unsafe sexual intercourse	192(23.4)	152(18.5)	234(28.5)	243(29.6)
EC is sign full contraceptive method	172(21.0)	272(33.1)	212(25.8)	165(20.1)
EC may cause infertility	47(5.7)	188(22.9)	250(30.5)	336(40.9)
If I had unintended sexual intercourse I would use EC	41(5.0)	80(9.7)	237(28.9)	463(56.4)
I would advise using EC for close friends if they had unintended sexual intercourse	70(8.5)	108(13.2)	313(38.1)	330(40.2)
EC promotes promiscuity	148(18)	298(36.3)	196(23.9)	179(21.8)
EC is one way of abortion	143(17.4)	173(21.1)	313(38.1)	192(23.4)
EC affect the regular contraceptive method	101(12.3)	279(34.0)	2264(32.2)	17(21.6)
Unplanned sexual intercourse is a problem for all young females	229(27.9)	390(47.2)	99(12.1)	103(12.5)
EC can be used for a long time	145(17.7)	198(24.1)	300(36.5)	178(21.7)
Attitude (summary index)				
Good Attitude	364 (44.3%)			
Poor Attitude	457 (55.7%)			

Table 5 Emergency contraceptive practice among female college students, Debre Tabor Town, northwest Ethiopia, October 2017

Variables	Frequency	Percent
Ever used EC among those who had sex (n = 263)		
yes	74	28.1
No	189	71.9
Ever used EC among unprotected sex (*n* = 111)		
Yes	37	33.3
No	74	66.7
Methods used as EC (*n* = 37)		
OC pills	26	70.3
IUCD	1	2.7
Condom	7	18.9
Withdrawal	2	5.4
Calendar	1	2.7
Place obtained (n = 37)		
Pharmacy	11	29.7
Government health institutions	3	8.1
Private clinics	23	62.2
How many times used (n = 37)		
One dose	6	16.2
Two and above	18	48.6
I don't remember	1	2.7
As necessary	12	32.4
Time EC was used (n = 55)		
Within 72 h for pills	14	37.8
Within 120 h for IUCD	12	32.4
I used as I want	10	27.0
I don't remember	1	2.7

Discussion

This study result showed that the utilization of EC was low. Knowledge of female students, age at present, and the marital status of the students were the major predictors of EC utilization.

In this study, we found that 33.3% (95% CI: 25.2, 42.3%) of those who had unprotected sexual act used EC, which is similar to the report of the studies done at Adama University (Ethiopia) 26.7% [14], Ghana 39.9% [10] and China 29% [11], but was lower than studies done in Ethiopian universities like Mizan Tepi 46.3% [13] and Adds Ababa 75% [15]. The difference might be due to low awareness, accessibility of EC methods, being in campus dormitory for those university students whereas in the private dormitory for college students; there is gender base and sexual health education in the colleges and universities by using gender clubs and clinics in the universities,but there may be difference in performance among the organizations. However, our study was higher than the study done in Ethiopia like Adama University 4.7% [16], Hawasa 10.8% [17], Jima 6.8% [18] and abroad Nigeria (10 &13.3%) [8, 19] and South Africa 21.2% [7]. The possible explanation for this might be a difference in socio-demographic and cultural background characteristics of the respondents and time-lapse.

A statistically significant association was obtained between the age of respondents and their EC utilization. Respondents whose age category is 20–24 years (AOR = 2.3, 95% CI: 1.21, 4.49) were two times more likely to use EC as contraception compared to those within the age range of 15–19 years old. The finding is similar to studies done in Ethiopia [13, 14, 16] and South Africa [7]. The probable reason for this could be younger students might have less information about the proper use of EC due to the fact that they were newly enrolled in the college and might not have received information in their prior schooling.

Another statistically significant association was also obtained between marital status and emergency contraceptive utilization of students. Respondents who were ever married (AOR = 2.8, 95% CI: 1.22, 1.21) and divorced (AOR = 4.9, 95% CI: 1.12, 21.08) were three and five times more likely to use emergency contraceptive respectively as compared to single ones. The finding is similar to studies done at Adama University (Ethiopia) [14, 16]. The possible justification for this might be access to current information; married students might get current information on EC from their partners. Besides, the effect of marital status and increment in age on EC utilization could also be linked to issues like minimizing the fear of being seen by others.

Finally, another significant association was also found between respondents having good knowledge of EC and EC utilization. Respondents who had good knowledge (AOR = 2.3, 95% CI: 1.20, 4.25) were two times more likely to use emergency contraceptives as compared to those having poor knowledge. This finding was consistent with studies conducted in Ethiopian Universities like Mizan Tepi [13], Arba Minch [20], and Adama [14]. The possible reason for this might be a good knowledge. Students who had good knowledge would help them to identify where, when, and how to use EC in preventing unintended pregnancy and abortion that could result from unprotected sex.

Although the finding of this study may not be generalized to students who are out of colleges, it has demonstrated the sexual and reproductive health problems faced by students in colleges found at Debre Tabor. Since an anonymous self-administered questionnaire was used, the possibility of social desirability bias cannot be eliminated as the study touches sensitive issues.

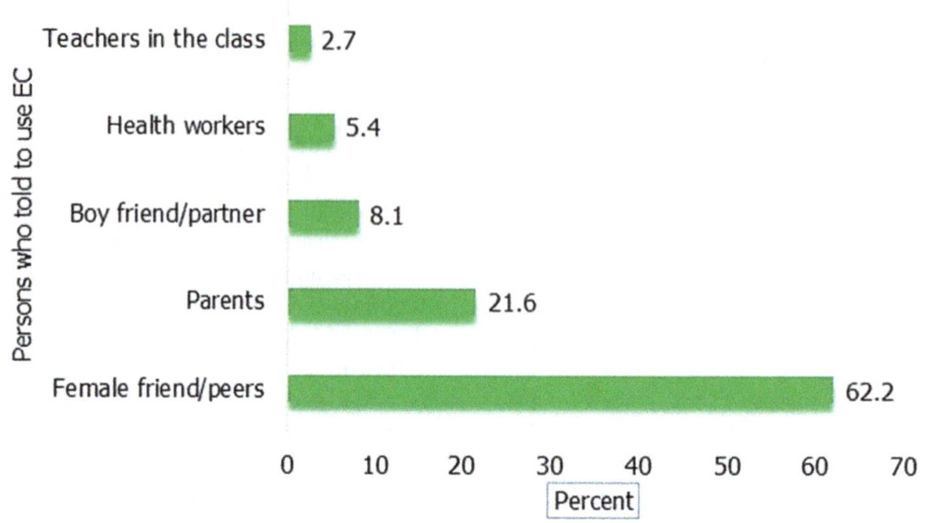

Fig. 2 Number of students who got advice to use EC after unprotected sex, Debre Tabor Town, Northwest Ethiopia June 2017 (n = 37)

Table 6 Bivariate and multivariate analysis on emergency contraceptive utilization among female college students in Debre Tabor Town northwest Ethiopia, October 2017 (n = 263)

Variables	EC used		Crude OR (95% CI)	Adjusted OR (95% CI)
	No (%)	Yes (%)		
Age (in years)				
15–19	91(48.2)	21(28.41)	1.00	1.00
20–24	90(47.6)	45(60.8)	2.2(1.19, 3.93)	**2.3(1.21, 4.49)***
> =25	8(4.2)	8(10.8)	4.3(1.46, 12.87)	1.9(0.52, 7.32)
Marital Status				
Never married	169(89.4)	49(66.2)	1.00	**1.00**
Married	16(8.5)	19(25.3)	4.1(1.96, 8.56)	**2.8(1.22, 6.21)***
Divorced	4(2.1)	6(8.1)	5.2(1.40, 19.07)	**4.9(1.12, 21.08)***
Extra Job				
Yes	11(5.8)	12(16.2)	3.1(1.32, 3.46)	2.5(0.98, 6.62)
No	178(94.2)	62(83.8)	1.00	1.00
Ever Pregnant				
Yes	6(3.2)	14(18.9)	7.1(2.62, 19.34)	3.7(0.50, 27.99)
No	183(96.8)	60(81.1)	1.00	
Unintended pregnancy				
Yes	4(2.1)	11 (14.9)	8.1(2.48, 26.27)	1.7(0.16, 17.17)
No	185(97.9)	63(81.1)	1.00	01.0
Field of Study				
Non-Health science	91(48.1)	25(33.8)	1.00	1.00
Health science	98(51.9)	49(66.2)	1.8(1.04, 3.19)	1.3(0.69, 2.49)
Knowledge				
Good knowledge	79(41.8)	47(63.5)	2.4(1.39, 4.22)	**2.3(1.20, 4.25)***
Poor knowledge	110(58.2)	27(36.5)	1.00	

N.B: 1 = reference,*= significantely associated factor Hosmier and lemesho Goodness of fit test = 0.591

Conclusion

The study finding pointed out that the proportion of emergency contraceptive utilization among female college students was low. Knowledge of students on EC, age at present, and marital status were found to be major determinants. Educating adolescents about emergency contraceptives to give attention to available methods, correct time of use, and promoting emergency contraceptives using formal and informal education like health education sessions gender club sensitization and peer education about sexual health and contraception so as to increase knowledge on EC and to enhance utilization and to make emergency contraceptive methods readily accessible.

Abbreviations

EC: Emergency Contraceptive; HIV/AIDS: Human Immune Deficiency Virus/ Acquired Immune Deficiency Syndrome; IUCD: Intra-Uterine Contraceptive device N.B: 1.00=reference, * =significantly associated factor Hosmier and Lemesho Goodness of fit test=0.591; STI: Sexually Transmitted Infection

Acknowledgments

We sincerely acknowledge the Amhara Public Health Institute for giving permission letters to conduct this research. Our next appreciation goes to study participants, coordinators, data collection facilitators, and the staffs of the respective colleges.

Authors' contributions

Tadesse Wuletaw (TW) designed the study, participated in the data quality control, analyzed the data, and drafted the paper, Araya Mesfin (AM) and Getnet Mihretie (GM) assisted with the design, approved the proposal, and revised drafts of the paper. The authors read and approved the manuscript.

Author details

[1]Department of Nursing, Debre Tabor Health Science College, Debra Tabor, Ethiopia. [2]Department of Health Informatics, Institute of Public Health, University of Gondar, Gondar, Ethiopia. [3]Department of Nursing, Debre Tabor University, Debra Tabor, Ethiopia.

References

1. Health WHOR. Family planning: a global handbook for providers: evidence-based guidance developed through worldwide collaboration. World Health Organization & Johns Hopkins Bloomberg School of Public Health: Johns Hopkins Ccp-Info; 2007.
2. Glasier A, Gülmezoglu AM, Schmid GP, Moreno CG, Van Look PF. Sexual and reproductive health: a matter of life and death. Lancet. 2006;368(9547):1595–607.
3. Mosher WD, Jones J. Use of contraception in the United States: 1982-2008. Vital Health Stat Ser 23, Data Nat Survey Family Growth. 2010;(29):1–44.
4. Palermo T, Bleck J, Westley E. Knowledge and use of emergency contraception: a multicountry analysis. Int Perspect Sex Reprod Health. 2014;40(2):79–86.
5. Sabo L, Schrager S. Emergency contraception in Wisconsin: a review. WMJ-MADISON-. 2006;105(5):40.
6. Cleland J, Bernstein S, Ezeh A, Faundes A, Glasier A, Innis J. Family planning: the unfinished agenda. Lancet. 2006;368(9549):1810–27.
7. Hoque ME, Ghuman S. Knowledge, practices, and attitudes of emergency contraception among female university students in KwaZulu-Natal, South Africa; 2012.
8. Ojule JD, Oriji VK, Georgewill KN. Awareness and practice of emergency contraception among students of University of Port Harcourt, south-South Nigeria. Nigerian Health J. 2008;8(1–2):6–9.
9. Worku A. Knowledge, attitude and practice of emergency contraceptives among female college students in Arba Minch town, southern Ethiopia. Ethiop J Health Dev. 2011;25(3):176–83.
10. Amalba A, Mogre V, Appiah MN, Mumuni WA. Awareness, use and associated factors of emergency contraceptive pills among women of reproductive age (15-49 years) in tamale, Ghana. BMC Womens Health. 2014;14(1):114.
11. Wang H, Long L, Cai H, Wu Y, Xu J, Shu C, et al. Contraception and unintended pregnancy among unmarried Female University students: a cross-sectional study from China. PLoS One. 2015;10(6):e0130212.
12. Commission FDRoEPC. Summary and statistical report of the 2007 population and housing census. Addis Ababa: Federal Democratic republic of Ethiopia Population Census Commission; 2008.
13. Shiferaw BZ, Gashaw BT, Tesso FY. Factors associated with utilization of emergency contraception among female students in Mizan-Tepi University, south West Ethiopia. BMC Res Notes. 2015;8(1):817.
14. Tilahun D, Assefa T, Belachew T. Predictors of emergency contraceptive use among regular female students at Adama University, Central Ethiopia. Pan Afr Med J. 2010;7(1).
15. Seife M. Assessment of level of awareness and utilization of emergency contraception, among college female students in Oromia regional state, Arsi zone, Asella town south-East Ethiopia: aau; 2007.
16. Tilahun D, Assefa T, Belachew T. Knowledge, attitude and practice of emergency contraceptives among Adama University female students, Ethiopia. Ethiop J Health Sci. 2010;20(3).
17. Tolossa E, Meshesha B, Abajobir AA. Assessment of level of knowledge and utilization of emergency contraception among female students of Hawassa University, South Ethiopia. Adv Reprod Sci. 2013;1(03):51.
18. Tajure N. Knowledge, attitude and practice of emergency contraception among graduating female students of Jimma University, Southwest Ethiopia. Ethiop J Health Sci. 2010;20(2).
19. Adinma ED, Adinma JIB-D, Eke NO, Iwuoha C, Akiode A, Oji E. Awareness and use of contraception by women seeking termination of pregnancy in south eastern Nigeria. Asian Pacific J Trop Dis. 2011;1(1):71–5.
20. Worku A. Knowledge, attitude and practice of emergency contraceptives among female college students in Arba Minch town, southern Ethiopia. Ethiop J Health Dev. 2012;25(3):176–83.

3

Influences on contraceptive method choice among adolescent women across urban centers in Nigeria

Elynn Kann Sanchez[1*], Courtney McGuire[1], Lisa M. Calhoun[1], Gwyn Hainsworth[2] and Ilene S. Speizer[1,3]

Abstract

Background: Despite calls to increase contraceptive use among adolescents and youth, large gaps still exist, creating an unmet need for family planning. Past research has focused on barriers to seeking a method. There is less understanding of the types of methods young women want and who and what influences these decisions. This study examines what method characteristics young Nigerian women prioritize when choosing a method to inform future family planning programming.

Methods: In 2018, eight focus group discussions (FGD) were conducted in the Nigerian cities of Ilorin and Jos with 83 young women ages 15–24. Participants were identified by community contacts and separated into groups by religion and marital status. The discussion guide utilized a vignette structure to understand the participants' perceptions on contraceptive behavior and attitudes and misconceptions surrounding different types of methods. The FGDs were undertaken and analyzed by collaborative teams from the University of Ibadan and the University of North Carolina-Chapel Hill. A thematic analysis of the transcripts was performed using Atlas.ti, including two rounds of coding, and multiple reviews by the research team.

Results: The method characteristics associated with young women's contraceptive decisions include: side effects, reliability, length of coverage, privacy, cost, and accessibility. Side effects, reliability, and privacy were described as negatively linked to short-acting methods whereas easy accessibility and low cost were positive characteristics of these methods. Long-acting methods were generally viewed as positive. Participants' focus on side effects commonly resulted from concerns about the impact on future fertility. The characteristics prioritized by individuals change throughout their adolescence and as their marital status changes. Providers, peers, parents, and partners were all found to have an influence over method choice in different ways. The role of these influencers also changes over the adolescent years.

Conclusion: This study demonstrates that programs should prioritize expanding method choice to increase the number of available options to ensure all young women can access a method that fits their desired method characteristics. Programming should ensure that medically accurate information is widely distributed to harness providers, peers, parents and partners as a resource for information about specific methods.

Keywords: Contraception, Adolescents, Sub-Saharan Africa, Method choice, Qualitative

* Correspondence: elynn@live.unc.edu
[1]Carolina Population Center, University of North Carolina-Chapel Hill, Chapel Hill, USA

Background

As of 2014, adolescents and youth ages 15–24 years accounted for 25% of the global population. Yet despite the size of this population, adolescents and youth experience barriers at the policy, service delivery point, and community levels affecting their access to the sexual and reproductive health services they need, particularly in low and middle income countries [1]. It is estimated that in Sub-Saharan Africa about 16% of births occur among women ages 15–19 years while 25% occur among those ages 20–24 years [2]. With maternal mortality remaining the leading cause of death among adolescent women, it is critical that adolescents and youth have access to the resources that will allow them to avoid an unintended pregnancy and/or plan for and remain safe throughout a pregnancy [1].

Nigeria, the setting for this study, faces similar reproductive health challenges as seen across Sub-Saharan Africa. Over half of Nigeria's population is below the age of 24 years, with over half of this young population living in urban settings [3]. In 2018, the total fertility rate in Nigeria was 5.3 children per woman [3], and urban adolescents and youth have a median 5.7 year gap between first sexual experience and first contraceptive use [3, 4].

Data from recent PMA surveys demonstrate that at the national level, the prevalence of modern contraception among women ages 15–24 years was 8.8% in 2017. About a third (36%) of unmarried, sexually active young women report using a modern method while only 7% of young women in union report the same. Notably, among those young women using a method, the types of methods used vary widely by marital status [3]. Unmarried women use short-acting methods such as male condoms (56.6% of users), oral contraceptive pills (25.2%), and emergency contraception (8.4%) [3]. Among women in union, the main methods used are injectables (30.2%), oral contraceptive pills (23.0%), and male condoms (20.1%) [3]. In Ilorin and Jos, the sites of this study, the dominant methods used by adolescents and youth closely mirror these country-wide trends [5]. Despite being effective and long-acting, the use of long-acting reversible contraceptives (LARCs), such as the IUD or implant, are still limited in Nigeria, particularly among unmarried and young populations [3].

Past research has identified barriers to adolescents and youth accessing contraceptive methods. These barriers include unsupportive social norms, lack of information on methods and sources of methods, physical barriers, and youth-specific barriers like provider bias when seeking care due to their age [6–9]. However, gaps exist in the understanding of factors that influence the choice of method among young women [10, 11]. The objective of this research is to better understand how method-specific characteristics and social influencers affect method choice among adolescents and youth in two cities in Nigeria.

Methods

This qualitative research analysis was performed using data collected as a part of a larger study on the sustainability of the Nigerian Urban Reproductive Health Initiative (NURHI). NURHI sought to increase access to and demand for contraceptive methods in urban centers of Nigeria through demand generation, service improvement, infrastructure strengthening, and advocacy. The first phase of NURHI was implemented in Ilorin, Kaduna, Ibadan, Benin City, Zaria, and Abuja from 2009 to 2015, all of which saw an increase in the modern contraceptive prevalence rate with an overall baseline percentage of 23.1% to an endline percentage of 34.2% [12]. The second phase of NURHI included implementation in Kaduna and Lagos States from 2015 to 2020 and Oyo State from 2015 to 2018. The NURHI Sustainability Study was undertaken in the cities of Ilorin (a city where programming ended in early 2015), Kaduna[1] (a city where programming continued), and a comparison city of Jos. The study sought to understand what program elements have been sustained over time, and what barriers there are to the sustainability of programming [12]. Prior to data collection, ethical approval for the study was sought and obtained from the Nigerian National Health Research Ethics Committee (#NHREC/01/01/2007) and University of North Carolina Institutional Review Board (#17–1215). To ensure compliance with this approval, informed consent was collected verbally from each participant in her primary language, and a data management plan was followed to protect the identify of participants.

In June 2018, 18 focus group discussions (FGDs) were held with participants recruited through convenience sampling by community contacts. The focus group participants were grouped by age (15–24 and 25–39 years), religion (Christian and Muslim), and marital status (married and unmarried). To identify the social norms surrounding contraceptive use and choice, the interview guide utilized a vignette structure to understand what social norms and attitudes exist and how they either facilitate or create barriers for young women's behavior in the community. Vignettes are a research tool that has been used in previous studies for their ability to identify community attitudes, beliefs, knowledge and social norms and create a space for the participants to share their own experiences through the characters in the story [13, 14]. For this study, the focus group participants were provided with the following vignette of a fictitious

[1]FGD were also held with young women in Kaduna, however, relevant questions required for this analysis were not included in the Kaduna FGD. For this reason, Kaduna data are not included in this analysis.

young woman at the beginning of the discussion and asked questions about perceptions of contraceptive use and contraceptive seeking behavior in their community:

> *"A 16-year-old girl from your community is dating her boyfriend who is 17 years old. They decide to start having sex together. Then the girl learns that her friend is pregnant. She learns about modern contraception, such as condoms, daily pill, injectables, and implants, and is thinking about starting to use modern contraception since she doesn't want to get pregnant like her friend."*

After establishing and discussing this context, later in the conversation with the younger participants (15–24 years) the facilitator posed the following set of follow-up questions to gain an understanding of adolescent and youth-specific beliefs and preferences related to method characteristics and availability:

> *"She seeks out advice on modern contraception from her health care provider. Her provider recommends two options: combined oral contraceptive pill, which she must take each day and can purchase from a patent medicine vendor (PMV) or a Pharmacy, or an implant, which is inserted [by a provider] in a health facility and is effective for 3-5 years and can be removed at any time if she wants to become pregnant.*

- *Which method do you think she will choose?*
- *Why would she choose that method?"*

The participants' perspectives and knowledge on contraceptive method choices throughout the FGDs are captured in the results below. The majority of the results were in response to this extension of the original vignette. This analysis focused on the FGDs with participants ages 15–24 years. In total, this analysis analyzed eight FGDs in the two cities with nine to thirteen participants each, equaling 83 participants whose demographics are included in Table 1.

The FGDs were led, transcribed, and translated by members of the University of Ibadan Centre for Population and Reproductive Health (CPRH). The resulting transcripts were shared with the research team from the University of North Carolina-Chapel Hill's Carolina Population Center. A thematic analysis was performed that began with reading the transcripts while creating notations of the emerging themes. These themes were combined with research question specific codes to create the original codebook that was uploaded to Atlas.ti and applied to the transcripts in the first round of coding. A second round of coding was performed to incorporate emerging themes that were not captured in the first codebook. Atlas.ti's analysis tools and an Excel matrix were utilized to identify trends across subgroups using the themes captured through both rounds of coding. A specific analysis was also performed to look at mentions of specific contraceptive methods in comparison to comments about method features generally.

Results

This analysis identified important influencing features that adolescent women consider when they are selecting a contraceptive method. The presence or absence of side effects and concerns about the impact on future fertility were the most frequently discussed factors influencing method choice, with the reliability of the method closely following. Lifestyle fits such as privacy, cost, and accessibility were also considered as influential in the overall decision of what method to choose. These influences were attached throughout to specific methods with short-acting methods being more likely to be associated with features that would detract from use, while implants were more frequently associated with features that would encourage use. Participants discussed providers, peers, parents and partners as people who would play a

Table 1 Focus group discussion demographics: participants ages 15–24 years

FGD number	Location	Marital status	Religion	Number of participants	Average age of the participants (by city)
1	Ilorin	Married	Christian	12	20.4 years
2	Ilorin	Married	Christian	9	
3	Ilorin	Unmarried	Muslim	9	
4	Ilorin	Unmarried	Christian	13	
5	Jos	Unmarried	Christian	10	20.9 years
6	Jos	Unmarried	Muslim	10	
7	Jos	Married	Muslim	10	
8	Jos	Married	Christian	10	
Total				83 (10.4 average)	

role in influencing the character's decision, though they described these roles differently.

From the start of each discussion, it was clear that consideration of contraceptive choice existed within a larger context where sexual activity and contraceptive use broadly was not fully supported for adolescent populations. The resistance to the character's sexual activity was inherently associated with the character's use of a contraceptive method, creating hesitancy toward talking about certain methods. This was particularly true when discussing unmarried adolescents, as a young woman's marital status served as an important filter by which to view her actions around sexual activity and contraceptive method use through. However, once the participants acknowledged likely contraceptive use due to the storyline of the vignette, the participants discussed how the predominant influences are considered within this social context. Throughout this results section, the influencing factors will be discussed starting with the most frequently mentioned (side effects) through the least frequently mentioned (accessibility). Then we will more thoroughly describe the influencers of a young woman's decision on what method to use. When appropriate, the regional or demographic differences in responses will be included.

Method specific features

Side effects

One of the most widely discussed reasons for contraceptive choice was the potential side effects caused by a method. The broad term, 'side effects' was the most frequently mentioned term by participants, while, less frequently, participants discussed specific side effects including loss of menstruation and weight gain.

A method's impact on the character's future fertility was widely discussed across all but one of the FGDs. However, any quantification of these discussions would result in a conservative estimate as the young women's general use of the word "side effect" may have also been referring to fear of infertility. For example, participants never specifically mentioned a delay in the return to menstruation after stopping a method as a concern, though in previous studies, it has been identified as a concern by women of all ages, specifically with injectable [10]. While this side effect was not stated as a concern specifically, it would fall within the scope of "concerns around future fertility." Lack of probing on the distinction between general and specific side effects may have led to this potential discrepancy.

The participants' prioritization of avoiding side effects in the long term was illustrated by an unmarried, Muslim, young woman from Ilorin who pointed to side effects as the reason for her resistance to contraceptives broadly in this interaction with the moderator,

> *"Participant: I think it is not good for her because she is too young.*
>
> *Moderator: In this situation, are you saying it is not good for her to use modern contraceptives?*
>
> *Participant: Yes, because it could have side effects when she's grown up."*

There were participants in all of the FGDs that expressed the general lack of support for contraceptives exhibited by the participant above. However, in this example, it was only when probed that side effects were described as the reason for this general concern. Additionally, this participant's use of the word "side effects" in the long term supports the possibility that participants' use of "side effects" could truly be connected to fertility concerns.

For some young women, concerns about side effects were not attached to a particular method, like one married, Christian, young woman from Jos who said,

> *"I will not advise her to go for it [contraceptive use] because, in as much as they are safe to be used as contraceptive that is used for preventing pregnancy, they all have their side effect ... "*

This young woman makes her recommendation based on prioritizing avoiding side effects over pregnancy prevention, a sentiment shared by many. The most frequent reason condoms were recommended as a contraceptive method was due to their lack of side effects. Participants commented on the side effects of specific methods, including much discussion of oral contraceptive pills; the discussion revolved around infertility and other side effects of oral contraceptive pills, including irregular bleeding and weight gain, in over half of the FGDs. Side effects of implants were also infrequently mentioned.

Reliability & length of coverage

Method reliability was a method-specific feature mentioned frequently by participants and framed as the general likelihood for user error, not the specific failure rate once used. For example, participants commonly described that oral contraceptive pills can be easily forgotten, or highlighted barriers to getting another injection, which in turn creates an opportunity for unintended pregnancy. Participants referred to the process of taking oral contraceptive pills daily as "unreasonable," like this unmarried, Christian, young woman from Ilorin, who responded to the moderator's question about if the character would choose the implant or oral contraceptive pill by replying,

> *"I think me as a person, I will advise her to go for the other one in which they will inject because you*

taking pills every day it's not reasonable and then sometimes something might happen probably forget or something might happen."

Like this example, participants were more likely to indicate that they believed the character in the vignette would choose the implant because once placed, it could be forgotten until she wanted to become pregnant. In five of the eight discussions, participants directly talked about the effectiveness of the implant, and their trust in the method was discussed in combination with the implant's simple insertion. An example of this was when an unmarried, Christian, young woman from Jos shared her support for the implant by stating,

"To me, it's better she uses the implant because she can remove it at any time that she feels like and as far as it is in her body, she won't get pregnant but she can remove it when she wants to get pregnant."

The number of participants that recommended the implant to the character indicates that participants prioritized selecting a method with a low potential for user error, which they also connected with a low level of interaction with the method itself.

Connected to this, we see that this participant and others valued the length of time that the implant would provide pregnancy protection, while also linking that length of coverage with flexibility. Participants commonly framed their discussions on the length of coverage around how often it would require them to interact with their method or seek care. As discussed above, participants commonly found taking oral contraceptive pills daily to be a concern, while acknowledging that it might be hard to access a new pack once the first pack was finished. Alternatively, the length of coverage provided by the implant's 3–5 year lifespan limits the participant's interaction to just the insertion and removal, which many viewed as a positive feature of the method. In two of the FGDs, participants showed support for the 3-month length of coverage provided by an injectable, though a few participants did discuss the challenge of remembering when to go for the next shot. Participants discussed flexibility with a method both through the frame of not having to interact with the method as well as being able to quickly decide to stop using the method should reproductive priorities change.

Privacy

The prioritization of privacy, meaning that others do not know about her contraceptive use, was a factor that was considered by the participants for all discussed methods, especially when there is a lack of social support for a young woman seeking a method. All of the participants who discussed privacy did so with the concern that the character's parents would find out about her method use. These mentions associated oral contraceptive pills negatively with privacy, while implants were positively connected with this factor. For example, one unmarried, Christian participant from Ilorin said,

"If I'm to recommend for her, I will surely want her to go for the implanol [implant] because you said it will be inserted around her arm and obviously it will be small it won't be something heavy, she could always put on a long sleeve unlike her taking pills every day. It's absurd and at a point, the parents will want to know what the drugs are for."

The participant indicates that the implant allows for the character to use a method covertly while avoiding the social pressures that accompany other methods. There were no observed differences in mentions of privacy across marital status or religion; however, mentions were concentrated among participants in Ilorin.

Cost

Unlike other factors, there was a divide in the participants on if the cost would be a consideration for the character. The cost of a method was raised in half of the discussions as a potential barrier, while the cheap price of oral contraceptive pills was mentioned as a benefit of the method less frequently. A few participants did acknowledge that the one-time payment for a long-acting method may be preferred, like one married, Christian participant from Jos who said,

"that one [implant] will be the easiest because she will just put it there and it will remain there as much as she wants and there will be no problem, but that other one will be stressful for her going to buy it, if there is no money it will be another problem."

For this participant, shorter-acting methods require a young woman to have consistent access to money. For adolescents and youth, the cost of oral contraceptive pills can be what initially attracts them to the method; however, this participant is arguing that the monthly payment may also be a disadvantage.

Alternatively, moderators in almost all of the FGDs specifically asked if the cost would be a barrier to accessing a method, and participants widely indicated that it was not. As one married, Christian, young woman from Jos said, *"as far as she is desperate, to have it, she would at any cost, she would go for it."* This participant is making a general statement that cost will not be a barrier due to the girl's determination. Additionally, other participants indicated that a partner would pay the cost. There were no differences in these beliefs between group demographics (marital status and religion), indicating that the role that cost plays in a young woman's decision varies widely depending on the individual young woman's situation.

Accessibility

The final factor that a handful of participants mentioned as a benefit of short-acting methods was that they were easily accessible. Participants discussed the accessibility of condoms and oral contraceptive pills, both of which can be purchased at the local pharmacy. For example, in this exchange with the moderator, an unmarried, Christian participant from Ilorin raises two main reasons for her belief that the character will choose the oral contraceptive pills,

> *"Participant: the implanol, it will have to be implanted in her so she will feel it will be more difficult than the pill she will feel it's easier and of non-stress. So she will want to go for the pills*
>
> *Moderator: So you are saying that she will go for the pills because it's easy?*
>
> *Participant: yeah it is easier disputing the fact that she's going to take it every day but the implantation stuff, she will feel it's too dangerous or something that's somehow for her to do it because you have to implant it then if you want to remove it, you still have to remove it."*

In this interaction we see the participant talks about accessibility in two different ways. First, she supports oral contraceptive pills for the character's ability to conveniently access them within her community. But we also see another idea of accessibility, which is that this quote appears to reflect fear surrounding the insertion process and provider bias which could also be a factor among this population [6]. Other participants supported this sentiment and indicated that in an environment where contraceptive use for young people is not fully supported by societal norms, being able to access oral contraceptive pills and condoms outside of facilities could be a supportive factor for these short-acting methods. It is important to note that this participant's mention of fear surrounding the insertion process of an implant was one of only two mentions of this concern. If this fear is a barrier for adolescents, it was not widely discussed in these FGDs.

Influencers of method selection

Provider

The most frequently mentioned influencer on the character's method choice was a doctor or nurse, as participants mentioned them more than twice as often as any other influencer throughout the FGDs. These mentions were intrinsically linked to the value participants placed on avoiding side effects. Participants saw medical professionals as a source of information on methods that would best "fit one's blood," with some young women discussing tests that could be run to find the best option. Others discussed how doctors could give information on multiple options from which the character could choose. An unmarried, Christian, young woman from Ilorin shared one example of this idea,

> *" ... she can seek medical advice because when she gets there she will know the different types of pills they use that can help her, that will not damage her womb ... "*

This participant reflects the overwhelming sentiment that the avoidance of side effects is a key influence on a young woman's decision when selecting a method; a process a provider can help to inform.

That said, the influence that doctors and nurses have on a young woman's decision was framed quite differently than the role of other influencers such as friends or family members. Unlike other influencers, the character's decision to seek care at a hospital or clinic was discussed as something she *should* do versus something that she *would* do. For example, one unmarried, Muslim participant from Jos said,

> *"I think she should go and see a doctor, they are the ones that will lead her on family planning so they can check which is better for her."*

Within the context of the participants' prioritization of avoiding side effects, this language on what the character should do is in line with the community's priorities. However, it does raise the question of if the participants' responses reflect what they think the character would actually do. On average, unmarried participants were three times less likely to discuss the role of a provider on influencing the contraception decision than married participants; this hints that there may be barriers to visiting providers that went undiscussed in the FGDs. This is supported by 2017 PMA2020 data that found that in Nigeria only 6.7% of unmarried adolescent family planning users accessed a method from a public facility as compared to 28.4% of married adolescent users [4]. It is notable that while pharmacies and patent medicine stores can be a place to access contraceptives without having to see a provider, only a small number of participants mentioned these as an option for young people. The majority of the FGD moderators did ask whether the character would face any challenges during a clinic visit. A few participants indicated that she would face some provider bias or disqualifying questions because of her age. However, this sentiment was not expressed widely, with many participants disagreeing that these types of challenges would occur.

Peers & parents

Peers were referenced almost two times more than parents, though both were discussed as playing a similar role in providing information to the character. While providers were discussed as helping the character find the method that would be the best medical fit through tests, peers' influence on method choice came in the form of stories that relayed information about characteristics of different methods as experienced by themselves or friends. It was quite common for participants to anticipate the character's friends to use personal experiences as a way of introducing these preferences of a method. For example, one unmarried, Christian, young woman from Jos stated,

> *"Yes her friends can influence her because maybe they will say I've used it, oh and it last so you can also go for it so it will also last."*

This short example shows how the speaker grounded her response in her perspective of friends sharing stories. In another example from Jos, a married, young woman describes general side effects from using contraceptives.

> *"It really has so many effects, many people bleed a lot. Those who have received it are those who tell us that they did it and it was not a pleasant experience, so they give advice. That is why people refuse to do it because there are so many side effects."*

This example echoes many others, like a young woman from Ilorin who had a friend who gained weight on oral contraceptive pills, or a young woman from Jos whose sister developed low blood pressure after receiving an implant. As the participants shared the stories that they had heard from friends, it indicated that these stories directly influence one's views on certain methods. Though this can be positive, the majority of these examples throughout the FGDs were about negative experiences with methods. The misconceptions about side effects as well as real side effects experienced by individuals are shared within peer groups, which can feed into the fertility concerns discussed above. Overall, participants saw peers' experiences as an introduction to new methods and as a litmus test for their safety.

Parents were discussed in a similar role, as people the character could turn to for stories (both positive and negative) about certain methods, in turn influencing views of the mentioned contraceptive. Additionally, parents were described as being able to bridge the gap between the character and a provider by bringing the character to a clinic. However, some participants cited privacy concerns in discussions about parents due to some parents' resistance to contraceptive use. In this way parents were seen as potentially wanting to influence the character away from use, leading to a young woman not seeking a parent's advice if she wanted to avoid this pressure. Similar to the described influence of providers, seeking support from parents was more likely described as something the character should do, versus would do. Because of this, participants indicated that the influence of parents is complicated and dependent on the type of relationship that each young woman has with her parents.

Partners

Partners were not discussed frequently as directly influencing contraceptive decision-making, however, when mentioned, their reference highlighted a different type of influence on a young woman's method choice than that of the provider, peers or parents. Partners were discussed as potentially covering the cost of a method. Additionally, a few participants mentioned that partners might have a preference over the type of method that is chosen. For example, in every FGD, participants discussed that a male partner would not want to wear a condom, particularly if a young woman was using another contraceptive method for pregnancy prevention. One group highlighted the risk of sexually transmitted infections associated with this trade off, however, this concern was not discussed widely by the groups.

Though this may not always be the case, when partners were mentioned, they were discussed as influencing the character's method choice decision by playing a key role in making the decision for her, while other influencers were simply providing information that would lead the character to a certain decision.

Navigating pathways

How one prioritizes different qualities of a method may vary depending on one's current physical and social situation. Further, the method chosen may change over time. This idea of method fluidity is particularly well captured by an unmarried, Christian, young woman from Ilorin who, in the below exchange, highlights a young woman's changing method choice over time:

> *"Participant: I think for starter, she will get a cheap one [family planning method] then maybe later she might upgrade and go for the expensive ones that will last longer.*

Moderator: some long-lasting ones are actually free. So what do you think she will go for? Is it because they are easy, I am not talking about money, I'm talking about easy to get and easy to use or injectable, you will go and get injectable after two months or three years or five years. Which one do you think she will use?

Participant: that's what I'm saying, for starter she might get the easier ones [pill or injectable] then maybe later when she's free and have enough time or when she's confident enough to go to the hospital then she will go for the ones that will stay longer."

The wide range of factors that participants discussed through the FGDs closely mirrors this quote, as the participant acknowledges that each person will have a different feature that they are prioritizing when choosing a method. These priorities will also change for an individual with experience, resulting in different method choices as individuals ages or goes through life changes. Throughout these discussions, the participants discussed cost, reliability, length of coverage, and accessibility. While side effects and future fertility are overwhelmingly important factors for adolescents and youth, young people will also factor in accessibility and cost when making a final decision.

Discussion

Overall, the results of this study find that short-acting methods, specifically oral contraceptive pills, were more frequently associated with factors that would deter from use, though were discussed as the more accessible and affordable method option. Alternatively, long-acting methods were discussed more positively and were preferred among respondents who desired a method that required little follow-up at health facilities and was less user-dependent. Providers, peers, parents, and partners were all found to have an influence over the character's method choice in different ways, highlighting that successful interventions for young people require the support and mobilization at multiple levels.

The results indicate that young people prioritize a sense of control, which can look different to different people. For example, oral contraceptive pills were frequently associated with convenience and cost, both of which a young person may see as factors they can control, while the majority of participants indicated that a method that was reliable and long-lasting was preferred, giving them greater control over their reproduction due to the effectiveness. The role of the provider also highlights this sense of control as participants wanted the character to gain trustworthy information about methods to make an informed decision. Both parents and partners were discussed with hesitance as both parties were mentioned as potentially taking the control out of the character's hands, with unsupportive parents limiting access while partners were described as the decision maker in the choice of method. Having control of one's own reproduction was a priority for the participants and ensuring access to an expanded choice of methods ensures she has the control to choose the method that would be the best fit.

This study did find some misunderstandings around the proper usage of the oral contraceptive pill. There were multiple occurrences of participants believing that oral contraceptive pills only need to be taken when the young woman wants to have sex, and this inaccurate feature was highlighted as a positive characteristic related to the method's flexibility. This potentially could be due to a confusion between the oral contraceptive pill and emergency contraception, a distinction that was not made in any of the discussions. Some participants did acknowledge that for young women who are accessing their short-acting methods through drug shops, they may not be receiving all the proper information about the method, or potential side effects. The improper use of short-acting methods can lead to side effects and unplanned pregnancy, which are outcomes that may be discussed with friends and dissuade them from using these methods in the future. This possibility for misinformation must be addressed with programming that ensures the distribution of medically accurate information. The WHO has resources available that relay the most current information on each contraceptive method, and how to properly counsel someone when choosing a method [15, 16]. Many of these resources focus on providers, though they should guide the creation of community materials and programming to ensure this information is distributed more widely.

Our results are supported by global data which finds that unmarried young women are more likely to use traditional methods or condoms while married young women are more likely to access methods such as injectables; LARC use is still low among both groups [17]. Nigerian PMA2020 data from 2017, supports these usage trends as well, and the factors identified by the participants in this study highlight why certain individuals are drawn to certain methods [3]. One area where the results diverged from global research was the dominance of providers as reported influencers when looking at the data collectively. Despite the support by the participants, previous research shows providers can play a restricting role on access to the use of contraception [5]. Our results did potentially support these restrictive roles when the data was analyzed by marital status, though direct mentions of provider restrictions within the data were limited. The findings around peers align with previous work. For example, one study among Nigerian youth found that 85% of female participants interviewed based their contraceptive decisions off of their peers [17]. The findings of our study were also in line with previous research about method-specific features that are desired by young women. Two previous studies found that participants ranked a lack of side effects and effectiveness as the most important features for them, which was supported by our findings though a lack of side effects and concerns of future fertility were the most mentioned factors among our participants [10, 11]. That said, privacy, which has been identified by several other studies as a concern, was minimally discussed by our participants [11, 18].

This study has some limitations as a result of the use of a vignette structure in the discussion guides. Vignettes are a form of priming and can have two possible influences. First, the vignette sets the scene that the character is accessing a method at a doctor. Due to this framing, we had limited ability to analyze participants' views on pharmacies and drug shops as they were not frequently discussed in the FGDs. Though young women can face barriers of negative social norms around adolescent and youth use of contraception and provider bias at a facility as well as a pharmacy or drug shop, proximity, and other convenience factors may lead young women to access contraception at these alternative non-health facility-based locations if choosing between a health facility and a pharmacy or drug shop. However, the findings of this study are unable to determine if this is the case. Because of this limitation, a more open-ended analysis of the pathways to a method should be considered for future research. Additionally, in the follow-up questions, by limiting the choices for participants to choose from to oral contraceptive pills or an implant, it limited the responses that participants provided on their believed method the character would select. Based on the Nigerian PMA2020 data on adolescent method mix, we know that implants account for only 14.4% of use among married adolescents compared to 30% for injectables [6]. Among sexually active, unmarried adolescents, these numbers fall below 5% for both methods, with condoms accounting for over 50% of use [3]. Additionally, the 2013 Nigerian Demographic and Health Survey found that among all women surveyed, only 24.7% had knowledge of implants while 70.9% had knowledge of pills [4]. By limiting the methods the participants were meant to discuss, it created an image of high implant use that is not supported by population data. This approach provided more detailed look at these two methods that offered perspectives on hormonal methods that required daily reminders versus a longer-term, less user dependent method. This study demonstrated an interest in certain features of implants or LARC methods, but this may ignore the fact that for young people these methods are potentially inaccessible. Future research would be needed to determine whether the use of LARCs among young women would increase if availability and accessibility of these methods was ensured.

Conclusion

The results of this study can be used by programs seeking to increase expanded method choice for adolescents and youth. In particular, this study demonstrates that young people are concerned about side effects and health effects and programs need to address these issues as part of strategies to increase use in this population. Further, programs should continue to prioritize expanding method choice by ensuring that accurate information is available on all available methods and addressing misinformation about methods that may cause hesitancy toward use, or use of some methods in certain contexts. Providers, peers, parents, and partners can be harnessed as a resource for information about specific methods and this may lead to these influencers being more supportive of young people's contraceptive use. Programming should ensure that medically accurate information is widely distributed to potentially reach these influencers and that providers are trained on youth friendly services that includes provision of a range of methods to young people. Further, promoting parent-child communication as well as normalizing contraceptive use among sexually active young people can help reduce barriers to use for this group.

Acknowledgements

This research was made possible by a grant from the Bill & Melinda Gates Foundation (BMGF) under the terms of the Full Access, Full Choice Project and the Measurement, Learning & Evaluation for the Urban Reproductive Health Initiative Project (MLE). This research was also supported by a Population Research Infrastructure Program (P2C HD050924) awarded to the Carolina Population Center at the University of North Carolina at Chapel Hill by the Eunice Kennedy Shriver National Institute of Child Health and Human Development. The views expressed in this paper do not necessarily represent the view of the foundation. The authors of this paper are grateful for the contribution and support of the University of Ibadan Centre for Population and Reproductive Health team throughout this research.

Authors' contributions

EKS performed coding, data analysis and drafted the manuscript. CM assisted with study design and manuscript review. IS supervised the design of the study and contributed to manuscript review. GH provided manuscript review. LC provided additional supervision to the design and implementation of the study and contributed to manuscript review All authors approve the final manuscript.

Author details

[1]Carolina Population Center, University of North Carolina-Chapel Hill, Chapel Hill, USA. [2]The Bill & Melinda Gates Foundation, Seattle, USA. [3]Gillings School of Global Public Health, Department of Maternal and Child Health, UNC, Chapel Hill, USA.

References

1. United Nations Population Fund. The power of 1.8 billion: adolescents, youth and the transformation of the future: United Nations Population Fund; 2014. http://www.unfpa.org/sites/default/files/pub-pdf/EN-SWOP14-Report_FINAL-web.pdf.

2. Speizer IS, Guilkey D, Calhoun LM, Corroon M, O'Hara R. Examination of youth sexual and reproductive health transitions in Nigeria and Kenya using longitudinal data. BMC Public Health. 2017. https://doi.org/10.1186/s12889-017-4039-8.
3. PMA 2020. Adolescents & young adults health brief. Nigeria: PMA 2020; 2017. p. 1–2.
4. National Population Commission. Nigeria demographic and health survey 2013. 2013.
5. Measurement, Learning & Evaluation (MLE) Project; Data, Research and Mapping Consult, Ltd. NURHI Sustainability Study: Women's Survey Descriptive Findings. MLE Technical Working Paper. Chapel Hill: Measurement, Learning & Evaluation; 2018.
6. Calhoun LM, Speizer IS, Rimal R, Sripad P, Chatterjee N, Achyut P, et al. Provider imposed restrictions to clients' access to family planning in urban Uttar Pradesh, India: a mixed methods study. BMC Health Serv Res. 2013;13: 532. https://doi.org/10.1186/1472-6963-13-532.
7. Sinai I, Nyenwa J, Oguntunde O. Programmatic implications of unmet need for contraception among men and young married women in northern Nigeria. Open Access J Contracept. 2018;9.
8. Schwandt HM, Speizer IS, Corroon M. Contraceptive service provider imposed restrictions to contraceptive access in urban Nigeria. BMC Health Serv Res. 2017. https://doi.org/10.1186/s12913-017-2233-0.
9. Tumlinson K, Okigbo CC, Speizer IS. Provider barriers to family planning access in urban Kenya. Contraception. 2015;92(2):143–51. https://doi.org/10.1016/j.contraception.2015.04.002.
10. Ngabo F, McKenna K, Tolley EE, et al. Preferences for a potential longer-acting injectable contraceptive: perspectives from women, providers, and policy makers in Kenya and Rwanda. Glob Heal Sci Pract. 2014. https://doi.org/10.9745/ghsp-d-13-00147.
11. Raidoo S, Kaneshiro B. Contraception counseling for adolescents. Curr Opin Obstet Gynecol. 2017. https://doi.org/10.1097/GCO.0000000000000390.
12. Measurement, Learning & Evaluation (MLE) Project; National Population Council (NPC); Data, Research and Mapping Consult, Ltd.; End of Project Report: The Measurement, Learning and Evaluation (MLE) Project for the Urban Reproductive Health Initiative, 2011 – 2017. Chapel Hill: Measurement, Learning & Evaluation Project; 2017.https://tciurbanhealth.org/wp-content/uploads/2017/12/mle_end_of_project_report_final_updatedlinks.pdf
13. Bailey A. Let's tell you a story: use of vignettes in focus group discussions on HIV/AIDS among migrant and mobile men in Goa, India. In: Doing cross-cultural research: ethical and methodological perspectives: Springer; 2008.
14. Gourlay A, Mshana G, Birdthistle I, Bulugu G, Zaba B, Urassa M. Using vignettes in qualitative research to explore barriers and facilitating factors to the uptake of prevention of mother-to-child transmission services in rural Tanzania: a critical analysis. BMC Med Res Methodol. 2014;14(1):1–11. https://doi.org/10.1186/1471-2288-14-21.
15. World Health Organization Department of Reproductive Health and Research (WHO/RHR) and Johns Hopkins Bloomberg School of Public Health/Center for Communication Programs (CCP), Knowledge for Health Project. Family planning: a global handbook for providers (2018 update). Baltimore and Geneva: CCP and WHO; 2018.
16. World Health Organisation 2015. Medical eligibility criteria for contraceptive use Fifth edition 2015: Who; 2015. www.who.int/reproductivehealth/topics/family_planning.
17. Iyoke C, Ezugwu F, Lawani O, Ugwu G, Ajah L, Mba S. Peer-driven contraceptive choices and preferences for contraceptive methods among students of tertiary educational institutions in Enugu, Nigeria. Patient Prefer Adherence. 2014;8:1043–50. Published 2014 Jul 31. https://doi.org/10.2147/PPA.S67585.
18. Tibaijuka L, Odongo R, Welikhe E, et al. Factors influencing use of long-acting versus short-acting contraceptive methods among reproductive-age women in a resource-limited setting. BMC Womens Health. 2017. https://doi.org/10.1186/s12905-017-0382-2.

4

Sex differences in family planning knowledge, attitudes and use in Uganda

Afra Nuwasiima[1*†], Agnes Watsemba[1†], Allan Eyapu[1], Peter Kaddu[1] and Justin Loiseau[2]

Abstract

Background: Literature is satiated with studies focusing on knowledge, attitude, and practices of family planning (FP) among the female population, conversely, the gaps in sex-disaggregated data on FP continue to exist. This study sought to report sex differences existing in FP knowledge, attitude, and use in Uganda.

Methods: This study uses data from a household survey that covered 16 districts in Uganda. Multi-stage cluster randomized sampling was employed for participant selection. Bivariate analysis for categorical data was conducted. Multilevel logistic regression model was applied to model the effects of socio-demographic characteristics on the use of modern FP methods.

Results: Data from 4,352 respondents in the ratios of 70 % females and 30 % of males were analyzed. The mean age was 28.7 SD (8.5) and was not significantly different between males and females. More male respondents had secondary or higher level of education (44 %) than females (36 %). Knowledge of at least one modern FP method was high, but small significant differences were revealed between males (96 %) and females (98 %). Significant knowledge differences were seen in specific FP methods. A higher proportion of females (71 %) than males (67 %) perceived modern FP methods as always available in the community whereas more males (40 %) believed that modern FP methods can result in infertility than females (35 %). There was high self-efficacy about family planning methods use in both males and females. The proportion of married females that reported using or their partner using a modern FP method was 39 % compared to 45 % reported by the married males. Approx. 53 % of the males compared to 37 % of the females that reported condom use also cited STI/HIV prevention as the main reason for condom use suggesting dual protection as a driver for use. Males, young adults, the more educated, and those in marriage or active relationships were more likely to use modern FP methods.

Conclusions: Our study found significant sex differences in knowledge, attitudes, and use of FP methods. The young adults and more educated respondents were more likely to use FP methods. The high self-efficacy observed for both males and females is a signal that both sexes can use FP methods. Project strategies and implementation should take into consideration the existing differences by sex and devise sex-tailored approaches to improve FP knowledge, attitudes, and use in this population. There was increased reporting of condom use as an FP and STI/HIV prevention method, follow-up studies aiming at succinctly measuring dual protection, and its drivers for both sex should be done.

Keywords: Family planning, sex, knowledge, attitudes, use, community health, Living Goods, Uganda

* Correspondence: anuwasiima@livinggodds.org
[1]Living Goods, Kampala, Uganda

Background

Use of family planning (FP) methods by women and men can improve the health, economic, and social domains of their lives [1]. As such, FP continues to be a key focus of the global agenda for improving maternal, sexual and reproductive health. According to the Uganda Demographic and Health Survey (UDHS) report 2016, some knowledge of FP methods is nearly universal in Uganda, with 99 % of both women and men having heard of at least one method of FP [2]. However, the use of modern FP and any form of FP among married women in Uganda stood at only 35 and 39 % respectively. FP methods use among sexually active unmarried women was slightly higher with 51 % using any FP method and 47 % using a modern method, and the total unmet need for FP among the sexually active women of reproductive age stood at 28 % among currently married women, and 32 % among the sexually active unmarried women.

In the FP Costed Implementation Plan 2015–2020 [3], the Uganda Ministry of Health (MoH) acknowledged that several innovative FP service delivery models have been successfully implemented by Non-Governmental Organizations (NGOs) in Uganda in an effort to remove access barriers for FP. For instance, community-based distribution of certain FP commodities has been successful at expanding access, and task shifting of injectable FP to Village Health Teams (VHTs)/Community Health Workers (CHWs). Over the past 2 decades, government-supported VHTs have provided a broad service package including family planning. However, key challenges still exist, limiting the effectiveness of the community health program; CHWs not adequately equipped with commodities and skills to deliver FP, absence of supervision, no compensation, and suboptimal use of reporting and decision support tools. In 2018, Living Goods, an international organisation piloted the implementation of comprehensive CHW led FP services model while addressing these gaps in the two districts of Wakiso and Mpigi in Uganda. The FP services provided to the clients mainly comprised of counseling, and provision of condoms, DMPA-SC (commonly known by the brand Sayana Press® or simply Sayana) and oral FP and as well as referral for long-term methods. The pilot program results suggested that by working through CHWs, it is possible to address the binding constraints to the uptake and utilization of FP including social opposition, misinformation and fear of side effects, among others[4].

Men's knowledge, attitudes, and behaviors around FP impact uptake and unmet need because men are not only women's partners, but individuals with distinct reproductive histories and desires of their own. A 2020 Tanzania study [5] found that knowledge of modern contraception was a crucial factor in influencing the use of modern FP among men and suggested that targeting of men with FP awareness programs would improve the use of FP among men. The UDHS 2016 findings [2] showed that 12 % of married women were refused to use FP by their partners while 44 % made the decision jointly with their husbands. The literature on the role and attitude of men in decision-making is mixed. A study in Uganda revealed that men were greatly interested in modern contraception, albeit they possessed little knowledge about it [6] while a related study in Tanzania showed that men expressed little interest in the use of modern FP methods, and yet were considered by women as key decision-makers in their use of FP[7]. Another study conducted in Uganda using nationally representative data revealed that the use of FP was significantly higher among men that had discussions with a health worker, desired for few children, belonged to a higher wealth index, and highly educated [8], and these factors are similar to factors that affect FP among women. Male inclusion in FP has been encouraged by various international and national initiatives including providing incentives for men who escort their partners for FP. However, gaps in data continue as FP data in programs and reports is rarely disaggregated by sex if men are included at all [9]. Where data on utilization of modern contraception were reported among men, FP methods use was found to be high[5].

Whereas there is paucity of literature on men's statistics, collection, analysis, and reporting of sex-disaggregated data are critical to fully understand the specific needs of men and women. This study sought to explore sex variations existing in the knowledge, attitudes, and use of FP services in selected districts of Uganda.

Methods

Study design

This was a cross-sectional survey, conducted as a baseline to a larger research project. The paper focuses on the results from the quantitative household survey. Data collection was conducted in August 2019.

The study setting

Data collection was undertaken in sixteen (xvi) districts of Uganda. The study did not seek to be nationally representative as the selection of study districts took into consideration Living Goods Uganda's current catchment area for the FP intervention. Figure 1 shows a map of Uganda with survey districts marked "Yes" with a pink color.

Study population

Participants in the household (HH) baseline survey comprised of women and men in the reproductive age of 15 to 49 years.

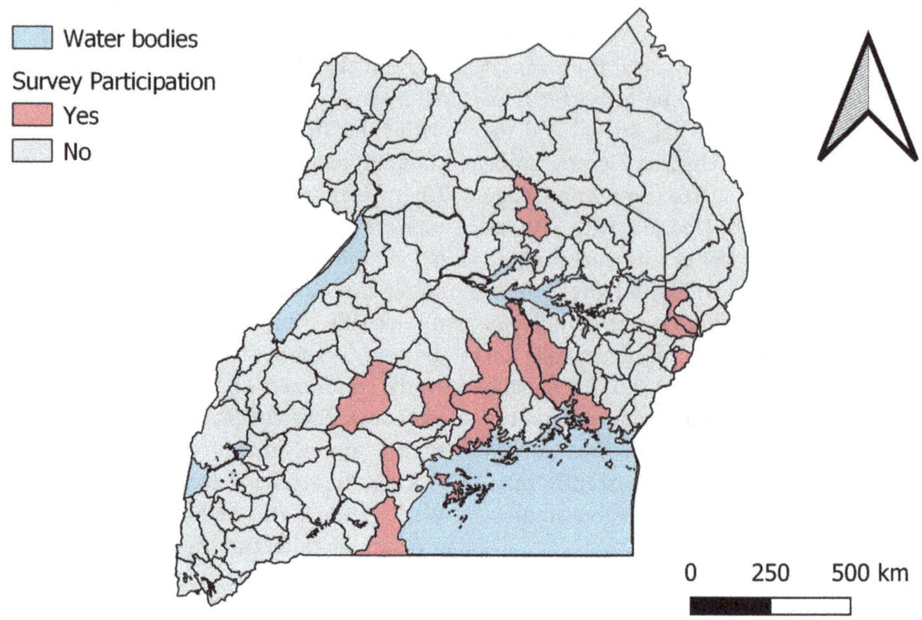

Fig. 1 Map showing the survey districts in Uganda

Sample size

The Cochran (1963) formula for two independent samples with a dichotomous outcome was used to determine the sample size (n). To achieve a maximum sample size, a proportion of 0.5 per sample group was used. A sample of 4,380 respondents was derived with a statistical power of 90 %, a precision level of 5 %, a design effect is 1.5, and a 95 % confidence level. The sample was distributed equally among sampled districts and villages.

Household sample selection

The selection of the households for the survey utilized a four-stage sampling approach. The first stage involved a purposive selection of districts for the survey and the second stage involved a random selection of sub-counties per district (2 to 6 sub-counties per district). The third stage involved the random selection of four villages within each sub-county using the computer-based Random Draw Method. The fourth and last stage involved systematic random sampling of households to be interviewed. To ensure all eligible households had an equal chance of participating in the survey, the survey team worked with local leaders to conduct a household listing of households with persons in the age range of 15–49 years (male and female). The desired ratio of 3 females to 1 male was used. The sample size was not adjusted for non-response and consequently, the household replacement was assumed to be feasible where a HH refused to participate or was not available at the time of interview. For the latter non-response, the replacement was done after making three [3] call-backs to the household. For each HH selected, only one person was needed for an interview. Therefore, simple random sampling using the raffle/lottery method without replacement was used to select a respondent from all eligible members of the desired sex in the household. The sex of the respondent was predetermined before arriving at the household.

Data collection methods

The quantitative household survey data collection was done through face-to-face interviews using a structured questionnaire. The questionnaire was programmed using the Open Data Kit (ODK) software and uploaded on electronic devices (smartphones).

Quality assurance

Before the study was started, a data quality assurance protocol was developed and this included constituting a strong and dynamic team with experience in conducting similar assignments, recruiting and training experienced research assistants and field supervisors to handle data collection. The ODK data collection tool was also designed with controls to limit data entry errors. Field supervisors did spot checks on 5 % of the respondents to validate the information collected by the interviewers and feedback was analyzed to improve the process. Also, the research team organized routine internal meetings to review progress on the data collection against set targets per district per cluster.

Data analysis

Descriptive analysis using proportions was conducted to show the distribution of FP knowledge, attitudes, and use of FP. Bivariate analysis using Pearson's Chi-square and Fisher's exact tests for categorical data was done. Additionally, a multilevel logistic regression model [10] was used to model the effects of socio-demographic characteristics on the use of family planning methods. The sex of the respondent was included in the model as a fixed factor to model sex differences. To model the associations of respondents within the different districts, sub-counties, and villages, the study considered a four-level analysis model with three high-level cluster variables (random effects equations) i.e. district, sub-county, and village treated as random effects factors to account for within-cluster correlations (intra-cluster correlation). This assumes that observations nested in a cluster share common characteristics in terms of access to community services and this may affect the use of family planning methods. All quantitative analysis was done in STATA version 15 software and statistical significance was considered at 5 %.

Ethical considerations

The study received ethical clearance from Mildmay Uganda Research and Ethics Committee (MUREC) and Uganda National Council for Science and Technology (UNCST). All members of the survey team were trained on the protection of human subjects. In the field, all members of the survey team obtained written informed consent, upheld the principles of voluntary participation, confidentiality, anonymity, and respect of the privacy of respondents, and the obligation to not do any harm. Identifiers such as names of respondents were not tagged on an interview recorded on the smartphones further improving the privacy and confidentiality of survey data.

Results

The quantitative study achieved an overall response rate of 99 % (100 % for women and 99 % for men) by reaching 4,352 respondents out of the targeted 4,380 respondents. The study managed to achieve the ratios of 70 % female and 30 % male representation in the quantitative survey. All 4,352 respondents had complete data on socio-demographic characteristics and main outcomes hence no missing data handling approaches were used.

Socio-demographic characteristics of respondents

Table 1 shows the distribution of the socio-demographic characteristics of the study participants disaggregated by sex. The distribution of respondents differed by sex on the following variables; age group, education level, marital status, the main source of income, and the number of children. Although there were observed significant differences in age groups for males and females starting at the age of 30, the overall mean age of respondents was 28.7 SD (8.5) and was not significantly different between males and females. Overall 39 % of the respondents had not achieved at least a primary leaving certificate with a higher proportion of females (41 %) than males (35 %). Approximately one-quarter of respondents were not married, with the percentage unmarried was higher among males (44 %) than females (21 %). A significantly lower percentage of females (16 %) than males (38 %) reported having no children.

Knowledge of FP methods

Table 2 shows the results of the respondent's knowledge of FP methods. Both sexually active and inactive respondents were included in the analysis. The findings revealed that overall 97 % of the respondents had heard of at least one modern FP method and there was a small, but significant difference between males (96 %) and females (98 %). There were also significant differences in knowledge of specific FP methods by sex. Women were most likely to know injectables, pills, implants, and IUDs. Male knowledge was highest for male condoms, followed by the same three methods as for females. Overall, the study observed higher levels of knowledge in hormonal birth control FP methods (implant, IUD, Injectable, Pills) than the natural methods (Lactational Amenorrhea, Withdrawal, Periodic abstinence) and permanent methods (female and male sterilization). Knowledge of male condoms was higher for both males and females than the female condoms.

Use of contraception methods

Use of contraception was assessed by looking at the proportion of sexually active respondents that were not currently pregnant that reported using the different FP methods (84 % of the total respondents). Table 3 shows the proportion of respondents that reported the use of FP methods. The use of modern FP stood at 38.7 % overall and this was significantly higher among the males (45 %) than the females (36 %). The main methods of FP reported by females were Depo (37 %), withdrawal (22 %), and male condoms (9 %) compared to male condoms (46 %), Depo (19 %), and withdrawal (12 %) reported by males. Overall the use of the permanent FP methods was higher (6 %) than long-term methods (3 %). For permanent use, there were significant differences between males and females, but, no significant sex differences were observed among the long-term methods.

Figure 2 shows the use of modern FP methods among women by marital status and sex. The findings indicated that the proportion of married/cohabiting females that reported

Table 1 Socio-demographic characteristics of respondents by sex

Characteristic	Distribution			P value
	Overall n = 4,352	Females n = 3,061	Males n = 1,291	
Mean Age (SD)	28.7 (8.5)	28.7 (8.5)	28.5 (8.5)	0.915
Age group (%)				
15–19	14.2	13.9	14.9	0.000*
20–24	24.6	24.7	24.4	
25–29	19.2	19.4	18.7	
30–34	14.7	15.3	13.3	
35–39	12.8	13.7	10.6	
40–44	10.8	9.7	13.5	
45–49	3.6	3.3	4.5	
Highest education level attained (%)				
None/ no education	5.6	6.5	3.5	0.000*
Primary incomplete	33.7	34.8	31.1	
Completed primary	21.9	22.1	21.4	
Secondary or higher	38.8	36.6	44.1	
Religious affiliation (%)				
Muslim	18.7	18.2	20.1	0.208
Roman Catholic	36.7	36.5	37.1	
Protestant	31.9	32.5	30.5	
Born again/Pentecostal	10.2	10.5	9.2	
None/Others	2.6	2.3	3.1	
Marital status (%)				
Single	14.2	10.9	22.0	0.000*
In a relationship	12.8	10.5	18.2	
Married / cohabiting	64.3	68.3	54.9	
Separated / divorced	7.1	8.0	4.7	
Widowed	1.6	2.2	0.2	
Residence of respondent (%)				
Urban	29.1	28.7	29.8	0.593
Trading Center	12.7	12.5	13.2	
Rural	58.7	58.2	57.0	
Main source of household income				
Crop farming/Cattle keeping	47.1	46.4	48.9	0.007*
Fishing	1.8	1.7	2.1	
Salary/Wage	14.0	14.1	13.7	
Business	28.1	29.5	24.6	
Boda-Boda / Other transport	4.4	4.3	4.6	
None	0.5	0.5	0.7	
Others	4.1	3.6	5.3	
Number of children (%)				
0	22.9	16.4	38.3	0.000*
1	15.6	16.5	13.3	
2	14.2	16.0	9.9	

Table 1 Socio-demographic characteristics of respondents by sex *(Continued)*

Characteristic	Distribution			P value
	Overall n = 4,352	Females n = 3,061	Males n = 1,291	
3	11.7	13.0	8.5	
4	9.8	10.7	7.7	
5+	25.7	27.2	22.1	

* Implies statistically significant results at 5 % level of significance

using or their partner using a modern FP was 39 % lower than 45 % reported by the male counterparts. Modern FP use was highest for both males and females that were in a relationship but married/ cohabiting and lowest for both males and females that were single or separated.

Condom use as a dual protection method

Figure 3 shows that half of the males and a third of the female respondents that reported condom use as the current method of FP used it as a prevention measure of STI/HIV infection. The study did not establish whether the primary objective was STI/HIV protection or protection against pregnancy or both, and this is a limitation to accurately measure the differentiated effect of condom use on the results reported among males.

Respondent perceptions, beliefs, and self-efficacy about FP services

Table 4 shows the respondent's perceptions on the availability, affordability, self-efficacy, and beliefs about the FP methods disaggregated by sex. The results in this section were restricted to men (92 %) and women (96 %) respondents that were in-union or sexually active singles. The results are explained in the following sub-sections.

Perceived availability of FP services

Overall, more than half of the respondents (69.9 %) perceived modern FP as always available in the community whenever they were needed, and this was significantly higher among the females (71.1 %) than the males (66.7 %).

Table 2 Knowledge of different FP services by sex of respondent

Measure	Distribution (%)			P-value
	Overall n = 4,352	Females n = 3,061	Males n = 1,291	
Ever heard of any family planning method	97.4	97.8	96.4	0.006*
Ever heard of any modern family planning method	97.2	97.6	96.2	0.012*
Aware of all modern FP methods	0.97	1.08	0.70	0.240
Knowledge of specific FP methods				
Injectables	83.6	89.5	69.5	0.000*
Pills	74.8	79.2	64.4	0.000*
Implants	66	73	49.3	0.000*
Male condoms	60.3	53.3	77.1	0.000*
IUD	53.9	60.6	38	0.000*
Periodic abstinence	16.6	18.1	13	0.000*
Withdrawal	15	14	17.2	0.008*
Female condoms	14.2	14.5	13.7	0.429
Female sterilization	13.5	14.7	10.7	0.000*
Male sterilization	11.7	9.9	16	0.000*
Emergency FP pills	9.2	9.8	7.7	0.024*
Lactational Amenorrhea	6.4	7.9	2.7	0.000*

* Implies statistically significant results at 5 % level of significance

Table 3 Proportion of respondents reporting use of FP methods

FP methods use	Distribution (%)			P-value
	Overall (n = 3,677)	Females (n = 2,614)	Males (n = 1,063)	
Currently using any FP method	50.3	48.6	54.7	0.001*
Currently using a modern FP method	38.7	36.0	45.3	0.000*
Main FP method used				
Short-term				
Pills	4.5	4.7	4.1	0.558
Injectable (Depo)	31.1	36.5	19.1	0.000*
Injectable (Sayana Press)	5.9	7.7	2.0	0.000*
Emergency FP	0.7	1.0	0.0	0.013*
Male condoms	20.3	8.6	45.7	0.000*
Female condoms	0.1	0.1	0.0	1.000
Long-term				
IUD	2.6	2.9	1.9	0.196
Implants	0.2	0.1	0.5	0.095
Permanent				
Male sterilization	1.6	2.0	0.7	0.029*
Female sterilization	4.0	4.8	2.0	0.004*
Natural				
Lactational Amenorrhea	5.5	5.2	6.1	0.393
Periodic abstinence	4.1	4.0	4.3	0.785
Withdrawal	18.8	21.7	12.4	0.000*
Others	0.7	0.5	1.2	0.134

* Implies statistically significant results at 5 % level of significance

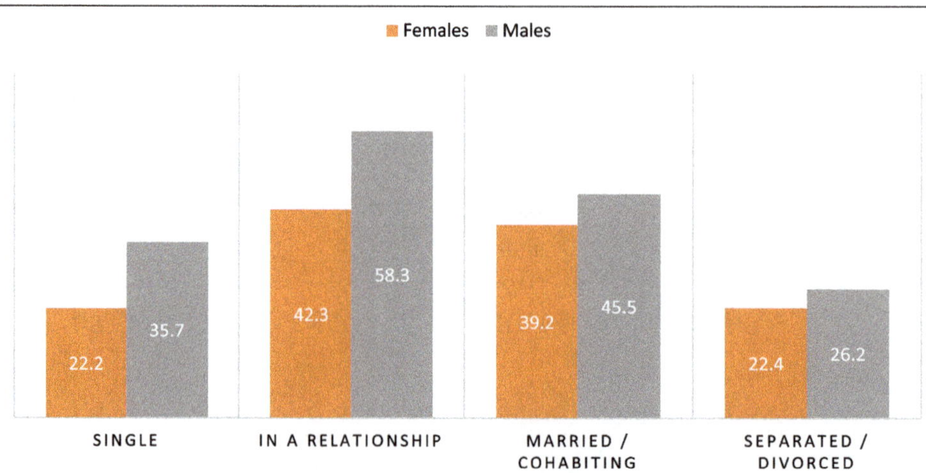

Fig. 2 Modern FP use by marital status and sex

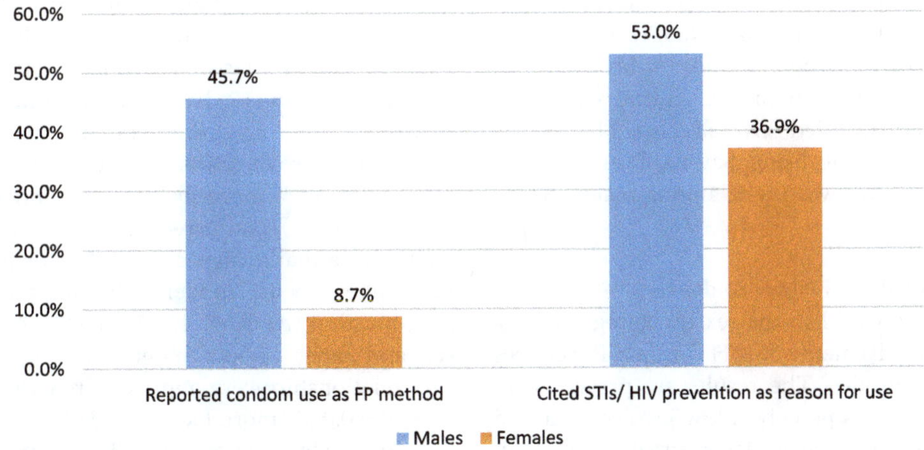

Fig. 3 Proportion of respondents that reported condoms use as an FP method and a form of protection against STIs/HIV infection (males = 268 and females = 111)

Perceived affordability of FP Services

The results in Table 4 further suggest that over half of the respondents (53 %) perceived modern FP methods to be affordable within their communities. There were no significant sex differences.

Perceived quality of FP services

The study results also revealed that overall almost three-quarters (73 %) of the respondents perceived public health facilities to be providing high-quality FP services, and this was significantly higher among the females (75.0 %) than males (68.5 %).

Beliefs about FP services

Beliefs about FP were assessed by exploring the respondent's perceptions about the side-effects of FP considering; beliefs about modern FP and infertility, cancer, and the effects of FP use on sexual pleasure. Table 4 shows

Table 4 Perceptions of community members on FP services by sex

Perception/Attitude	Overall (n = 4,128)	Female (n = 2,936)	Male (n = 1,192)	P-value
Perceived availability of FP services in the community				
• *Agree that modern FP are always available in my community when I need them*	69.9	71.1	66.7	0.005*
Perceived affordability of FP services in the community				
Modern contraceptives are affordable in my community	52.6	52.3	53.5	0.457
Community perception of the quality of FP services				
• *Agree that FP services provided in public health facilities are of high quality*	73.1	75.0	68.5	0.000*
Beliefs about FP services				
• *Believe that using modern FP can result in infertility*	36.4	35.1	39.7	0.005*
• *Believe that using IUDs can result in cancer*	41.9	41.6	42.5	0.590
• *Believe that using Sayana Press reduces sexual pleasure*	11.4	12.5	8.6	0.000*
Self-efficacy about FP services				
• *I am embarrassed to get/ask about FP from a health facility*	11.3	11.2	11.5	0.816
• *I would be embarrassed if people found out that I am using FP*	10.0	9.9	10.0	0.790
• *It is ok for a woman/girl to suggest to her male partner that they use a condom or another method to avoid pregnancy*	87.5	87.9	86.4	0.198
• *My partner would be annoyed with me if they discovered I was asking for condoms, pills or other FP methods*	29.8	34.2	18.7	0.000*
• *My friends would laugh at me/ tease me if they found out that I was asking for condoms, pills or other FP services*	12.6	13.9	12.1	0.108

* Implies statistically significant results at 5 % level of significance

that more males (40 %) significantly perceived modern FP to result in infertility than females (35 %). For specific methods, overall 42 % of the respondents believed that the use of IUDs can result in cancer, and no significant sex differences were revealed. Overall, also, 11 % of the respondents believed that using Sayana Press reduces sexual pleasure, and this was lower among males (8.6 %) than females (12.5 %).

Perceived role of CHWs in FP service delivery

The study sought to establish the sex-disaggregated perception of the involvement of CHWs in FP services provision in communities. The results are presented in Fig. 4. Overall, there was perceived low involvement and quality of CHWs in FP services. Approximately only 3 in 10 of the respondents agreed that CHWs were available in the community to offer FP services and agreed that FP services provided were of high quality. There were no significant sex differences observed.

Decision-making regarding FP use

Decision-making regarding FP use is a critical factor in the adoption of FP services. The results presented in Fig. 5 suggested that a larger proportion of females (53 %) decided for the couple to take on FP than 33 % reported by males. More males reported that the decision for the couple to use FP was joint compared to females. Even though half of the women reported deciding to use FP themselves, majority of them indicated that their partners were aware of the FP use.

Effect of socio-demographic characteristics on modern FP use

Table 5 shows findings from the adjusted multilevel logistic regression to assess the effect of socio-demographic characteristics on modern FP use. The findings indicated that females were 35 % less likely to use FP compared to males (Adjusted odds ratio (AOR) = 0.65, P = 0.000). Respondents aged 40–44 and 45–49 were 36 and 69 % less likely to use modern FP compared to those aged 15–19. No significant differences were observed for other age groups in comparison to the 15–19 age group. For education level, those that completed primary were 43 % more likely to use modern FP (AOR = 1.43, P = 0.041) compared to those with no education while those that achieved secondary or higher were 45 % more likely to use modern FP compared to those with no education (AOR = 1.45, P = 0.030). After adjusting for sex and other socio-demographic characteristics, those in a relationship were approximately two times (AOR = 2.48, P = 0.000) more likely to use FP compared to those in no/ single relationships. The married respondents were also 88 % more likely to use modern FP compared to those in no relationship. No significant differences were revealed for religion, place of residence, source of income, and the number of children.

Discussion

Literature is replete with studies focusing on knowledge, attitude, and use of FP services among the female population, conversely, the disaggregation of results by males and females has been less of a focus and not emphasized in reporting [9]. This paper's findings add to a growing body of literature on sex-disaggregated FP knowledge and use. The results from the study revealed significant sex differences in the knowledge, attitudes, and use of FP services in selected districts in Uganda.

The finding that knowledge of FP was equally high for both males and females, despite the small differences is an indication that males and females have been equally targeted and engaged with information on FP in Uganda. It is not surprising that men were more aware of condoms as an FP method than any other method while women were more aware of the longer-term FP

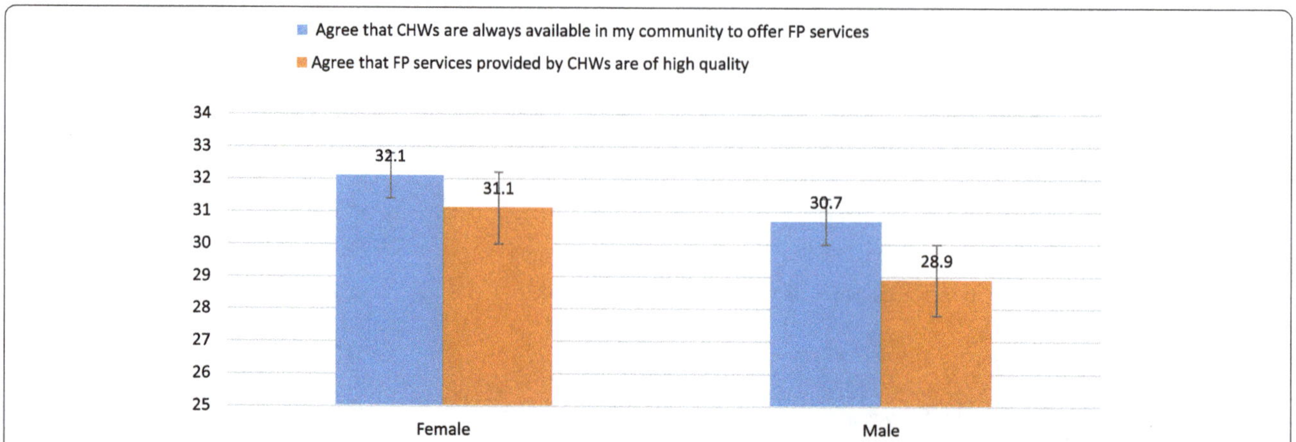

Fig. 4 Perceived role of CHWs in FP service delivery

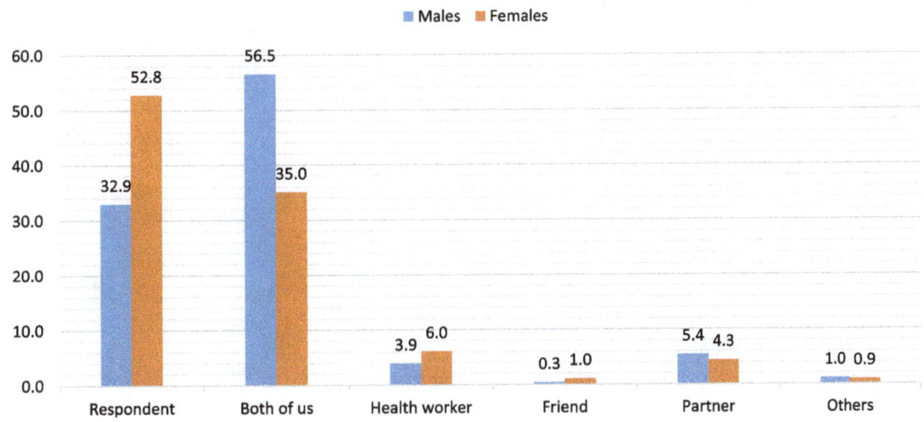

Fig. 5 Decision making in FP uptake

methods. It may be argued that whereas men may be more focused on the dual protection they can get from condoms, women are usually more concerned about the prevention of unplanned pregnancy and this explains why men may be more informed more about condom use. These findings contradict those found in Mwanza region Tanzania [7], Mpigi district Uganda[6], Mbeya region Tanzania [11], and Nigeria [12] which all found that men had little knowledge on the subject.

Whereas females had more knowledge on FP and its availability within their communities, their attitudes, and fears about the possible side effects were significantly different from those of males. The study found out that more males were worried that modern FP methods can result in infertility while females were on the other hand more concerned about reduced sexual pleasure or their partners being angry if they found out. Whenever such fears exist, it becomes difficult for people to embrace FP methods. The mismatch in fears between men and women related to FP may also affect couples' communication on FP matters and result in lower uptake of FP and or discontinuation. The negative effect of fear of side effects on FP uptake has been reported by previous research studies [6, 7, 13–16].

Findings revealed that half of the males that reported condom use as the current FP method also cited STIs/HIV prevention as the reason for its use. This finding revealed that most of the males preferred condom use dual protection compared to a third of the females resulting in a potential overestimation of reported FP use among males. Whereas almost half of the males in this study commonly reported condoms as their FP method of use, other studies have associated condom use with HIV prevention and protection efforts [17] or casual sexual relationships rather than as an FP method [18]. Future research should establish the primary use of condoms whenever they are reported as the FP method to avoid overstating its use as an FP method. The findings further suggested that the use of short-term modern FP methods accounted for more than three-quarters of the total modern FP methods in this study and recent studies associated short-term methods use with high odds of discontinuation and switching affecting uptake and retention of clients on FP [2, 16]. Our study findings from the regression model suggested that males, the young adults, the highly educated, and those in marriage or active relationship were more likely to use modern FP services. These findings are consistent with other research studies that reported high FP among the educated [8], and the married [19]. Contrary to the recent studies [8, 20] our study finding revealed no significant variations in uptake of modern FP among respondents with no child and those with an increasing number of children.

Results from a recent randomized controlled trial study found that where CHWs were active in the provision of low-cost health products and basic child health services to low-income families, there were improved health outcomes among the community members like reduced morbidity and mortality [21]. Our study findings revealed low involvement of CHWs in the delivery of family planning services. Learning from findings on the RCT study [21], we think that there is a potential opportunity for research on how CHWs can be leveraged to provide FP services and follow-up of clients. The Living model that addresses some of the bottlenecks to effective CHW services delivery like inadequate tools, lack of supervision, and compensation is a learning opportunity on how CHWs can be supported to drive impact in the community in the sexual and reproductive health services domain.

Our findings are not indicative of the national picture and should not be decisively used to generalize the entire country's situation since they are largely biased to a few selected districts where Living Goods Uganda has a presence. Albeit, the findings provide important sex-disaggregated insights into the knowledge, attitudes,

Table 5 Multilevel multiple logistic regression model findings on modern FP use

Characteristic	Modern FP use	
	AOR (95 % CI)	P value
Sex of respondent: *Ref = Male*		
Female	0.65 (0.55,0.76)	0.000*
Age of respondent: *Ref = 15–19*		
20–24	0.98(0.75,1.29)	0.908
25–29	1.12(0.83,1.51)	0.469
30–34	1.01(0.721.42)	0.960
35–39	0.88(0.61,1.27)	0.504
40–44	0.64(0.44,0.95)	0.028*
45–49	0.39(0.23,0.66)	0.000*
Highest education level: *Ref = None/ no education*		
Primary incomplete	1.21(0.87,1.69)	0.253
Completed primary	1.43(1.01,2.03)	0.041*
Secondary or higher	1.45(1.04,2.04)	0.030*
Religion: Ref = Muslim		
Roman Catholic	1.01(0.82,1.24)	0.894
Protestant	0.90(0.73,1.11)	0.345
Born again/Pentecostal	0.79(0.60,1.05)	0.108
None/Others	0.80(0.38,1.66)	0.545
Marital status: Ref = *Single*		
In a relationship	2.48(1.85,3.32)	0.000*
Married / cohabiting	1.88(1.39,2.54)	0.000*
Separated / divorced	0.85(0.57,1.27)	0.434
Widowed	0.64(0.30,1.37)	0.250
Residence: *Ref = Urban*		
Trading Center	0.92(0.70,1.20)	0.519
Rural	1.06(0.87,1.30)	0.552
Household main source of income: *Ref = Crop farming/Cattle keeping*		
Fishing	0.90(0.52,1.56)	0.711
Salary/Wage	1.05(0.83,1.31)	0.690
Business	0.99(0.83,1.18)	0.918
Boda Boda/ Other transport	1.13(0.79,1.60)	0.501
None	2.54(0.95,6.80)	0.062
Others	0.95(0.66,1.37)	0.791
Number of children: *Ref = No child*		
1	0.84(0.64,1.12)	0.237
2	1.30(0.95,1.78)	0.098
3	1.31(0.93,1.84)	0.119
4	1.33(0.91,1.92)	0.137
5+	1.23(0.86,1.86)	0.252

* Implies statistically significant results at 5 % level of significance

beliefs, and use of FP and are thus important for improving the programming of future FP interventions. The results showed that females had a higher positive attitude and beliefs on availability, affordability, and beliefs of FP methods than males. Overall both males reported high self-efficacy and this can be leveraged to promote use of FP methods. The study couldn't succinctly establish the reasons for condom use or the differentiated effect of condom use on modern contraception as a dual protection method for STIs/HIV and pregnancy. Follow-up studies will aim to measure this accurately. Given that this study was conducted as part of a baseline to an FP project, project strategies and implementation will take into consideration the existing differences by sex as documented in this paper and devise sex-tailored approaches to improve FP knowledge, attitudes, and use in this population.

Conclusions

Our study found out that knowledge of at least one modern FP method was high, but small significant differences were revealed between males (96 %) and females (98 %). Large differences were however observed in FP-specific methods. There was high self-efficacy about family planning methods use in both males and females. Significantly, more males (40 %) believed that modern FP methods can result in infertility compared to females (35 %). A significantly lower proportion of married females reported using or their partner using a modern FP method (39 %) compared to 45 % reported by the married males. The young adults and more educated respondents were more likely to use FP methods. Project strategies and implementation should take into consideration the observed sex differences in attitudes, beliefs, and knowledge and devise sex-tailored approaches to improve FP uptake. There was increased reporting of condom use as an FP and STI/HIV prevention method, follow-up studies aiming at succinctly measuring dual protection, and its drivers in both males and females should be done.

Abbreviations

AOR: Adjusted Odds Ratio; CHW(s): Community Health Worker(s); CI: Confidence Interval; FGDs: Focus Group Discussion; FP: Family Planning; HH: Household; IUDs: Intra-Uterine Device; LG : Living Goods; MCH: Maternal and Child Health; MOH: Ministry of Health; MUREC: Mildmay Uganda Research and Ethics Committee; ODK: Open Data Kit; UBOS: Uganda Bureau of Statistics; UDHS: Uganda Demographic and Health Survey; UNCST: Uganda National Council for Science and Technology

Acknowledgements

The authors for this study would like to acknowledge the Socio-Economic Data Centre Ltd Uganda consultants led by Professor Narathius Asingwire that designed the evaluation protocol, acquired ethical clearance and conducted data collection from which this study draws the data. The consultants however have no role in the manuscript writing for this paper.

Authors' contribution

AW and AN conceived the study. AN conducted the data analysis. AW and AN wrote the first draft. AE, PK, JL reviewed the draft manuscript. All authors reviewed and approved the final manuscript.

Author details

[1]Living Goods, Kampala, Uganda. [2]Global Research & Evidence Strategy Living Goods, Nairobi, Kenya.

References

1. Guttmacher Institute BMGF. ADDING IT UP: Investing in Contraception and Maternal and Newborn Health. Guttmacher Inst [Internet]. 2017;(June):1–4. Available from: http://www.gatesfoundation.org/What-We-Do/Global-Development/Family-Planning%0Ahttps://www.guttmacher.org/fact-sheet/adding-it-up-contraception-mnh-2017.
2. Uganda Bureau of Statistics and ICF. Uganda Demographic and Health Survey 2016 [Internet]. Kampala; 2018. Available from: https://dhsprogram.com/pubs/pdf/FR333/FR333.pdf.
3. Uganda Family Planning. Costed Implementation Plan, 2015–2020. Uganda: Kampala; 2014.
4. Allan E, Frank N, Phionah K. DIGITAL HEALTH PILOT. PROJECT IN UGANDA EXTENDS THE REACH OF FAMILY PLANNING CARE IN THE COMMUNITY [Internet]. 2021. Available from: https://knowledgesuccess.org/2021/01/15/digital-health-pilot-project-in-uganda-extends-the-reach-of-family-planning-care-in-the-community/.
5. Msovela J, Kessy AT, Rumisha SF, Simba DO, Urassa DP. Male partner approval on the use of modern contraceptive methods : factors determining usage among couples in Kibaha district, Tanzania. 2020;8:1–7. Available from: https://contraceptionmedicine.biomedcentral.com/articles/https://doi.org/10.1186/s40834-020-00107-8.
6. Kaida A, Kipp W, Hessel P, Konde-Lule J. Male participation in family planning: Results from a qualitative study in Mpigi District, Uganda. J Biosoc Sci. 2005;37(3):269–86.
7. Mosha I, Ruben R, Kakoko D. Family planning decisions, perceptions and gender dynamics among couples in Mwanza, Tanzania: A qualitative study. BMC Public Health [Internet]. 2013;13(1):1. Available from: BMC Public Health.
8. Kabagenyi A, Ndugga P, Wandera SO, Kwagala B. Modern contraceptive use among sexually active men in Uganda: does discussion with a health worker matter?. BMC Public Health. 2014;14(1):1-8.
9. The importance of gender in family planning and reproductive health data [Internet]. 2017. Available from: https://www.measureevaluation.org/resources/publications/fs-17-205b/at_download/document.
10. Khan M, Shaw J. Multilevel Logistic Regression Analysis Applied to Binary Contraceptive Prevalence Data. J Data Sci 2011;9(No.1):93–110.
11. Mwageni EA, Ankomah A, Powell RA. Attitudes of men towards family planning in Mbeya region, Tanzania: A rural-urban comparison of qualitative data. J Biosoc Sci. 1998;30(3):381–92.
12. Blanc AK. The Effect of Power in Sexual Relationships on Sexual and Reproductive Health: An Examination of the Evidence. Stud Fam Plann. 2003;32(3):3–4.
13. Campbell M, Potts M. Barriers to Fertility Regulation: A Review of the Literature. Stud Fam Plann [Internet]. 2006;37(2). Available from: https://doi.org/10.1111/j.1728-4465.2006.00088.x.
14. Castle S. Factors Infuencing Young Malians' Reluctance to Use Hormonal Contraceptives. Stud Fam Plann [Internet]. 2004;34(3). Available from: https://onlinelibrary.wiley.com/doi/abs/10.1111/j.1728-4465.2003.00186.x.
15. Hall MAK, Stephenson RB, Juvekar S. Social and logistical barriers to the use of reversible contraception among women in a rural Indian Village. J Heal Popul Nutr. 2008;26(2):241–50.
16. Nuwasiima A, Nuwamanya E, Babigumira JU, Nalwanga R, Asiimwe FT, Babigumira JB. Acceptability and utilization of family planning benefits cards by youth in slums in Kampala, Uganda. 2019;2:1–11. Available from: https://rdcu.be/bXQnM.
17. Green EC, Halperin DT, Nantulya V, Hogle JA. Uganda's HIV prevention success: The role of sexual behavior change and the national response. AIDS Behav. 2006;10(4):335–46.
18. Pranitha M, John C. Risk Perception and Condom Use Among Married Or Cohabiting Couples in KwaZulu-Natal, South Africa. Int Fam Plan Perspect. 2005;31(1):24–9.
19. Asiimwe JB, Ndugga P, Mushomi J, Menyenye Ntozi JP. Factors associated with modern contraceptive use among young and older women in Uganda; a comparative analysis. BMC Public Health. 2014;Sep 8(14):926.

20. D. W AM, F A, B. M. Determinants of modern contraceptive utilization among married women of reproductive age group in North Shoa Zone, Amhara Region, Ethiopia. Reprod Health [Internet]. 2014;11(1):1–7. Available from: http://ovidsp.ovid.com/ovidweb.cgi?T=JS&PAGE=reference&D=emed12&NEWS=N&AN=2014111648.
21. Nyqvist MB, Guariso A, Svensson J, Yanagizawa-Drott D. Reducing child mortality in the last mile: Experimental evidence on community health promoters in Uganda. Am Econ J Appl Econ. 2019;11(3):155–92.

5

Long-acting reversible contraception utilization and associated factors among women in extended postpartum period in Hossana town, southern Ethiopia

Biruktawit Fekade Woldu[1*], Tadesse Lelago Ermolo[2], Lidiya Gutema Lemu[3] and Negeso Gebeyehu Gejo[1]

Abstract

Background: In low and middle-income countries, 95% of postpartum women want to avoid a pregnancy for 2 years, but 70% are not using contraception. Delay in use of contraception by couples during postpartum period can result in many unwanted pregnancies. Long-acting reversible contraception (LARC) is ideal for postpartum women. Therefore this study aimed at assessing the prevalence and factors associated with LARC use among postpartum women.

Methods: Facility based cross sectional study was conducted from July 23-Aug 25, 2018. Systematic random sampling technique was employed to recruit a total of 381 women in extended postpartum period visiting Child Immunization service in hosanna health institutions. Pretested structured questionnaire was used for data collection. Data was analyzed by SPSS version 20. Binary and multiple logistic regression analysis was done. The presence and strength of association was determined using AOR with its 95% CI. Variables with *P* value less than 0.05 were considered as statistical significant.

Results: The prevalence of LARC use was 36.5% (95%CI (33.05–39.95)). The main reason for not using LARC was fear of side effect and false information. Previous use of LARC (AOR = 3.3, 95%CI (1.7–6.5)) and have ever discussed with health providers on LARC (AOR = 2.5, 95%CI (1.1–5.74)) were found to be significantly associated with LARC use.

Conclusions: The utilization of LARC among postpartum women was found to be higher than other studies in Ethiopia. Provision of effective contraceptive counseling during Antenatal, delivery and postnatal care services with emphasis on LARC/Postpartum Intra-Uterine Device is important.

Keywords: Long-acting, Contraception, Postpartum, Prevalence, Factors, Hossana

* Correspondence: biruktifekade@gmail.com
[1]Department of Midwifery, College of Medicine and Health Sciences, Wachemo University, Hossana, Ethiopia

Background

After one-time placement of a device, Long-acting reversible contraception (LARC) methods provide reliable long-term highly effective prevention of pregnancy. LARC methods include subdermal hormonal implant and Intra-Uterine Devices (hormonal IUDs and non-hormonal copper-containing IUDs) [1]. Regardless of considerable advances in contraceptive technologies, unintended pregnancies remain a significant global public health issue. In developing countries 214 million reproductive age women who desire to avoid pregnancy are not using a modern contraceptive method [2, 3].

Modern contraceptive use has increased around the world. However, less than 15% of married women of reproductive age use a modern method in many of the poorest countries. The use of LARC among modern contraception users is still low [4]. In Ethiopia, Contraceptive prevalence rate among currently married women has increased steadily from 14% in 2005 to 41% in 2019. The largest increase is observed in the use of injectable. The use of LARC remains low at 11% (9%- Implants & 2%-IUD) [5]. In southern region, where the study area is located, 44.6% of currently married women were using a modern family planning. Among these only 9.2% use LARC (7.7%- Implants & 1.5%-IUD). Utilization of LARC was found to have significant association with women's socio-demographic and reproductive characteristics. Knowledge, attitude and previous LARCs use was also found to have significant association with its use [6–14].

In the first year after childbirth, 95% of women in low and middle-income countries want to avoid pregnancy within the next 2 years; however 70% are not using contraception. Delay in practice of contraception by couples during postpartum period can result in many unwanted or mistimed pregnancies. A woman conceives within/less than 24 months of delivery has higher chances of complications like abortions, pre-term labor, low birth weight babies, postpartum hemorrhage, neonatal morbidity and mortality [15]. Postpartum family planning is defined as the prevention of unintended pregnancy and closely spaced pregnancies through the first 12 months following childbirth [16]. Postpartum period is one of the important and crucial times when women and couples are highly motivated and receptive to family planning methods. LARC methods are safe for almost all women, including those in a postpartum period [2]. As they do not contain estrogen and have few contraindications, they are ideal for use in postpartum women [17]. According to a study in five low-income countries, almost all women wish to delay or prevent a future pregnancy at six weeks postpartum. Despite this, usage of modern contraceptive methods at 42 days post-partum varied widely. The uptake of the most effective LARC (IUDs) is very low even amongst users of modern contraceptives [18]. Different studies conducted in different parts of Ethiopia also indicated lower prevalence of postpartum LARC use [19–24]. Study on LARC use among postpartum women is lacking in the study area. Therefore the objective of this study was to assess the prevalence and factors associated with LARC use among women in extended postpartum period visiting child immunization in Hosanna health institutions, Southern Ethiopia.

Methods

Study setting and population

Facility based cross sectional study was conducted from July 23-Aug 25, 2018 in hosanna health institutions, Hadiya zone Southern Ethiopia. Hossana town comprises of three sub cities and eight kebeles(the lowest governmental administrative units). According to CSA population count of May 2007, the total number of Hossana town population was 69,959 for the year 2007/8. Among these 34,454 (49.25%) were females. There is 1 teaching referral hospital and 3 health centers in the town which provide postpartum family planning service. Women in extended postpartum period visiting child immunization service in the four health institutions during the study period were eligible for enrollment. Those women who are pregnant and unable to speak or hear were excluded from the study.

Sample size determination and sampling technique

Sample size was calculated using single population proportion formula by taking account of Proportion of LARC use among postpartum women in Durame town 36.7% [13], CI = 95% Margin of error = 5 and 10% non-response rate. A total of 392 women on extended postpartum period (6 weeks to 1 year after delivery) were invited to participate. Systematic random sampling technique was employed to select participants. The total number of women who visit child Immunization (N) was estimated by considering the immediate previous 1 month record of Expanded Program on Immunization chart. Then number of sampling intervals (k) was determined by dividing N by sample size ($n = 392$). Then lottery method was used to select the first participant. Then after every 3rd unit was included until the required sample reached. In case of refusal or not meeting inclusion criteria, the next person was selected. The sample size for each institution was distributed proportionally.

Data collection

Data were collected using pretested, interviewer administered structured questionnaire. The questionnaire was adapted from different literatures by considering the local situation of the study subjects. Information on participants' socio-demographic, reproductive characteristics, knowledge, attitude and practice towards LARC was collected. The data collection tool prepared in English was translated in to Amharic and then returned back to English to ensure accuracy. Before the actual data collection, Pre-test was done on 5% women in a health center located outside the town and necessary corrections made accordingly. Four trained diploma midwifery graduates collected the data supervised by one BSc midwife working in university. Completeness of the questionnaires was checked on the spot by supervisor.

Measurement

LARC use: was defined as utilization of any of LARCs (IUD or subdermal hormonal implant) by women on extended postpartum period.

The mean score was used to categorize women's knowledge towards LARC; women who scored above mean score were considered to have good knowledge and women who scored below the mean were considered to have poor knowledge.

Women's attitude towards LARC was categorized in the same approach. Those women who scored above the mean were considered to have positive attitude and scored below the mean considered to have negative attitude towards LARC.

Data analysis

Data was analyzed by using SPSS version 20. Descriptive statistics were computed. Binary logistic regression analysis was done and all explanatory variables with p value less than 0.2 were entered to multiple logistic regression model. The second analytical step used a stepwise backward model. Then association was assessed using AOR and its 95%CI. And p value of < 0.05 was considered as statistically significant. Goodness of model fitness was tested by using Hosmer and Lemeshow test.

Results

Data were analyzed from 381 women, making response rate of 97.1%. Mean age of participants were 27(SD ± 4.6). Majority of participants were urban resident (89%). Less than one fifth of respondents attend diploma and above level of education (17.1%). Half of the women were housewife (50.4%) (Table 1).

Table 1 Sociodemographic characteristics of postpartum women in Hossana health institutions, 2018($n = 381$)

Variable	Frequency	Percentage
Age (years)		
16–20	31	8.1
21–25	124	32.5
26–30	154	40.4
31–35	50	13.1
36–40	22	5.8
Residence		
Urban	339	89.0
Rural	42	11.0
Marital status		
Married	369	96.9
Single	7	1.8
Separated	5	1.3
Educational status		
Can't read and write	15	3.9
Can Read & Write	19	5.0
Primary	141	37.0
Secondary	141	37.0
Diploma & Above	65	17.1
Working status		
Housewife	192	50.4
Merchant	51	13.4
Government Employee	67	17.6
Private Employee	58	15.2
Other	13	3.4

Reproductive characteristics of respondents

More than two-third (71%) of participants had two or more births. Median number of alive children per women and birth interval were 2 IQR [1, 4] and 36 months IQR [24,48] respectively. Around one-third (28.3%) participants do not want any more children for the future.

Less than one fifth of respondents (18.1%) intended to give birth within 2 years. More than one-forth (28.6%) had never discussed with health professionals towards LARC and 52.4% were advised on LARC during the immediate postpartum period (Table 2).

Knowledge, attitude and previous LARC use

More than two-third (71.4%) of the women had good knowledge towards LARC. Around half of them (53.2%) had positive attitude towards LARC. Two-third (68.5%) of participant's partner had supportive attitude towards LARC. Two-third (66.4%) of respondents had ever used at least one type of modern contraception and one-fourth (26%) had ever used LARC before delivery of last child (Table 3).

Prevalence of postpartum LARC use

Two-third (66.6%) of postpartum women had started to use modern family planning method. LARC method use among participants was 36.5% (implant 34.1%, IUCD-

Table 2 Reproductive characteristics of postpartum women in Hossana health institutions, 2018($n = 381$)

Variable	LARC use	
	Yes n(%)	No n(%)
Parity		
1	72(65.5)	38(34.5)
2–4	137(61.7)	85(38.3)
≥ 5	33(67.3)	16(32.7)
Number of alive children		
1	75(65.8)	39(34.2)
2–4	135(60.8)	87(39.2)
≥ 5	32(71.1)	13(28.9)
Place of last birth		
Home	15(71.4)	6(28.6)
Health institution	227(63.1)	133(36.9)
Birth interval(in month) ($n = 272$)		
0–23	28(73.7)	10(26.3)
24–35	56(64.4)	31(35.6)
36 & above	87(59.2)	60(40.8)
Number of children want for the future		
0	74(68.5)	34(31.5)
1–3	131(59.8)	88(40.2)
4–6	37(68.5)	17(31.5)
Intended to give birth within 2 years ($n = 273$)		
Yes	49(71.0)	20(29.0)
No	119(58.3)	85(41.7)
Ever discussed with health professionals		
Yes	123(45.2)	149(54.8)
No	16(14.7)	93(85.3)
Advised during immediate postpartum		
Yes	95(47.5)	105(52.5)
No	44(24.3)	137(75.7)

Table 3 Knowledge, attitude and previous LARC use among postpartum women in Hossana health institutions, 2018($n = 381$)

Variable	LARC use	
	Yes	No
Knowledge towards LARC		
Good	121(44.5%)	151(55.5%)
Poor	18(16.5%)	91(83.5%)
Attitude towards LARC		
Positve	77(41.8%)	107(58.2%)
Negative	61(38.4%)	98(61.6%)
Previous LARC use		
Used before	58(59.2%)	40(40.8%)
Never used	81(28.6%)	202(71.4%)

2.4%). The main reason for not using LARC was fear of side effect (39.3%) followed by false rumors towards LARC (it cause harm to uterus, infertility, interfere with work, fly/lost in the body) (21.9%) (Table 4).

Factors associated with LARC use

In the multiple logistic regression analysis Previous LARC use and ever discussed with Health Professionals on LARC were found to be significantly associated with LARC use. Those women who have ever used LARC before were 3.3 times more likely to use LARC on postpartum period (AOR = 3.3, 95%CI(1.7–6.5). Postpartum women who have ever discussed with health professionals on LARC were 2.5 times more likely to use LARC (AOR = 2.5, 95% CI (1.1–5.7)) (Table 5).

Discussion

In this study the prevalence of LARC use among postpartum women was found to be 36.5% (95%CI (33.05–39.95)), which is similar with a study done in Durame [13]. However it is higher than a study in Northern Ethiopia [24]. The difference can be due to variation in participants' characteristics and institution based nature of our study.

Majority of LARC users opted for Implant (93.5%) and very few used IUCD (6.5%). Which is consistent with different studies [6, 14] where strong preference for implants over IUCD were observed. These can be due to prevailing misinformation towards IUCD.

The main reason for not using LARC among postpartum women was fear of side effect (39.3%) followed by false information towards LARC (it cause harm to uterus and infertility, interfere work, fly/lost in the body) (21.9%) which is consistent with other study [8]. This indicates the need of community based health education and awareness creation programs.

In this study previous LARC use was found to be significantly associated with postpartum LARC use (AOR = 3.34 (1.70–6.55)). Similar finding were indicated by other studies [10, 13]. The possible explanation can be women possibly will have adequate information on the contraception method they used before, which can motivate them to use the same method repetitively.

Table 4 method-mix adopted among postpartum women in Hossana health institutions, 2018($n = 381$)

Contraception method	Frequency	Percentage
Injectable	98	25.7
Implants	130	34.1
IUCD	9	2.4
Pills	15	3.9
Condom	2	0.5
Non users	127	33.4

Table 5 Logistic regression analysis of factors associated with LARC use among postpartum women in hossana health institutions, 2018 ($n = 381$)

Variable	LARC use		COR (95%CI)	AOR (95%CI)
	Yes (n%)	No (n%)		
Residence				
Urban	130(38.3)	209(61.7)	1	
Rural	9(21.4)	33(78.6)	0.43 (.20–.94)	0.53 (0.19–1.42)
Intention to give birth within 2 years				
Yes	20(29.0)	49(71.0)	1	
No	85(41.7)	119(58.3)	1.75(.97–3.15)	1.82 (0.94–3.54)
Knowledge towards LARC				
Good	121(44.5)	151(55.5)	4.01(2.31–7.08)	0.95 (0.43–2.10)
Poor	18(16.5)	91(83.5)	1	
Partner attitude				
Supportive	118(45.2)	143(54.8)	2.59 (1.48–4.54)	0.50 (0.24–1.03)
Not supportive	20(24.1)	63(75.9)	1	
Previous LARC use				
Yes	58(59.2)	40(40.8)	3.61 (2.24–5.83)	3.34(1.70–6.55)*
No	81(28.6)	202(71.4)	1	
Adviced during immediate postpartum				
Yes	95(47.5)	105(52.5)	2.81 (1.81–4.36)	1.26 (0.66–2.42)
No	44(24.3)	137(75.7)	1	
Ever discussed on LARC with professionals				
Yes	123(45.2)	149(54.8)	4.79 (2.68–8.58)	2.56 (1.14–5.74)**
No	16(14.7)	93(85.3)	1	

*Significant at < 0.05 ** significant at < 0.001

Those postpartum women who ever discussed with health professionals on LARC were found to be more likely to use LARC (AOR = 2.569(1.148–5.7470)). It is in line with another study [6]. This can possibly explained by the fact that access to clear factual information on the benefits and limitations of contraceptive methods is imperative to promote informed choice and to overcome misperceptions and myths more broadly perpetuated in the community.

Limitation

Quantitative nature of the study hinders indepth exploration of women's perception and barrieres for LARC use. As this study was conducted in urban facilities, the finding might not be representative for the rural communities.

Conclusion

The utilization of LARC among postpartum women was found to be higher than other studies done in Ethiopia. Majority of participants opted for implants over IUCD. The main reason for not using LARC was fear of side effect and rumors. Provision of effective contraceptive counseling during Antenatal, delivery and postnatal care services with emphasis on LARC/ PPIUDs is important. Further studies need to be conducted to assess women's knowledge, perceptions and attitudes towards PPIUDs.

Acknowledgements

We are indebted to data collectors and all women who agreed to participate in this study. We want to thank health institution administrators for their great collaboration.

Authors' contributions

BFW, TLE, and LGL contributed to the initiation of the study, design, organizing the data collection process and analysis of the result. BFW, TLE, LGL and NGG involved in writing of the manuscript. All authors read and approved the final manuscript.

Author details

[1]Department of Midwifery, College of Medicine and Health Sciences, Wachemo University, Hossana, Ethiopia. [2]Department of Nursing, College of Medicine and Health Sciences, Wachemo University, Hossana, Ethiopia. [3]Department of Midwifery, College of Health Sciences, Mizan Tepi University, Mizan Aman, Ethiopia.

References

1. Winner B, Peipert JF, Zhao Q, Buckel C, Madden T, Allsworth J, et al. Effectiveness of long-acting reversible contraception. N Engl J Med. 2012; 366:1998–2007.
2. WHO. Family planning/Contraception Fact sheet. In: WHO, editor. 2017.
3. Curtis KM, Peipert JF. Long-acting reversible contraception. N Engl J Med. 2017;376:461–8. https://doi.org/10.1056/NEJMcp1608736.
4. Family Planning Worldwide 2019 Data Sheet www.prb.org/pdf19/familyplanning-2019-datasheet_eng.pdf, Accessed 11 Dec 2019.
5. Central Statistical Agency (CSA) [Ethiopia] and ICF. 2019. Ethiopia mini demographic and health survey 2019: key indicators report. Addis Ababa, Ethiopia, and Rockville, Maryland, USA. CSA and ICF. https://dhsprogram.com/pubs/pdf/PR120/PR120.pdf.
6. Taye A, Woldie M, Sinaga M. Predictors of Long Acting Reversible Contraceptive use among Married Women Visiting Health Facilities in Jimma Town. J Women's Health Care. 2014;4:217. https://doi.org/10.4172/2167-0420.1000217, https://www.researchgate.net/profile/Mirkuzie_Woldie2/publication/273128776_Predictors_of_Long_Acting_Reversible_Contraceptive_use_among_Married_Women_Visiting_Health_Facilities_in_Jimma_Town/links/550749090cf2d7a28123bea4/Predictors-of-Long-Acting-Reversible-Contraceptive-use-among-Married-Women-Visiting-Health-Facilities-in-Jimma-Town.pdf.
7. Shegaw G, Mohammed AA, Nadew K, Tamrat K, Zeru G, Desta H, Yinager W. Long acting contraceptive method utilization and associated factors among reproductive age women in Arba Minch Town, Ethiopia. Greener J Epidemiol Public Health. 2014;2(1):023-031.
8. Gebremichael H, Haile F, Dessie A, Birhane A, Alemayehu M, Yebyo H. Acceptance of long acting contraceptive methods and associated factors among women in Mekelle City, Northern Ethiopia. Sci J Public Health. 2014; 2(4):239-45.
9. Kabalo MY. Utilization of reversible long acting family planning methods among married 15-49 years women in Areka town, Southern Ethiopia. Int J Sci Rep. 2016;2(1):1-6. http://www.sci-rep.com.
10. Melka AS, Tekelab T, Wirtu D. Determinants of long acting and permanent contraceptive methods utilization among married women of reproductive age groups in western Ethiopia: a cross-sectional study. Pan Afr Med J. 2015;21:246.
11. Austad K, Shah P, Rohloff P. Correlates of long-acting reversible contraception uptake among rural women in Guatemala. PLoSONE. 2018; 13(6):e0199536. https://doi.org/10.1371/journal.pone.0199536.
12. Teferra AS, Wondifraw AA. Determinants of Long Acting Contraceptive Use among Reproductive Age Women in Ethiopia: Evidence from EDHS 2011. Sci J Public Health. 2014;3(1):143-9. https://doi.org/10.11648/j.sjph.20150301.33.
13. Tamrie YE, Hanna EG, Argaw MD. Determinants of long acting reversible contraception method use among mothers in extended postpartum period, Durame Town, Southern Ethiopia: a cross sectional community based survey. Health. 2015;7:1315-26. https://doi.org/10.4236/health.2015.710146.
14. Gudaynhe SW, Zegeye DT, Tarekegn A, Kibret GD. Factors affecting the use of long-acting reversible contraceptive methods among married women in Debre Markos Town, Northwest Ethiopia 2013. Glob J Med Res. 2014;14(5). https://medicalresearchjournal.org/index.php/GJMR/article/view/783.
15. Shoupe D. LARC methods: entering a new age of contraception and reproductive health contraception and reproductive medicine. 2016;1(4). https://doi.org/10.1186/s40834-016-0011-8, http://creativecommons.org/publicdomain/zero/1.0/.
16. World Health Organization. Programming strategies for postpartum family planning 2013. https://www.who.int/reproductivehealth/publications/family_planning/ppfp_strategies/en/.
17. Parks C, Peipert F. Eliminating Health Disparities in Unintended Pregnancy with Long-Acting Reversible Contraception (LARC) Am J Obstet Gynecol. 2016;214(6):681688. https://doi.org/10.1016/j.ajog.2016.02.017, https://www.ncbi.nlm.nih.gov/pmc/articles/PMC4884485/.
18. Pasha O, Goudar SS, Patel A, Garces A, Esamai F, Chomba E, et al. Postpartum contraceptive use and unmet need for family planning in five low-income countries. Reprod Health. 2015;12(2):S11. https://www.ncbi.nlm.nih.gov/pubmed/26063346.
19. Abera Y, Mengesha ZB, Tessema GA. Postpartum contraceptive use in Gondar town, Northwest Ethiopia: a community based cross-sectional study. BMC Womens Health. 2015;15(1):19.
20. Gebremedhin AY, Kebede Y, Gelagay AA, Habitu YA. Family planning use and its associated factors among women in the extended postpartum period in Addis Ababa, Ethiopia. Contracept Reprod Med. 2018;3(1):1.
21. Abraha TH, Gebrezgiabher BB, Aregawi BG, Belay DS, Tikue LT, Welay GM. Predictors of postpartum contraceptive use in rural Tigray region, northern Ethiopia: a multilevel analysis. BMC Public Health. 2018;18(1):1017.
22. Gebremariam A, Gebremariam H. Contraceptive use among lactating women in Ganta-Afeshum District, Eastern Tigray, Northern Ethiopia, 2015: a cross sectional study. BMC Pregnancy Childbirth. 2017;17(1):421.
23. Demie T, Demissew T, Huluka T, Workineh F, Libanos H. Postpartum family planning utilization among postpartum women in public health institutions of Debre Berhan town, Ethiopia. J Women's Health Care. 2018;7:2. 2018; 7(426):2167-0420.
24. Mengesha ZB, Worku AG, Feleke SA. Contraceptive adoption in the extended postpartum period is low in Northwest Ethiopia. BMC Pregnancy Childbirth. 2015;15(1):160. https://bmcpregnancychildbirth.biomedcentral.com/articles/10.1186/s12884-015-0598-9.

6

Factors affecting demand for modern contraceptives among currently married reproductive age women in rural Kebeles of Nunu Kumba district, Oromia, Ethiopia

Alemu Kebede[1], Sileshi G. Abaya[2], Elias Merdassa[1] and Tariku Tesfaye Bekuma[1*]

Abstract

Background: Family planning plays a key role in improving the health of the mother and the child. Yet there are still significant levels of demand for family planning that are unmet and these can lead to unintended pregnancy. So, women's demand for contraceptive utilization to limit, space, or delay the number of family size can be increased by integrating family planning service at each service delivery points.

Objective: The main aim of this study was to assess the demand for modern contraceptive and associated factors among currently married women of the reproductive age group in rural kebeles of Nunu Kumba District, 2015.

Methods: A community-based cross-sectional study design was conducted from January 15–30, 2015 among 584 systematically selected currently married women of reproductive age in six rural kebeles of Nunu Kumba District. A pre-tested and interviewer-administered questionnaire was used to collect the data. Data were analyzed using SPSS version 20. Descriptive statistics were done to summarize the data. A multivariate logistic regressions analysis method was employed and odds ratio with 95% confidence interval was used to control for possible confounders. *P*-value < 0.05 was used to declare a significant association.

Results: The total demand for modern methods of contraceptive was 450 (77.1%) of which 325 (55.7%) of them were current user and 125 (21.4%) of them were had unmet need for modern contraceptive methods. Being in the younger age group (15–24 and 25–34 years [AOR = 0.196; 95% CI: 0.055, 0.692] and [AOR = 0.179, 95% CI: 0.043, 0.745] respectively, husband having no intention for more children [AOR = 4.124, 95% CI: 1.891, 8.996], number of children alive [AOR = 2.617, 95% CI: 1.056, 6.486], and couples ever not discussed on family planning [AOR = 0.340, 95% CI: 0.187, 0.619] were factors associated with demand for modern methods of contraception.

Conclusion: The total demand for modern methods of contraceptive was high in the study area except for long-acting and permanent methods with high unmet need for spacing than for limiting. Therefore, any program aimed at promoting family planning at the district level should look for ways and means of increasing demand for long-acting and permanent family planning methods and encouraging husband involvement to increase its utilization.

Keywords: Demand, Family planning use, Unmet need, Nunu Kumba, Married women

* Correspondence: tarii2007@gmail.com
[1]Department of Public Health, Institute of Health Sciences, Wollega University, P. O. Box: 395, Nekemte, Ethiopia

Introduction

The need or demand for contraceptives, and meeting the demand or the supply of contraceptives are dependent on each other. As women's demand for contraception increases, the need for governments, donors, manufacturers and other stakeholders to supply the demand becomes increasingly critical [1]. Improvements in meeting the demand for family planning require not only data on overall levels and trends in contraceptive prevalence and unmet need for family planning but also an assessment of the diversity of contraceptive methods used [2].

Researchers have shown that Reproductive age women have varying contraceptive needs. Because of side effects, daily intake and similar complain, many women do not use oral contraceptives effectively which can lead to unintended pregnancy. Rather, they choose long-term reversible contraception lik Intra Uterine Devices (IUDs) and implants [3]. The total demand for family planning is currently defined as the percent of married or in union women aged 15–49 years who want to delay or limit childbearing (i.e. the combination of women with unmet need and women using family planning constitutes the total demand for family planning) [4].

Yet there are still significant levels of demand for family planning that are unmet. If this unmet need were met, unintended pregnancies would be reduced, women's health and lives would be improved, can prevent an estimated 2.7 million infant deaths globally and the consequent impact on fertility would result in lower population growth [5]. The growing use of contraception around the world has given couples the ability to choose the number and spacing of their children and has tremendous lifesaving benefits. But, contraceptive use is still low and the need for contraception high in some of the world poorest and most populous places [6]. Contraceptive use was increased worldwide over the last decade but, Africa has stilla high unmet need for family planning that approximately 25% of women and couples in Sub-Saharan Africa who wanted to space or limit their births are not using any type of contraception [7].

Half of the married women worldwide now use a modern method of contraception, but 200 million women still have an unmet need that they would like either to stop having children or delay their next birth for at least 2 years but are not using an effective contraceptive method. This unmet need is fueled by lack of information, fear of social disapproval or a husband's opposition, religious or cultural beliefs, and concern for contraceptive side-effects or impacts on health. This could lead to increased unwanted pregnancy and induce abortion [8–10].

In many resource-poor settings, the growing unmet need for contraception is astounding. So, couples who wish to have fewer children are unable to determine the size of their families as funds for family planning continues to be scarce and existing programs and services fail to meet the concerns and desires of their users [11].

In Ethiopia, the strategy was emphasized on delivery of short-acting methods, especially pills where the probability of an adult woman dying from a maternal cause during her reproductive lifespan is about one in 40 [12, 13]. EDHS 2011 indicated that unmet need for contraceptives was about 25% with a total demand of 54% [14].

Although family planning use among women of reproductive age has been increased from its virtual nonexistence level, it is still low in Ethiopia. This is as a result of low availability of a variety of contraceptive methods [15]. Availability of quality family planning services, diversity of the methods and correct information enable women to make informed choices. This study has determined the level of family planning and identified factors associated with demand for family planning and hoped to be used as an input for program and health policymakers in designing family planning service delivery strategies in Ethiopia in general and in the study area specifically.

Conceptual framework

The framework is conceptualized by using two groups of variables, the dependent and independent variables. The independent variables are those that influence demand for modern family planning (dependent variables) which include socio-economic, reproductive history and client-related factors (Fig. 1).

Methods

Study area and period

The study was conducted in Nunu Kumba District from January 15–30/ 2015. Nunu Kumba is 68kms away from Nekemte town, the capital of the zone, and 381kms from Addis Ababa, the capital city of Ethiopia. It is one of the 17 Districts in the East Wollega Zone. It is bordered on the Southwest by Jimma Arjo District, on the Northwest by Wayu Tuka District, on the Northeast by Wama River which separates it from Wama Hagalo District, and on the Southeast by Ilu Ababora zone. The administrative center of this District is Nunu. The data from District health office (2014) indicated that the district has 22 Kebeles; of which 2 were urban and 20 were rural and had an estimated total population of 78,541, of which 39,585 were males and 38,956 were females. In this District, there were 4 health centers and 20 rural health posts. Also, there were two secondary schools [9, 10] and one preparatory school (Nunu Kumba district Health office report, 2015).

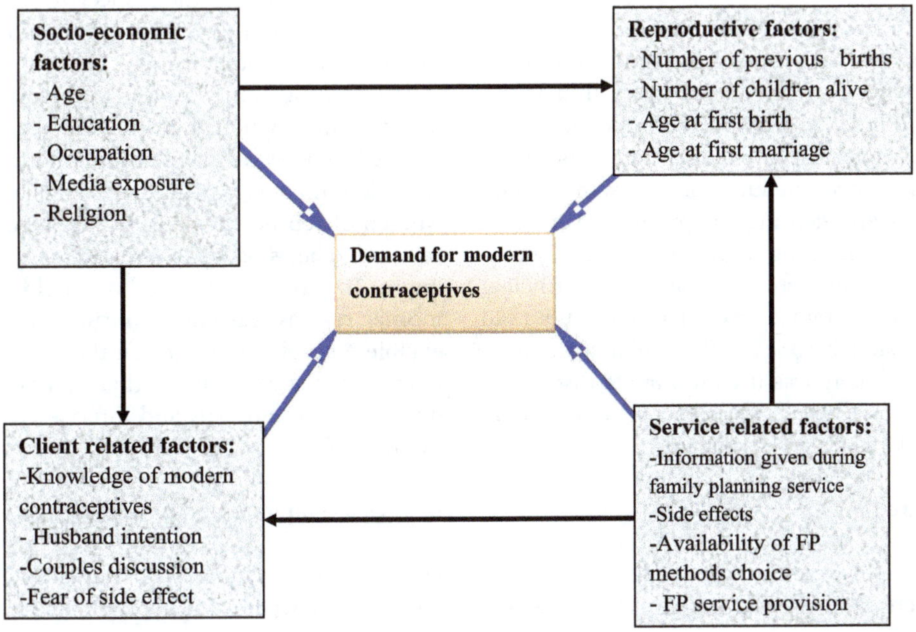

Fig. 1 Conceptual Framework of demand for modern contraceptives of respondents in Nunu Kumba woreda, January 2015 (Adopted from Jane Bertrand framework, 2006).

Study design

A community-based cross-sectional study design was employed using both quantitative and qualitative methods.

Source population

All currently married women of the reproductive age group in rural kebeles of Nunu Kumba district were the source population.

Study population

Randomly selected married women between 15 and 49 years of age who were living in selected rural kebeles of Nunu Kumba district.

Inclusion and exclusion criteria

Inclusion criteria

- All married women of the reproductive age group in selected kebeles.
- Being a resident of selected kebeles at least for 6 months

Exclusion criteria

Married women of the reproductive age group who were critically ill, unable to talk or hear during the study period were excluded from the study.

Sample size determination

Quantitative method

The sample size was determined using the formula for a single population proportion:

$$n = \frac{\left(Z_{\alpha/2}\right)^2 \times \mathrm{pq} \times \mathrm{DE}}{\mathrm{d}^2}$$

Where: - α - the level of confidence

p - Percentage of total demand for family planning among currently married women of Butajira district, which is 77.8% [15]

q - (1-p);

n - Sample size.

Z - Standard normal distribution curve value for 95% CI which is 1.96 (where α = 0.05).

d - Tolerable margin of error = 5%

Hence

$$\mathrm{n} = \frac{(1.96)^2 \times 0.778 \times 0.222}{(0,05)^2} \times 2 = 530.8$$

DE - design effect of the study due to its multi-stage nature

Additional 10% allowance (non-response) for absenteeism and refusal to participate in the study was considered. Thus, 530.8 + 53.08 = 583.88; 584 married women were interviewed.

Qualitative part

Four sessions of focus group discussions were carried out among model married mothers and model husbands other than those who took part in the study. Individuals of similar backgrounds: age group, educational status, occupation, and residents of the study area for more than 6 months have been included in the same group. After participants were identified, appropriate time and comfortable place of meeting were selected and organized. All the discussions were moderated by a principal investigator with one trained recorder and one note taker health professionals (BSc). A The semi-structured, open-ended questionnaire was used to initiate discussion and all the discussions were undertaken in *Afan Oromo* which is the local language of discussants.

Sampling procedure

Quantitative study

Firstly, 20 rural kebeles were listed and using simple random sampling technique, 6 rural kebeles were selected. Then, the sample for the respective selected kebeles was allocated proportionally to their population size of mothers in reproductive age groups. Using a sampling frame fromthe family folder in the health posts and any updated information that was added from HEWs in the selected kebeles, actual sample for each selected kebele was determined. Accordingly, 584 currently married women of reproductive age group were selected from all selected kebeles using systematic random sampling technique. In case, when the household in which eligible mother resides was closed during data collection or the eligible mother was absent on the date of data collection, interviewers were revisited that household three times at different time intervals and interviewed (included) these mothers (Fig. 2).

Data collection tools and data collection procedures

Data collection tools Data was collected by interviewing married women of reproductive age group face to

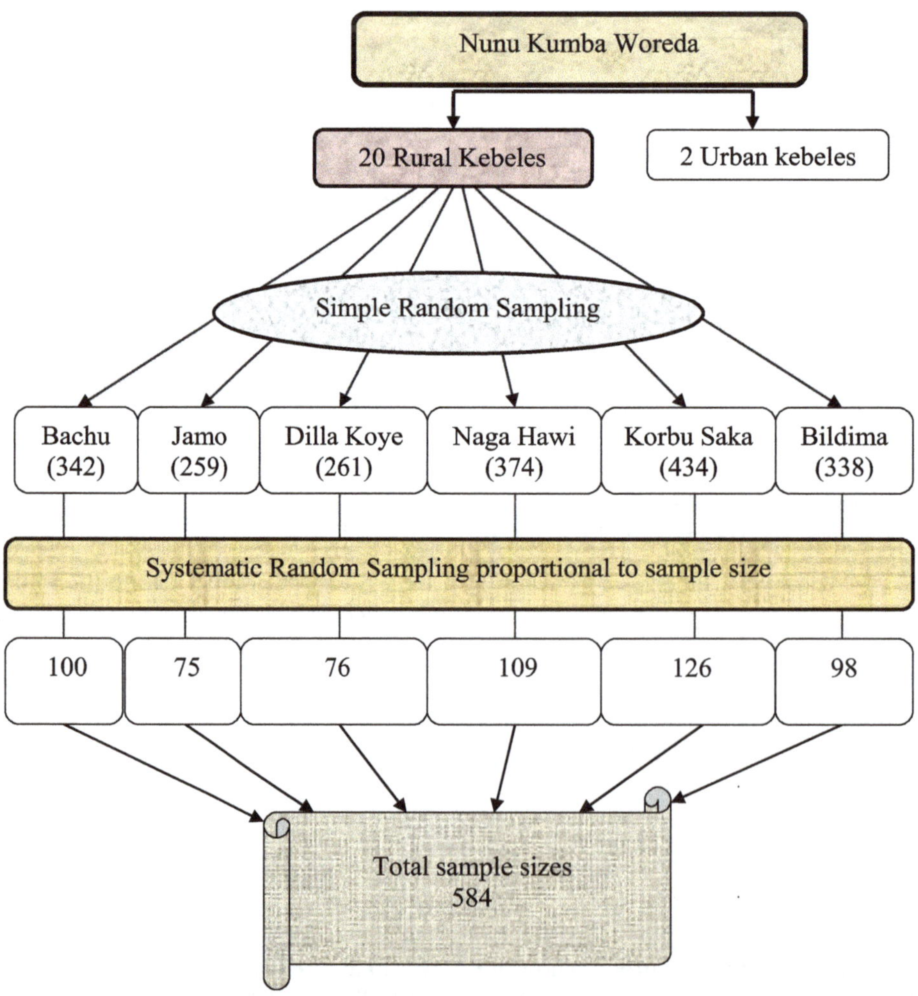

Fig. 2 Schematic presentation of sample size (for quantitative study) selection procedure of Nunu Kumba Woreda, January 2015

face using structured, standardized and interviewer-administered questionnaire adapted from EDHS and modified based on the objective of the study. The questionnaire contains questions addressing the demand for modern contraceptive methods and factors associated with contraceptives need among married women of the reproductive age group in the study area. It was prepared in English and translated to Afan Oromo, and back-translated to English by different experts (high school Language teachers) to ensure consistency. In addition, FGD guide was prepared in English and translated to Afan Oromo was used directly as a guide for the FGD.

Data collectors Data was collected by six female grade 12 completed students and supervised by three health professionals (degree holders). Both the interviewers and supervisors were given two-day training before the actual work about the aim of study which was assessed the level of modern contraceptives demand and associated factors that were helped for the amendment of the identified gap with the concerned body; and data collection techniques by going through the questionnaires question by question.

Operational definitions

- **Total demand for family planning:** percent of married or in union women aged 15–49 years who want to delay or limit childbearing
- **Long-acting and permanent methods of contraception (LAPMs):** those methods that prevent pregnancy for three and more years per application (Implants, IUCD, male and female sterilizations).
- **Demand for modern contraceptives:** current use of modern contraception plus the unmet need for modern contraception
- **Unmet need for family planning:** women who want to avoid a pregnancy but are not using an effective method of family planning
- **Postpartum amenorrhoeic:** Women whose menstrual period has not returned since their most recent birth, and who gave birth in the last 2 years (0–23 months).
- **Infecund:** Women, who had first married five or more years ago, never used contraception, and have not had a birth in the past 5 years.

Variables

Dependent variables

- Demand for modern contraceptives

Independent variables

- Socio-demographic (economic) characteristics - such as the age of woman, religion, Educational status of woman and husband, ethnicity, occupation, Parity
- Knowledge about modern contraceptives
- Husband/partner influence
- Choice of method
- Number of children alive
- Information is given to clients during family planning service
- Contraceptives side effects

Data processing and analysis

After data collection, each questionnaire was checked by the supervisors. Then, the actual data was entered and analyzed by SPSS version 20 statistical packages. To check missing values and outlier's frequency output was used and cleaning was done. Descriptive statistics were done to summarize the data. A bivariate analysis was used to identify candidate variables and a multivariate logistic regression model was used to control for possible confounding variables and predict population parameters. Crude and Adjusted Odds ratio with 95% confidence interval was used to assess the association of dependent and independent variables. All the assumptions of the models (normality of the data and multicollinearity) were checked to be satisfied. Regarding focus group discussions, the recorded audio was transcribed verbatim and the note was reviewed. Thematic content analysis was used in that texts were categorized into primary themes. Then it was compiled into broader concepts. Besides, quotes of participants that exemplify key concepts were used directly during analysis. Finally, the concepts were developed into major themes under each discussion guides.

Data quality management and control

The quality of data was assured by properly designing and pre-testing of the questionnaire; proper training of the interviewers and supervisors on data collection procedures: proper categorization and coding of the questionnaire. The questionnaire was reviewed every day and checked for completeness by the immediate supervisors and principal investigator, and the necessary feedback was given to data collectors in the next morning before data collection.

Pre-testing

The questionnaire was pre-tested in one of the kebeles other than the selected study area (in Jima Arjo District, Wayu Abayi kebele), but has similar socio-demographic characteristics with the study population. Accordingly, it was carried out among 5% of the total sample size and necessary modifications were made to the questionnaire before actual data collection.

Ethical consideration

Ethical clearance was obtained from the Research Ethics Committee of Wollega University. Then, support letter was written from the District Health Office and given to each Kebele administrators and verbal consent was taken from each eligible woman. Study subjects were informed that the study was not had any risks. In addition, the objective and benefits of the study were explained to them. Identifying information (like name, phone number, etc) was excluded from the questionnaire to ensure privacy and confidentiality. The right of individual not to participate in the study was also be respected.

Results

Quantitative study

Socio-demographic characteristics of respondents

A total of 584 currently married women in the reproductive age were responded for the study making the response rate of 100%. Majority of the respondents were between the ages of 35–39 years. The mean age of respondents was 31.26 years with $\pm$ 6.53 years standard deviations. Majority of the study subjects were Oromo in ethnicity 570 (97.6%) and 329 (56.3%) of them were Protestant followers. Concerning educational status, 29 (5%) of respondents were secondary school and above, and 367 (62.8%) of them were illiterate. On the other hand, majority 264 (45.2%) of respondents' husband were unable to read and write; and 108 (18.5%) of them were grade 5–8. Two hundred ninety-seven (50.9%) of respondents werehousewives and four of them were a governmental employee. About 50% of the respondents earned less than 1300 and 25% of them earned less than 950.00 ETB (Table 1).

Table 1 Socio-demographic characteristics of respondents in Nunu Kumba District, January 2015

Variables (n = 584)	Frequency	Percent
Age		
15–19	13	2.2
20–24	77	13.2
25–29	141	24.1
30–34	144	24.7
35–39	146	25.0
40+	63	10.8
Ethnicity		
Oromo	570	97.6
Amhara	12	2.1
Gurage	2	0.3
Religion		
Orthodox	211	36.1
Muslim	44	7.5
Protestant	329	56.4
Respondents educational status		
Unable to write and read	367	62.8
Read and write	29	5.0
Grade 1–8	159	27.2
Grade 9–12	25	4.3
College and above	4	0.7
Respondents occupational status		
House wife	297	50.9
Student	23	3.9
Farmer	260	44.5
Government employee	4	0.7
Family monthly income in quartile	Birr (ETB)	Frequency
First quartile	950	146
Second quartile	1300	292
Third quartile	1850	438

Reproductive history of the respondents

Out of the total respondents, 268 (45.9%) were married between the age of 15–19 years and 298 (51%) of the respondents were married between the age of 20–24 years old. Five hundred twenty-three (89.6%) of the respondents had ever been pregnant, out of which 391 (74.9%) of them were between 20 and 24 years of age at first birth. Three hundred seven (52.6%) respondents decided the total number of children they would like to have in their lifetime with TFR 5.1, out of which 120 (39.1%) and 186 (60.6%) of them would like to have 3–4 and above 4 children in lifetime respectively (Table 2).

Five hundred twenty-three (89.6%) women have given one or more births of which only two women have no live child duringthe data collection period. In addition, it was mentioned that 79 (15.1%) have a history of stillbirths and 51 (9.8%) have a history of abortion. Out of 523 nonpregnant women, 297 (56.8%) intended to have children in the future, 191 (36.5%) mentioned that they did not need children and 35 (6.7%) have not decided their future intention to have children. Similarly, 278 (53.2%) of them knew their husband intention while 71 (13.6) did not know (Fig. 3).

Among those who intended to have children in the future, 185 (62.3%) were because of few children they have, 73 (24.6%) of them wanted more sons and 33 (11.1%) wanted more daughters, while six (2%) of them were because of children died.

Table 2 Reproductive history of the respondents in Nunu Kumba district, January 2015

Variables (*n* = 584)	Frequency	Percent
Age at first marriage		
15–19	268	45.9
20–24	298	51.0
25–29	17	2.9
30–34	1	0.2
Age of mother at first birth (*n* = 523)		
15–19	72	13.8
20–24	391	74.7
25–29	59	11.3
30–34	1	.2
Number of live births (*n* = 522)		
< 5	412	78.9
> =5	110	21.1
Number of children alive (*n* = 521)		
1–2	145	27.8
3–4	188	36.1
5+	188	36.1
Number of children respondents would like to have in a lifetime (*n* = 307)		
2	1	0.3
3–4	120	39.1
> 4	186	60.6

Knowledge of women about modern contraceptive and source of information

Five hundred seventy-three (98.1%) of the respondents have heard at least one method of modern family planning. Health workers 573 (100%) and radio 201 (35.1%) were the most commonly mentioned source of information respectively. Public health facilities (99.5%) were the most common place where the information about family planning method can be gained. Regarding the advantage of family planning methods, 457 (79.9%), 386 (67.5), 92 (16.1%) knew/mentioned to limit family size, to protect unwanted pregnancy and to prevent STIs, respectively. The most commonly known family planning methods were injectables (96.2%), followed by pills (94.4%), implants (88%) and condom (22.2%). Five hundred nineteen (90.7%) respondents mentioned that modern contraceptive methods are the best method to prevent unwanted and mistimed pregnancy. Two hundred sixty-seven (46.6%) respondents had discussed about family planning with their husband in the last 12 months. Out of the total respondents, 206 (35.3%) discussed about family planning with health care providers and visited health facility in the last 12 months for different family planning related services (Table 3).

Attitude towards family planning utilization

Women were asked to reflect their opinion on certain attitude questions. Five hundred sixty (95.9) of them agreed that if the family uses contraceptives, children will have better opportunities for education, while 2.4% of them disagreed on the idea. Similarly, out of total respondents, 95.5% of them believed that family planning helps to improve one's standard of living and 11 (1.9%) of them were neither agreed nor disagreed. In the same

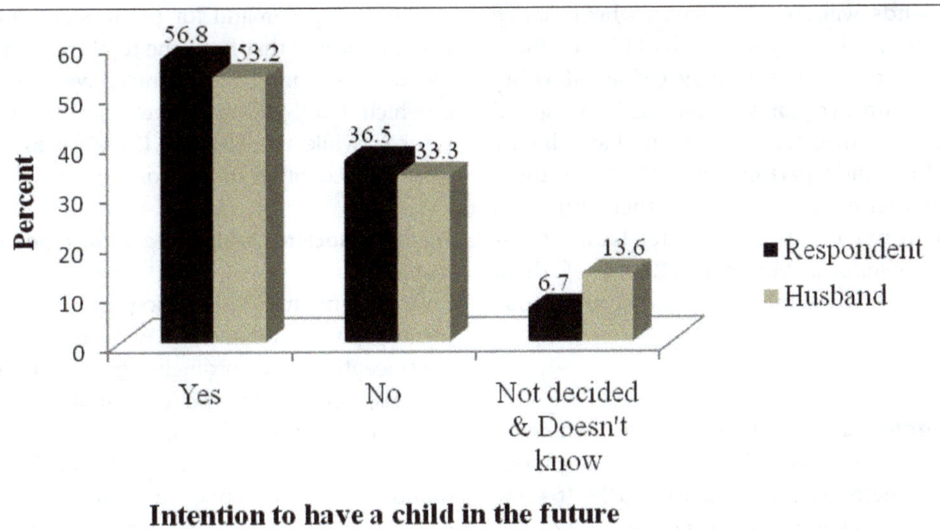

Fig. 3 Respondents' and their husbands' intention (as reported by the respondent) to have a child in the future in Nunu Kumba woreda, January 2015

Table 3 Knowledge/awareness of respondents on family planning in Nunu Kumba district, January 2015

Variables	Frequency	Percent
Heard about FP ($n = 584$)		
Yes	573	98.1
No	11	1.9
Source of contraceptives mentioned by respondents		
Public health facility	570	99.5
Private health facility	99	17.3
NGO health facilities	12	2.1
Contraceptives methods are known by respondents		
Pills	541	94.4
Injectables	551	96.2
Implants	504	88.0
IUCD	292	51.0
Permanent FP	134	23.4
Condom	127	22.2
Couples discussion about family planning within last 12 months ($n = 573$)		
Yes	267	46.6
No	306	53.4

NB: Percentage may not add up 100% as multiple responses are possible for the variables of sources of contraceptives mentioned and contraceptive methods known by respondents

way, 93.8 and 94.7% of the respondents agreed that family planning helps the mother to regain strength before her next birth of baby and child spacing helps protect the health of children and mothers, respectively. Sixty-nine (11.8%) of the respondents agreed that family planning causes loss of confidence between husband and wife. Fifty (8.6%) of the respondents agreed that husbands will abandon wives who practice family planning. More than three-fourths (458) of them believed that using contraceptive may cause infertility for women. Five hundred forty-seven (93.7%) agreed that a couple who practices family planning has a happy family. Out of the study participants, 71.6% of them discussed family planning issues with their husband and 82.9% of them made a decision about family planning with their husbands. Moreover, 22.1% of them agreed in having many children are advantageous (Table 4).

Contraceptive utilization among currently married women

From all respondents, 325 (55.7%) have been using modern contraceptive methods. The majority, 209 (64.3%) were using Implant followed by Injectable 75 (23.1%) and only three respondents were using permanent method (Fig. 4).

Unmet need for family planning was found to be 125 (21.4%) out which 77 (13.2%) was for spacing and 48 (8.2%) was for limiting (Fig. 5).

In this study, the total demand for modern contraceptives were 450 (77.1%), out of which 325 (55.7%) were family planning users, while 125 (21.4%) had unmet need for family planning. Out of the total family planning users, 203 (34.8%) were using contraceptives for spacing and 122 (20.9%) were using for limiting (Fig. 6).

Concerning current pregnancy status of the respondents, 61 (10.4%) were pregnant out of which 51 (83.6%) were intended and 7 (11.5%) were mistimed while the three (4.9%) were unwanted.

About eight out of ten respondents with unintended pregnancies stated that they became pregnant due to fear of contraceptive side effects. But, all respondents in postpartum amenorrheic mentioned that their last pregnancy was intended. From the total, 187 of non pregnant, non family planning user and not postpartum amenorrheic women, 184 (98.4%) replied that they were fecund and regarding their future intention to have a child, it was mentioned that 70 (37.5%) of them want later, 69 (36.8%) of them want soon and 45 (24.5%) of them want no more children. Three respondents have considered themselves as infecund.

Out of 256 non- family planning users, 160 (62.5%) of them have intended to use a contraceptive, 79 (30.9%) of them have not intended to use and the rest seventeen (6.6%) of them have not decided their future intention to use modern methods of contraceptives. Regarding intention on family planning utilization, out of those who have not intended to use family planning, 51 (64.6%) of them were as a result of fear of side effects and only one respondent was as a result of husband refusal (Fig. 6).

Concerning demand for the modern contraceptives, this result indicated that from the total mothers interviewed, demand for the modern contraceptives was 450 (77.1%) out of which 325 (55.7%) was met that they were using contraceptives while the rest 125 (21.4%) was unmet since they were in need either to limit or space child births (Fig. 6).

Factors associated with demand for modern contraceptive methods

Bivariate and multivariate logistic regression was used to identify variables associated with the demand for modern contraceptives. Accordingly, in the bivariate/unadjusted analysis, demand for modern family planning was associated with many variables like age, educational status, presence of communication materials in the house, estimated monthly income, number of children ever born, number of children alive, spousal discussion in the past 12 months about contraception, spousal ever discussed about contraception, and husband intention to have children. But, age at

Table 4 Attitude of respondents towards family planning in Nunu Kumba district, January 2015

Variables ($n = 584$)	Agree No. (%)	Disagree No. (%)	Neutral No. (%)
If family use contraceptive, children will have better opportunities for education	560 (95.9)	14 (2.4)	10(1.7)
FP helps to improve one's standard of living	558 (95.5)	15 (2.6)	11 (1.9)
FP helps the mother to regain strength before her next birth of a baby	548 (93.8)	28 (4.8)	8 (1.4)
Child spacing helps protect the health of children and mothers	553 (94.7)	26 (4.4)	5 (0.9)
FP causes loss of confidence between husband and wife	69 (11.8)	496 (84.9)	19 (3.3)
Husbands will abandon wives who practice FP	50 (8.6)	509 (87.2)	25 (4.3)
Contraceptive use may cause infertility in women	104 (17.8)	458 (78.4)	22 (3.8)
A couple who practices FP has a happy family	547 (93.6)	32 (5.5)	5 (0.9)

first marriage, number of pregnancy, age at first birth, number of living male female children, educational status of husband and decision maker on in the family on family planning were variables not associated with demand for modern methods of contraceptive (Table 5).

After adjusting for confounding by multivariate analysis, factors that remained significantly associated with demand for modern contraceptive methods were: age of respondents, number of children alive, husband intention to have children, spousal discussion in the past 12 months about modern contraceptive and respondent ever discussed about contraception with their husband.

Women whose age 15–24 years were 0.8 times less likely to have demand for modern contraception than women whose age were in between 35 and 49 years [AOR = 0.196, 95%CI: 0.055, 0.692]. Similarly, women whose ages were between 25 and 34 years were almost 0.8 times less likely to have demand for modern contraception than women whose ages were in between 35 and 49 years [AOR = 0.179, 95%CI: 0.043, 0.745]. This showed that age and demand for modern contraceptive methods have a positive association. This study revealed that women who had 2–3 children were almost three times more likely to have demand for modern methods of contraceptive than women who had no and one child. [AOR = 2.617, 95%CI: 1.056, 6.486].

Regarding future intention, women whose husband do not want more children were about four times more likely to have a demand for modern contraception than those who intended to have more children [AOR = 4.124; 95%CI: 1.891, 8.996]. Similarly, women who did not know their husbands' future intention to have children were more than four times more likely to have demand for modern methods of contraceptive than those who desired more children [AOR = 4.403;

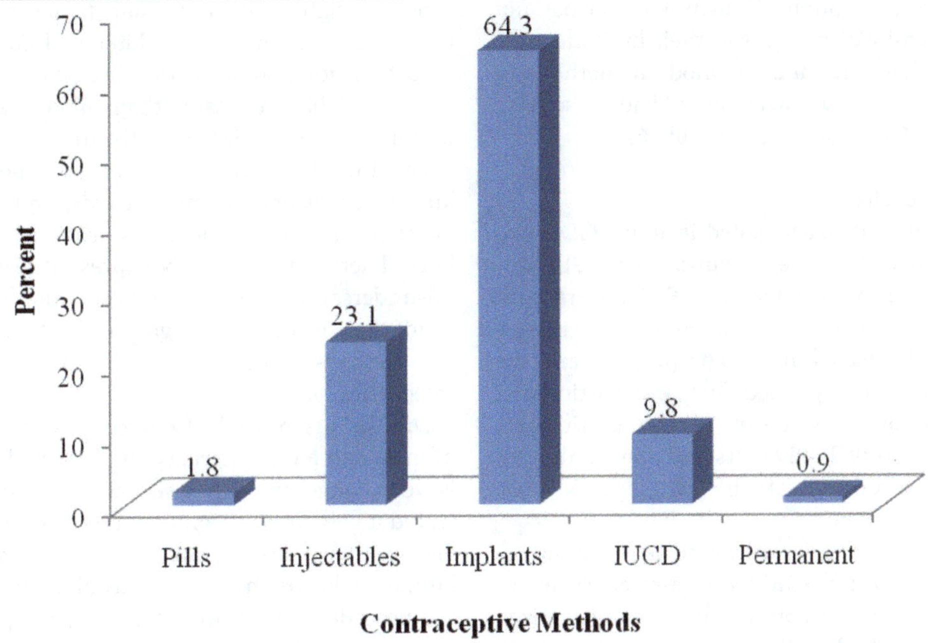

Fig. 4 Distribution of modern contraceptive methods being used by respondents in Nunu Kumba woreda, January 2015

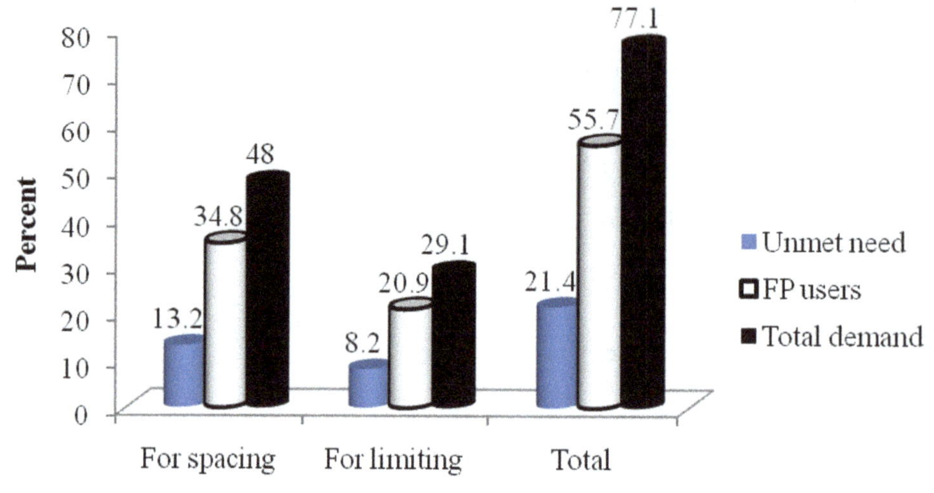

Total Demand = FP users (55.7%) + Unmet need for FP (21.4%)

Fig. 5 Total demand for modern contraceptives among respondents in Nunu Kumba woreda, January 2015

95%CI: 1.763, 10.995]. This result showed a negative association between future intention for more children and demand for family planning.

There was a positive association betweenthe demand for modern contraception and spousal discussion about family planning. However, the spouse who had not discussed about contraception in the past 12 months has-was 0.5 times less likely to have demand for modern contraception than those who had discussed about family planning [AOR = 0.472; 95%CI: 0.255, 0.874]. Furthermore, there was an association between the demand for modern methods of contraception and couples ever had discussed about contraception. Women whoever had not discussed about family planning with their husband were 0.7 less likely to have demand for modern methods of contraception than those who ever had discussed [AOR = 0.340; 95%CI: 0.187, 0.619] (Table 6).

Qualitative study results

A total of 33 discussants participated in four FGDs; two with men and two with women groups; each FGD containing 8 discussants on average. The FGDs were conducted separately for community members (women of reproductive age, husbands/men). The purpose and the content of FGDs were explained first and participants participated voluntarily. Nineteen of the participants were in the age group of 25–29 years and almost all were Protestants and seventeen of the participants were housewives by occupation.

In the group discussions, it was found that the majority of participants in the study had awareness about modern methods of contraception. They also recognized that the modern method of the contraceptive can protect unintended pregnancy and help to determine the number of children they want. They mentioned as they prefer to have 3–4 children in their lifetime. Some of the discussants using contraceptives were those having more than four children and they considered that having more than four children is not good.

Most of the discussants mentioned that older women are using family planning than younger women who want to have a child soon. In relation to this, a 32 years old, Para four women said that, "I knew many women in neighbor with older age and who have four and above children are using contraceptive methods to space or limit their family size, but women who have few children or no son or daughter are not using family planning because they need additional child." (Literate, Implant user).

Furthermore, some of the discussants also mentioned that Injectables are safer than other methods as it has minor side effects like gastritis, menstrual cycle disturbance, and dizziness; and some of them had limited knowledge of permanent methods; and relied highly on negative and intangible ideas from friends and neighbors. There was a strongly expressed fear of procedures, misunderstanding of procedures, and side effects like headaches, bleeding changes, and weight gain for modern methods of contraception, especially, Implants and Injectables.

One discussant said, "I did not have any understanding of male and female sterilization; how is that? The implant is very dangerous, I myself saw it on my friend, and I feared it very much. It moves in the body even to the head. Sterilization is alsoharmful, I want to do that, but I fear it because I heard that heavy bleeding can happen during the procedure and it may cause uterine problems. I want to stop birth, but it is said that it is not good for health and you should have an adequate diet. How would those

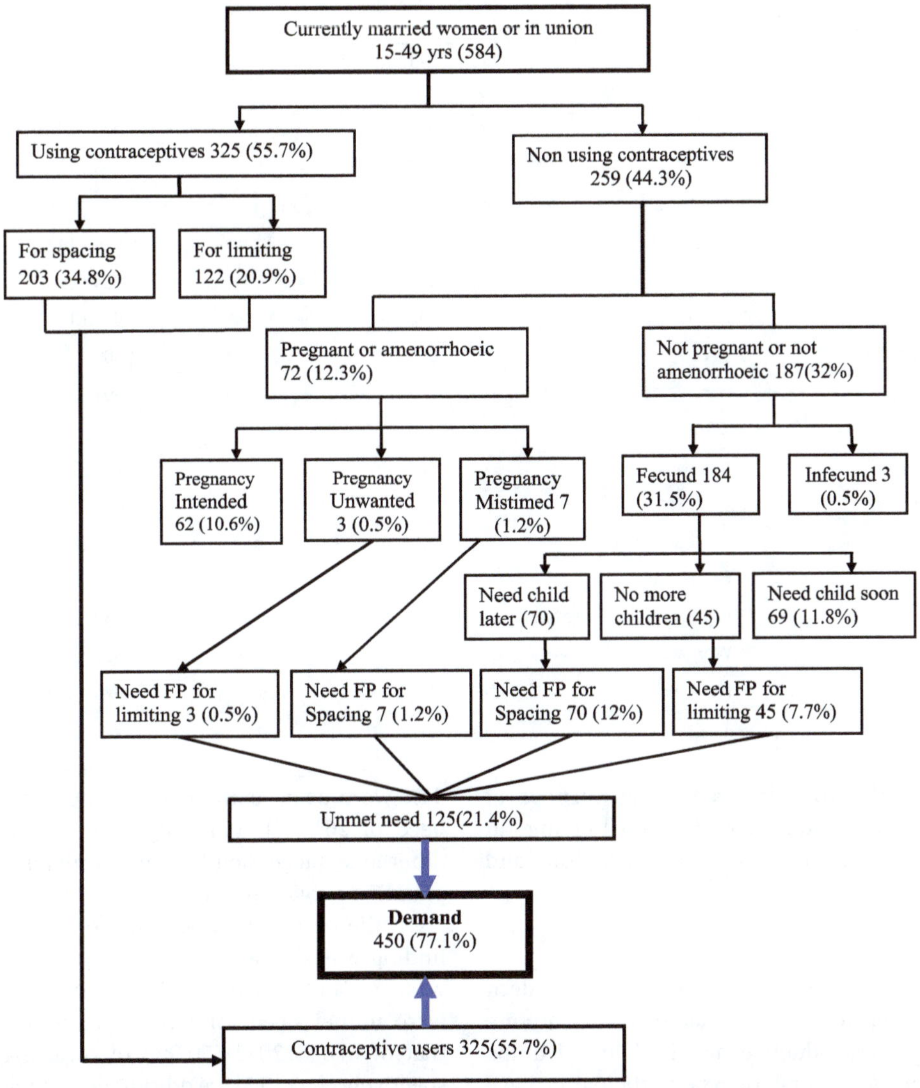

Fig. 6 Model for determination of demand for the modern contraceptive in Nunu Kumba woreda, January 2015 (Bradley and F. West off et al. 2012)

poor people, who couldn't eat well, use it?" (A 35 years' women, grade 2, Para 7, Injectable user).

Moreover, both women and men discussants said, "Couples should support each other and contraceptive use should be decided together by the couples." But, they were still concerned about the side effects, return of fertility after taking implants and IUCD, insertion and removal procedures and effect on physical activities as well. They also associate it with the type of food they were taking. In addition, they had a fear of resistance to ingimplants by the family planning service providers. Some women had concerns such as need for a vaginal examination, discomfort during sex, fear of privacy, side effects (infection), and effects on long-term fertility if used IUCD.

For example, a woman discussant said, "After using IUCD, you may not give birth even it is said that it can stop birth. IUCD can result in sterility and can move into the abdomen. The implant also has pain and may be difficult to remove if it is covered by muscle. I saw my friend suffered from this problem. The implant can make the injected hand numb and you can't rise and carry heavy things by that hand; how can they use these methods?" (A 33 years old, illiterate, Para 5, Injectable user).

In general, the discussants pointed out for the public to be interested in using modern contraception methods, especially long-acting and permanent methods in the future. They also indicated that further information on family planning service should be disseminated to the

Table 5 Bivariate analysis of factors not associated with Demand for modern methods of contraceptives among respondents in Nunu Kumba district, January 2015

Variables	Response	Demand for FP		Crude OR (95% C.I.)	*P*-value
		Yes	No		
Number of pregnancy	< 5	308	72	1.000	0.000
	> = 5	116	27	1.004 (0.625, 1.641)	0.986
Age at first birth	15–24	48	12	1.000	0.000
	25–34	376	87	0.926 (0.472, 1.816)	0.822
Number of living female children	< 5	5	2	1.000	0.000
	> = 5	346	74	0.535 (0.102, 2.09)	0.459
Number of living male children	< 5	3	1	1.000	0.000
	> = 5	386	76	0.591 (0.061, 5.755)	0.650
Age at first marriage	< 18	276	92	1.000	0.000
	> = 18	174	42	0.724 (0.480, 1.093)	0.124
Husband educational status	Can't read and write	147	48	1.000	0.899
	Read and write	62	18	1.009 (0.554, 1.837)	0.977
	Elementary	205	59	1.161 (0.472, 2.855)	0.745
	High school and above	36	9	0.889 (0.479, 1.649)	0.709
Decision maker on FP use	Woman	36	11	1.000	0.001
	Husband	414	123	1.028 (0.508, 2.081)	0.938

OR Odds ratio

community by health professionals for the purpose of continuous awareness creation and attitudinal change in the public towards family planning utilization and misconceptions.

Discussions

This study has attempted to assess demand for modern methods of contraceptive and associated factors among married women of reproductive age in Nunu Kumba district, rural kebeles. A total of 584 participants have been involved in the interview and 33 discussants participated in FGDs.

This study revealed that 77.1% of respondents had demand for modern contraceptive methods; of which 21.4% had an unmet need for modern contraceptives (13.2% for spacing and 8.2% for limiting) and 55.7% were currently using modern methods (34.8% for spacing and 20.9% for limiting). This finding is lower than the study conducted at rural part of Enemay district, Northwest Ethiopia reported 81.5%, but higher than the findings of the study conducted at Misha district, Southern Ethiopia reported 58.3% [16, 17]. These variations might be attributed to the expanding health services coverage and increased awareness of family planning and maternal health services.

Regarding demand for family planning, this finding is slightly lower than study done in Rwanda [13] (79%) of which 33% for spacing, 46% for limiting, but higher than that of study in Tanzania (2010) reported 60% of which 34% were using contraception methods and with unmet need of 26% [6]. This might be as a result of the time difference, accessibility, and availability of the family planning service provisions.

On the other hand, demand for family planning in this finding was similar to study conducted in Butajira which was 77.8% of which 25.4% were current users and 52.4% were unmet need for family planning, but greater than that of EDHS 2011 (50.9%) of rural married women respectively [14, 15]. Additionally, demand for modern contraception in this study was higher than the study done in Southern Ethiopia, Misha district (57.7%), of which 31.2% was contraceptive users (to space or limit their birth) and 26.5% had an unmet need for family planning [16]. This might be due to the difference in geographical and accessibility of a variety of family planning methods and the difference in time of investigation. Medias are also promoting modern contraception which can increase the acceptance and utilization of modern contraceptive methods.

Regarding the age of the respondents, this result indicated that women whose age were between 15 and 24 years and 25–34 years were less likely to have demand for modern contraception than women whose age were in between 35 and 49 years. Similar results from focus group discussion indicated that women of older age and multi Para have more demand for contraceptives in comparison with younger women who have few or no children. This showed that women age is positively

Table 6 Multivariate analysis of factors associated with demand for modern contraceptives among respondents in Nunu Kumba district, January 2015

Variables	Demand for FP		Crude OR (95% C.I.)	Adjusted OR (95% C.I.)
	Yes	No		
Age of women				
15–24	55	35	0.295 (0.167, 0.521)	0.196 (0.055, 0.692)*
25–34	219	66	0.622 (0.392, 0.988)	0.179 (0.043, 0.745)*
35–49	176	33	1.000	1.000
Women educational status				
Can't read and write	314	82	1.000	1.000
Elementary	112	47	0.622 (0.410, 0.946)	0.939 (0.515, 1.712)
High school and above	24	5	1.254 (0.464, 3.386)	1.416 (0.255, 7.850)
Exposure to media				
Yes	272	65	1.000	1.000
No	178	69	0.616 (0.418, 0.909)	0.630 (0.373, 1.064)
Number of children alive				
< =1	49	22	1.000	1.000
2–3	132	31	1.912 (1.011, 3.616)	2.617 (1.056, 6.486)*
> =4	243	44	2.480 (1.365, 4.503)	2.444 (0.707, 8.456)
Husband intention to have children				
Yes	205	73	1.000	1.000
No	156	18	3.086 (1.769, 5.383)	4.124 (1.891, 8.996)**
Don't know	63	8	2.804 (1.282, 6.134)	4.403 (1.763, 10.995)**
Couples ever discussion about FP				
Yes	352	66	1.000	1.000
No	98	68	0.270(0.180, 0.406)	0.340 (0.187, 0.619)**
Couples discussed about FP in last 12 months				
Yes	238	29	1.000	1.000
No	207	99	0.255 (0.162, 0.401)	0.472 (0.255, 0.874)*

NB: 1.000 Reference category, *OR* Odds ratio, *CI* Confidence Interval
*P-value < 0.05; **P-value < 0.01

associated with contraceptive prevalence. The reason for the age difference could be due to those women who were older were having more children and have more desire to limit or space the number of pregnancy than younger who had none or few children. This result is supported by studies done in Debre Markos and Goba, Bale Zone in which women who want more children were younger [3, 18]. Furthermore, a study done in most Sub-Sahara African countries showed that demand for family planning and patterns for unmet need by parity were similar to those by age because, as would be expected, age and parity are closely linked. This implies that unmet need for spacing decreases with age while unmet need for limiting increases, with slightly lower levels of unmet need among the oldest group of women, who have reached menopause, at which point they no longer need family planning at all [19].

Regarding future fertility intention, women whose husbands did not want more children were four times more likely to have demand for modern contraception than those who desire more children. This implies that those who have many children do not want more children and prefer to limit their number of children rather than spacing. So, as the number of children increases, the demand for modern methods of contraceptives utilization also increases. This result is consistent with the findings from a study done in Debre Markos [18].

This study also showed that women who had 2–3 children were almost three times more likely to have demand for modern methods of contraceptive than women who had no or one child. The reason for deference might be due to the more child the woman is having, the more likely she wants to space or limit the number of child and the more she was using contraceptive methods or had an unmet need. This study is in line with the study conducted in Debre Markos, north west Ethiopia which showed that women who have three and above children had more demand for family planning than those having less than three children [18]. Similarly, results from focus group discussion showed that women who had more than four children were using family planning to limit and space their children.

Regarding a couple discussions, 71.6% of them discussed family planning issues with their husband and 82.9% of them made a decision about family planning with their husbands. This study indicated that there was a positive association between the demand for contraception and spousal discussion about contraception. This result is supported witha study conducted in Misha district Southern Ethiopia in which discussion between couples on fertility issues was strongly associated with the use of contraceptives, indicating the importance of frequent discussions [16].

With regards to factors associated with the demand for modern contraceptives, the result from FGDs showed that couples discussion about family planning utilization is very important. Women who make the discussion about family planning with their husbands had more demand or lesser unmet need for contraception. This is due to the fact that husband-wife communications on family planning provide an enabling environment for women to implement their fertility desires and contraceptive needs.

Furthermore, women who had ever discussed family planning with their husband were more likely to discuss on the desired family size they want to have and know their husband's perception towards modern contraceptive methods than those who had no discussion with having unmet need for the methods. The result is in line with studies done in Goba, Debre Birhan District (North Shoa Zone) and Tanzania in which contraceptive practice was found to be associated with a spousal discussion about family planning and women's perception of husband's approval of contraceptive practices [3, 6, 18].

Strength

Using both quantitative and qualitative methods is the strength of the study.

Limitation

Since the study was cross-sectional, the temporal relationship between exposure and outcome variable could not be established. The study was conducted only in the rural part of the community. In addition, the study did not involve men in the quantitative data collection and the information about the husband which was indirectly obtained from women might have not represented them.

Conclusion

The total demand for modern contraceptive methods in the study area was found to be high. Though contraceptive use was high, the uses of long-acting methods like IUCD and permanent methods were seen to very low. Woman's age, number of children alive, couple's intention for more children and discussions about contraceptive use among the couple were significantly associated with demand for modern contraceptives among women. Therefore, any program aimed at promoting family planning at the district level should look for ways and means of increasing demand for modern contraceptive methods in the study area. Service providers in the district should also provide necessary information regarding all methods of contraceptives to minimize fears that exist among women particularly on long-acting and permanent methods of family planning. Male involvement should be encouraged as couples' discussion on family planning affected its utilization in the study area.

Abbreviations

CPR: Contraceptive Prevalence Rate; EDHS: Ethiopia Demographic and Health Survey; FGD: Focus Group Discussion; FP: Family Planning; HEWs: Health Extension Workers; IUCD: Intra Uterine Contraceptive Device;
LAM: Lactational Amenorrhea Method; LAPM: Long-Acting and Permanent Methods; MDGs: Millennium Development Goals; MOH: Ministry of Health; MWRA: Married Women of Reproductive Age; NGOs: Non-Governmental Organizations; OCP: Oral Contraceptive Pills; SSA: Sub-Saharan Africa;
TFR: Total Fertility Rate

Acknowledgments

First, we would like to acknowledge Wollega University, College of Health Sciences for bringing this research work opportunity. Our deepest gratitude also extended to Nunu Kumba Woreda Health Office staffs and Kebele leaders for their cooperation during the whole data collection period.

Authors' contributions

AK, SG, EM, and TT have equally participated in proposal writing, data collection process, data analysis, and interpretation, and report writing. In addition, TT and AK drafted and prepared the manuscript. All authors have read, reviewed, and approved the final version of the manuscript.

Authors' information

AK is working at Gute Health center, East Wollega, SG (Ph.D.) is Assistant Professor of Public Health, working at Adama Hospital Medical College, Ethiopia; while the rest two co-authors are from Wollega University Institute of health science, Department of Nursing.

Author details

[1]Department of Public Health, Institute of Health Sciences, Wollega University, P. O. Box: 395, Nekemte, Ethiopia. [2]Public Health, Adama Hospital Medical College, Adama, Ethiopia.

References

1. IPPF. Understanding demand and supply for contraception. United Kingdom: Portfolio Publishing.com; 2011. p. 1–4.
2. Kantorova ABV. Global trends in contraceptive method mix and implications for meeting the demand for family planning. New York; 2012.
3. Abulie Takele GDMY. Demand for long-acting and permanent methods of contraceptives and factors for non-use among married women of Goba Town, Bale Zone, South East Ethiopia: Madawalabu University; 2012.

4. Madeleine S, Fabic YC, Bongaarts J, Darroch JE, Ross JA, Stover J. Meeting demand for family planning within a generation: the post-2015 agenda. Washington DC: New York Office of Population and Reproductive Health, Bureau for Global Health, United States Agency for International Development; 2014.
5. Ferede T. Multilevel Modelling of Modern Contraceptive Use among Rural and Urban Population of Ethiopia. Am J Math Stat. 2013;3:1–16.
6. Michael EJ. Use of contraceptives methods among women in stable marital relations attending health facilities in Kahama District, Shinyanga region, Tanzania; Muhimbili University; 2012.
7. Haile A. Demand for long-acting and permanent contraceptive methods and associated factors among family planning service users. Batu town, Ethiopia: East Shoa Zone; 2009.
8. Gribble KRJ. Expanding contraceptive choice: five promising innovations. Washington DC: Population Reference Bureau; 2009.
9. Hatam Hosseini BB. Demand for using contraceptive methods among Kurdish women in the city of Mahabad. Med Sci. 2012;17:1–2.
10. Alem Gebremariam AA. Intention to use long-acting and permanent contraceptive methods and factors affecting it among married women in Adigrat town, Tigray, Northern Ethiopia. Reprod Health. 2014;11:1–9.
11. Prata N. Making family planning accessible in resource-poor settings. Philos Trans R Soc Lond B Biol Sci. 2009;364:3093–99.
12. USAID, CfDaPAC, Partners in Population and Development, Africa Regional Office (PPD ARO), Population Reference Bureau (PRB). Family Planning in Ethiopia; 2012. p. 1–4.
13. Rahman M. A potential contraceptive method mix for the Ethiopian family planning program. Health. 2008:1–12.
14. Central Statistical Agency [Ethiopia] and ICF International. Ethiopia Demographic and Health Survey 2011. Addis Ababa, Ethiopia and Calverton, Maryland, USA: Central Statistical Agency and ICF International; 2012.
15. Worku WMA. Determinants of low family planning use and high unmet need in Butajira District, south Central Ethiopia. Reprod Health. 2011;8:1–8.
16. Doyore KCF. Unmet Need for Family Planning and Associated Factors among Currently Married Women in Misha District. South Ethiop Public Health. 2014;3(4):1–9.
17. Getiye Dejenu MAAAA. Prevalence and associated factors of unmet need for family planning among married women in Enemay District, Northwest Ethiopia. Med Sci. 2013;13(4):1–11.
18. Gizachew Abdissa Bulto TAZTKB. Demand for long-acting and permanent contraceptive methods and associated factors among married women of the reproductive age group in Debre Markos town, North West Ethiopia. Women's Health. 2014;14:1–12.
19. Sarah EK, TNC B, Fishel JD, Westoff CF. Revising Unmet Need for Family Planning. Calverton, Maryland, USA: ICF International; 2012. p. 1–94.

7

Predictors of contraceptive discontinuation among postpartum women in Arusha region, Tanzania

Michael J. Mahande[1*], Ryoko Sato[2], Caroline Amour[1], Rachel Manongi[3], Amina Farah[3], Sia E. Msuya[1,3,4], Bilikisu Elewonibi[2] and Iqbal Shah[2]

Abstract

Background: Postpartum contraceptive discontinuation refers to cessation of use following initiation after delivery within 1 year postpartum. Discontinuation of use has been associated with an increased unmet need for family planning that leads to high numbers of unwanted pregnancies, unsafe abortion or mistimed births. There is scant information about contraceptive discontinuation and its predictors among postpartum women in Tanzania. This study aimed to determine predictors of contraception discontinuation at 3, 6, 12 months postpartum among women of reproductive age in Arusha city and Meru district, Tanzania.

Methods: This was an analytical cross-sectional study which was conducted in two district of Arusha region (Arusha city and Meru district respectively). A multistage sampling technique was used to select 13 streets of the 3 wards in Arusha City and 2 wards in Meru District. A total of 474 women of reproductive age (WRAs) aged 16–44 years residing in the study areas were included in this analysis. Data analysis was performed using STATA version 15. Odds ratios (ORs) with 95% confidence interval (CI) for the factors associated with contraceptives discontinuation (at 3, 6 and 12 moths) were estimated in a multivariable logistic regression model.

Results: Overall, discontinuation rate for all methods at 3, 6, and 12 months postpartum was 11, 19 and 29% respectively. It was higher at 12 months for Lactational amenorrhea, male condoms and injectables (76, 50.5 and 36%, respectively). Women aged 40–44 years had lower odds of contraceptive discontinuation at 3 months as compare to those aged 16 to 19 years. Implants and pills users had also lower odds of contraceptive discontinuation compared to injectable users at 3, 6 and 12 months respectively.

Conclusion: Lactational amenorrhea, male condoms and injectables users had the highest rates of discontinuation. Women's age and type of method discontinued were independently associated with postpartum contraceptive discontinuation. Addressing barriers to continue contraceptive use amongst younger women and knowledge on method attributes, including possible side-effects and how to manage complications is warranted.

Keywords: Contraceptive, Discontinuation, Determinants, Tanzania

* Correspondence: jmmahande@gmail.com
[1]Department of Epidemiology and Biostatistics, Institute of Public Health, Kilimanjaro Christian Medical University College, P.O Box 2240, Moshi, Tanzania

Introduction

Contraceptive discontinuation is defined as starting contraceptive use and then stopping for any reason while still at risk of an unintended pregnancy [1]. It has been reported to be higher for short-acting methods such as condoms, injectables, pills and traditional methods as they can be discontinued by the user herself compared to long-acting reversible methods such as implants and the Intrauterine device (IUD) which require a visit to facility to discontinue [1–3]. The method-related reasons and contraceptive failure have been reported as the predominant causes for contraceptive discontinuation [4].

Postpartum period in the first 12 months following childbirth has been associated with high unmet need for contraceptives coupled with unintended pregnancies [5]. Breastfeeding practices and beliefs about return of menses as a marker of fertility resumption during the postpartum period, makes it difficult for women to determine their fertility risk. Thus, women are less motivated to start contraceptive use while breastfeeding [6, 7]. Previous investigators have demonstrated that women who discontinue contraception use during the postpartum period may opt not to use any method (contraceptive discontinuation) or switch to different modern method (method switching) which is less effective than the previous method at preventing pregnancy, and thereby exposes women to risk of unintended pregnancy, abortions and mistimed pregnancies/births [7, 8].

Sustaining postpartum contraception use is important for woman's fertility because it ensures optimal birth spacing, prevents unintended pregnancies, abortion and has an impact on infant and child survival [9]. Examining postpartum contraceptive discontinuation will shed a light on the knowledge gaps in contraceptive use such as trends and determinants for contraceptive discontinuation, and will help in reducing unmet need for family planning [10]. It will also provide evidence for areas that require coordinated efforts between different stakeholders involved in family planning programs and the government. This will help to improvement quality of services for family planning and reduces the discontinuation postpartum contraception.

Previous studies from developing countries showed that, on average, 19–64% of women discontinued using reversible contraceptive methods by the 12th month of use [4, 11]; [12–15]. The discontinuation rate for condoms within the first 12 months is higher than intrauterine devices (50% vs 13%, respectively), and up to 40% higher for other methods such as pill, injectable, periodic abstinence and withdrawal [3, 4, 16]. Contraceptive discontinuation among women with no desire to get pregnant increases the risk for unwanted pregnancies [8]. This reflects a failure of family planning programs and services [3, 4, 17–19].

According to Tanzania Demographic and Health Survey, only 15.5 and 22.4% of women reported using modern contraceptive methods at 3 months and 12 months post-delivery respectively, especially during postnatal visit probably due to contraceptive counselling [20]. A cohort study conducted in Northern Tanzania among 5284 pregnant women who were followed from 6 to 15 months postpartum, reported that 34% of women initiated contraceptive use during the postpartum period and 25% of the participants started at 7 months postpartum [21]. Authors in this study noted that 18.8% of contraceptive users discontinued at 15 months postpartum. The reasons for contraceptive discontinuation include partner disapproval (32%), side-effects (6%), wanting a child (4%) and other reasons (37%) [21]. The most recent study in Tanzania reported that short contraceptive methods were associated with high rate of discontinuation compared to long term acting contraceptives [13].

There is scant information on contraceptive discontinuation rates, patterns and associated factors post-delivery. This study aimed to determine predictors of contraception discontinuation at 3, 6, 12 months postpartum among women of reproductive age in Arusha city and Meru district, Tanzania.

Methods

Study design and setting

This study was conducted in two districts of Arusha region (Arusha city and Meru district respectively) from December 2017–June 2018.

Study population, sample size and sampling method

The study sample included women of reproductive age (WRAs) aged 16–44 years who started to use family planning methods (modern/traditional) after a delivery (6 weeks) that occurred at least 12 months prior to the survey. Multistage cluster sampling with probability proportional to size was used to draw respondents from 13 streets (i.e. 3 wards) in Arusha City and 2 wards in Meru District. The details of the sampling procedures have been described elsewhere [15, 22]. A contraceptive calendar is a contraceptive history collected for each woman who, or whose husband, was not sterilized at the calendar's start. The data were recorded in a calendar matrix, consisting of rows and columns, with each row of the calendar representing a particular month. The sample size was estimated based on number of events included in the contraceptive calendar, which included retrospectively reported month-by-month during 31 months before the interview. A total of 12,203 contraceptive use events were recorded during the study period. We excluded 3216 episodes which started prior to the calendar period of 31 months before the survey;

2883 episode because no birth within 31 month; 2211 episode because the episode started before the latest birth; 2494 episode because no method used, birth, termination, or pregnancy; 184 events during 0-3 months before the survey [methods unknown ($n = 142$) & sterilization/other ($n = 42$)]. The remaining 1215 episodes of use within the last 3 to 28 months prior to interview constituted the final sample size (Fig. 1).

Study variables

The main outcome was contraceptive discontinuation after starting to use of contraceptive at three time points; 3 months, 6 months, and 12 months post-delivery. The independent variables were selected based on the previous studies. These include sociodemographic characteristics: maternal age, maternal education and wealth index. Women were asked of the number of antenatal care (ANC) visits during the last pregnancy, number of months since birth to first family planning use, received contraceptive counseling during ANC or PNC visits and attendance of postnatal care after last delivery. The type of contraceptive methods used were IUD, pills, male condoms, injectables, implant, rhythm and withdrawal. Women were also asked for the reasons related to discontinuation of modern contraceptive.

Data collection methods

Data collection was conducted through face-to-face interviews using questionnaire administered using tablets. A team of trained research assistants including medical doctors, statisticians, demographers and social scientist were used to collect information from the participants. A standardized questionnaire in Kiswahili language which was adapted from the Tanzania Demographic and Health Survey (TDHS) 2015–2016 [12] was used to collect information from the study participants for household survey to meet the WIE objectives. These variables includes women age, education level, marital status, area of residence, wealth index, utilisation of contraceptive methods, cost to access the family planning services, type of facility, distance to health facility, type of contraceptive used and availability of family planning commodities to mention a few.

Data analysis

Data analysis was performed using STATA version 15. Descriptive statistics were summarized using frequency and proportions for categorical variables. The percentage of women who had discontinued their method of contraception at 3, 6 and 12 months were reported. Adjusted Odds ratios (ORs) with 95% confidence interval (CI) for the factors associated with contraceptive discontinuation

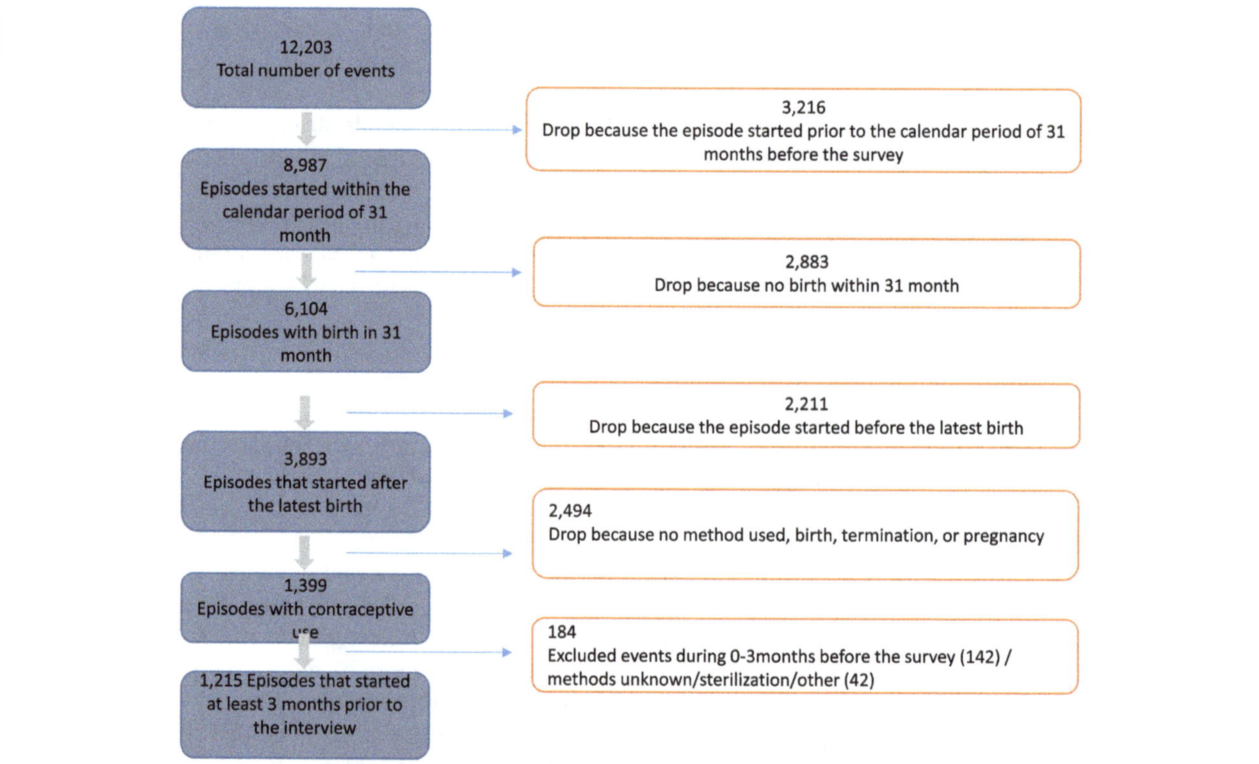

Fig. 1 Flowchart of Events included in Contraceptive Calendar

Table 1 Characteristics of study participants ($N = 1215$ episodes)

Characteristics	n	%
FP counselling at ANC (Yes)		
Yes	382	70.9
No	157	29.1
Family Planning counselling at postnatal care		
Yes	424	76.5
No	130	23.5
Mother age (year)		
16–19	10	1.7
20–24	161	28.0
25–29	181	31.5
30–34	111	19.3
35–39	80	13.9
40–44	31	5.4
Education level		
None	17	3.0
Primary	316	55.1
Secondary	209	36.4
Higher education	32	5.6
Wealth index (as per DHS)		
Poorest	112	19.5
Poorer	59	10.3
Medium	101	17.6
Richer	253	44.1
Richest	49	8.5
Method discontinued		
Injectables	175	30.5
Implants	153	26.7
Pills	61	10.6
Condom	22	3.8
Rhythm	79	13.8
Other	84	14.6
Sample = 574 women with some FP use that initiated at least 12 months prior to the survey		
Number of living children		
0	2	0.3
1	201	35.0
2	165	28.7
3	117	20.4
4	60	10.5
5	20	3.5
6	6	1.0
7	2	0.3
Desire to get pregnant		
No	176	30.6
Yes	398	69.34
Received FP counselling during their ANC or PNC		
No	460	80.1
Yes	114	19.9
Support from the husband/partner for contraceptive use		
No	125	21.8
Yes	449	78.2

were estimated in a multivariable logistic regression model. The correlation between discontinuation at certain time (3, 6, and 12 months) with sociodemographic characteristics were separately evaluated. We used the logistic regression because the dependent variable is a dummy variable (discontinued at 3, 6, or 12 months). Independent variables we used for the regression analysis were reported in Table 1. Only variables which were significant in the bivariate analysis were included in the final model.

Table 2 Contraceptive discontinuation rates and associated reasons (*N*=1,215 episodes)

At 3 months postpartum									
Reasons for discontinuation									
Contraceptive methods	**Method failure**	**Desire to become pregnant**	**Other fertility related reasons**	**Side effects**	**Wanted more effective method**	**Other method related**	**Other/ DK**	**All reasons**	**Unweighted N**
IUD	0.00	0.00	0.00	3.23	0.00	0.00	0.00	3.23	73
Injectables	0.29	0.27	1.96	10.89	0.80	1.12	1.12	16.45	351
Implants	0.00	0.00	0.00	1.55	0.00	0.00	0.00	1.55	359
Pill	0.00	0.00	1.05	8.67	1.13	4.16	1.37	16.37	147
Male condom	0.00	0.00	1.77	0.00	2.03	0.00	5.59	9.38	51
Rhythm	0.61	1.13	0.89	1.39	4.26	0.00	0.00	8.27	150
LAM	0.00	0.00	0.00	0.00	24.93	0.00	1.76	26.68	47
Withdrawal	3.93	0.00	10.26	0.00	18.33	0.00	0.00	32.52	37
All methods	0.33	0.24	1.30	5.08	2.97	0.84	0.73	11.50	1215

Results

Characteristics of study participants

We have a total of 1215 episodes from the calendar data (Table 1). About one third of all episodes (31%) were aged 25 to 29 years old. More than half (55%) of all episodes had primary education. Majority (71%) of all episodes were reported to have received family planning counselling during ANC visit and postnatal care visit (76.5%).

Contraceptive discontinuation at 3, 6 and 12 months postpartum

Overall, 11.5% of all episodes discontinued at 3 months. Of these, injectables, pills and male condoms were discontinued by 16, 16 and 9% of the sample respectively, while implants and IUD discontinued by 1.55 and 3.23% at 3 months. On the other hand, of the 11.5% episodes discontinued at 3 months, 27% were LAM users (Table 2). Likewise, there was 19.4% episodes discontinued at 6 months, where injectables, pills and male condoms were discontinued by 24.64, 25.44 and 20.37% of the sample respectively while implants and IUD accounted for 3.84 and 8.34% during the same period. At 6 months, 49% of those 19.4% episodes discontinued were LAM users (Table 3). Furthermore, about 29.4% episodes discontinued at 12 months, injectables, pills and male condoms accounted for 38.15, 36.48% and 50. 49% of the sample while implants and IUD contributed 5.11 and 9.06% at 12 months while 76.12% of 29.4% episodes discontinued at 12 months were LAM (Table 4).

Multivariable analysis for determinants of contraceptive discontinuation at 3, 6 and 12 months postpartum

The determinants for contraceptive discontinuation across time points are shown in Table 5 (focusing only on the first Family Planning use since the birth). In

Table 3 Contraceptive discontinuation rates at 6 months and associated reasons (*N*=574)

Discontinuation at 6 months postpartum									
Reasons for discontinuation									
Contraceptive method	**Method failure**	**Desire to become pregnant**	**Other fertility related reasons**	**Side effects**	**Wanted more effective method**	**Other method related**	**Other/ DK**	**All reasons**	**Unweighted N**
IUD	0.00	0.00	0.00	8.34	0.00	0.00	0.00	8.34	73
Injectables	0.40	0.37	2.41	16.91	1.40	1.48	1.68	24.64	351
Implants	0.00	0.42	0.00	3.42	0.00	0.00	0.00	3.84	359
Pill	0.00	0.00	2.47	14.23	2.90	4.47	1.37	25.44	147
Male condom	0.00	0.00	1.77	0.87	5.31	0.00	12.43	20.37	51
Rhythm	2.28	1.13	1.23	1.39	11.77	0.00	0.34	18.14	150
LAM	0.00	0.00	4.80	1.80	41.56	0.00	1.76	49.91	47
Withdrawal	3.93	0.00	10.26	0.00	35.13	0.00	0.00	49.32	37
All methods	0.64	0.38	1.87	8.35	6.04	0.99	1.15	19.41	1215

Table 4 Contraceptive discontinuation rates at 12 months and associated reasons (*N*=574)

Discontinuation 12 months postpartum									
Reasons for discontinuation									
Contraceptive method	Method failure	Desire to become pregnant	Other fertility related reasons	Side effects	Wanted more effective method	Other method related	Other/ DK	All reasons	Unweighted N
IUD	0.00	0.00	0.00	9.06	0.00	0.00	0.00	9.06	73
Injectables	1.66	0.88	3.37	21.09	3.77	4.53	2.86	38.15	351
Implants	0.00	0.42	0.00	4.69	0.00	0.00	0.00	5.11	359
Pill	2.53	0.00	2.47	18.48	6.06	4.47	2.47	36.48	147
Male condom	**0.00**	2.05	1.77	8.15	16.84	0.00	21.68	50.49	51
Rhythm	3.30	1.13	1.88	4.99	14.96	0.00	0.34	26.60	150
LAM	4.67	0.00	4.80	1.80	63.09	0.00	1.76	76.12	47
Withdrawal	3.93	0.00	10.26	0.00	54.70	0.00	2.85	71.74	37
All methods	1.81	0.59	2.26	11.26	9.58	1.97	1.94	29.40	1215

multivariable regression model, age and type of method discontinued were independently associated with postpartum contraceptive discontinuation. Women aged 40 to 44 years had significantly lower odds [(OR: 0.118, 95% CI: 0.016, 0.883)] of contraceptive discontinuation at 3 months postpartum compared to their counterparts aged 16 to 19 years of age. Furthermore, women who reported using implants had significantly lower odds of contraceptive discontinuation at 3 months, 6 months and 12 months postpartum (OR: 0.095; 95% CI: 0.051,0.176), (OR: 0.142; 95% CI: 0.073,0.276) and (OR: 0.218; 95% CI: 0.100,0.473) respectively, compared to those using injectables. Women who reported using pills had lower odds of contraceptive discontinuation at 3 months (OR: 0.527; 95% CI: 0.285, 0.975), 6 months (OR: 0.489; 95% CI: 0.246, 0.973) and 12 months (OR: 0.230; 95% CI: 0.068, 0.779) respectively compared to those who discontinued injectables. Other factors were not significantly associated with contraceptive discontinuation at 3, 6 and 12 months postpartum (Table 5).

Discussion

This study examined the determinants of postpartum contraceptive discontinuation at 3, 6 and 12 months postpartum. Overall, 11.5% of all episodes discontinued at 3 months, 19.4% discontinued at 6 months and 29.4% discontinued at 12 months. Women aged 40 to 44 years had significantly lower odds of contraceptive discontinuation at 3 months postpartum compared to their counterparts aged 16 to 19 years of age. Furthermore, women who reported using implants and pills had significantly lower odds of contraceptive discontinuation at 3 months, 6 months and 12 months compared to injectable users.

The average number of months since child birth to first family planning use was 3.8 months, this was similar to what was observed in rural Ghana [23] where the average time of first family planning use following child birth was 3.5 months and in contrast to what was observed in Nairobi slums where initiation of contraceptives following child birth occurred 7 months after delivery [11]. The fact that women initiate contraceptive use early in our setting may be encouraging, however the type of methods used must be borne in mind because short contraceptive methods have been associated with high rate of discontinuation compared to long term acting contraceptives [13]. Thus, short-acting contraceptive methods do not guarantee adequate birth spacing and the prevention of unwanted or mistimed pregnancies.

The most common methods discontinued after postpartum initiation in this study were LAM, pill and injectable. This is consistent with the previous reports from Tanzania Demographic and Health Survey and Health and Demographic Surveillance System (HDSS) in Magu district in Tanzania [13, 20]. Our finding was different from Malawian study, where women who reported long-acting methods and injectable use at 3 months post-delivery were more likely to continue compared to those using pills, condoms, traditional methods [2]. It also differs from the South Africa that reported high rate of implant continuation at 12 months at a rate of 86% [7]. The difference in findings could be explained by the differences in characteristics between the studied population especially the cultural barriers. Furthermore, the high contraceptives discontinuation rate in our population calls for a need to provide women with education on contraception, increase access to contraceptives as these will facilitate women to have informed choice and decision towards contraceptive use. However, there may be a possibility of some women experiencing forms of coercion to adopt a LARC the immediate postpartum period and choosing later to have the method removed.

The lower odds of postpartum discontinuation among women aged 40–44 years in our study is consistent with previous report in Kenya by [11] where higher odds of contraceptive discontinuation among adolescent women at 3 months, 6 months and 12 months compared with the adults counterparts. Previous studies in Tanzania and Nepal also reported the effect of age and type of contraceptive methods used on post-partum contraception discontinuation [13, 24]. The high contraceptive discontinuation among young women could be explained by their fertility desire to have more children. Unlike the short-term contraceptives, the lower discontinuation rate for long-acting methods could be explained by its difficulty to remove which requires health care professionals with cost implications [25, 26].

Strengths and limitations of the study

The strength of this study is that, being a community-based study may reflect the representation of what is happening at the ground in the general population. We also used a rigorous data collection methods to enhance validity for observed findings. Despite its strength, some limitations which need to be taken into account while interpreting our finding. First, being a cross-sectional in nature, the study cannot establish a causal effect. Secondly, we did not collect information on sexual resumption, menstrual resumption, partners and service related factors which would further explain the methods discontinuation during the course of time.

Conclusions

Lactational amenorrhea, male condoms, injectables and pills users had the highest rates of discontinuation compared with implants and IUD users. Women aged 40 to 44 years had lower odds of postpartum contraceptive discontinuation at 3 months while implants and pills had lower odds of contraceptive discontinuation at 3 months, 6 months and 12 months. Addressing barriers to prolonged contraceptive use amongst younger women and knowledge on attributes of contraceptive methods and their potential side-effects is warranted. In addition, the programs should assist women to timely switch to a method of their preference when they discontinue the method that fail, do not meet their expectations or cause side-effects.

Acknowledgements

The authors would like to thank the study participants for their valuable participation in this study. We also thank the Arusha Regional Medical Officer, District Medical Officers and other administrative staff in Arusha city and Meru district; for their cooperation and support during the study period. Furthermore, we would like to thank the research assistants for their positive participation and involvement in this study.

Authors' contributions

SEM, BE and IS designed the study. All authors were involved in data collection. RS and MJM conducted data analysis. MJM, RS and BE drafted the manuscript. MJM RS RM CA BE SEM and IS contributed to the final draft of the manuscript. All authors reviewed and gave their final approval to the manuscript.

Author details

[1]Department of Epidemiology and Biostatistics, Institute of Public Health, Kilimanjaro Christian Medical University College, P.O Box 2240, Moshi, Tanzania. [2]Department of Global Health and Population, Harvard T.H. Chan School of Public Health, Boston, USA. [3]Department of Community Health, Institute of Public Health, Kilimanjaro Christian Medical University College, P.O Box 2240, Moshi, Tanzania. [4]Department of Community Health, KCMC Hospital, P.O Box 3010, Moshi, Tanzania.

References

1. FP2020(2015) Contraceptive reasons, challenges, discontinuation: and solutions.
2. Kopp DM, Rosenberg NE, Stuart GS, Miller WC, Hosseinipour MC, Bonongwe P, Mwale M, Tang JH. Patterns of contraceptive adoption, continuation, and switching after delivery among Malawian women. PLoS One. 2017;12(1):1–12. https://doi.org/10.1371/journal.pone.0170284.
3. Thobani R, Jessani S, Azam I, Reza S, Sami N, Rozi S, Abrejo F, Saleem S. Factors associated with the discontinuation of modern methods of contraception in the low income areas of Sukh initiative Karachi: a community-based case control study. PLoS One. 2019;14(7):1–12. https://doi.org/10.1371/journal.pone.0218952.
4. Ali MM, Cleland JG, Shah IH, World Health Organization. Causes and consequences of contraceptive discontinuation: evidence from 60 demographic and health surveys. World Health Organization; 2012. https://apps.who.int/iris/handle/10665/75429
5. WHO. Postpartum family planning. Stud Fam Plann. 2015;22(5):294–307. https://doi.org/10.2307/1966684.
6. Borda M, Winfrey W. Postpartum fertility and contraception: an analysis of findings from 17 countries. Access-fp. 2010;1(March):11–50 Available at: http://reprolineplus.org/system/files/resources/ppfp_17countryanalysis.pdf.
7. Singata-Madliki M, Dekile-Yonto N, Hofmeyr GJ, Lawrie TA. Postnatal contraception discontinuation: different methods, same problem. BMJ Sex Reprod Health. 2018;44(1):66–7. https://doi.org/10.1136/bmjsrh-2017-101846.
8. Jain AK, Winfrey W. Contribution of contraceptive discontinuation to unintended births in 36 developing countries. Stud Fam Plann. 2017;48(3): 269–78. https://doi.org/10.1111/sifp.12023.
9. World Health Organization (2013): Programming strategies for Postpartum Family Planning. Available at: https://www.apps.who.int/iris/bitstream/10665/93680/1/9789241506496_eng.pdf. (Accessed on 20 Mar 2017).
10. Jackson E, Glasier A. Return of ovulation and menses in postpartum non-lactating women: a systematic review. Obstet Gynecol. 2011;117(3):657–62. https://doi.org/10.1097/AOG.0b013e31820ce18c.
11. Mumah JN, Machiyama K, Mutua M, Kabiru CW, Cleland J. Contraceptive adoption, discontinuation, and switching among postpartum women in Nairobi's urban slums. Stud Fam Plann. 2015;46(4):369–86. https://doi.org/10.1111/j.1728-4465.2015.00038.x.
12. TDHS. Tanzania Demographic and Health Survey 2015/16 Final Report. Tanzania Demogr Heal Surv Malar Indic Surv 2015-16. 2016.
13. Safari W, Urassa M, Mtenga B, Changalucha J, Beard J, Church K, Zaba B, Todd J. Contraceptive use and discontinuation among women in rural North-West Tanzania. Contracept Reprod Med. 2019;4(1):18. https://doi.org/10.1186/s40834-019-0100-6.
14. Barden-O'Fallon, Speizer IS, Calhoun LM, Corroon M, et al. BMC Womens Health. 2018;18:35. https://doi.org/10.1186/s12905-018-0529-9.
15. Sato R, Elewonibi B, Msuya S, Manongi R, Canning D, Shah I. Why do women discontinue contraception and what are the post-discontinuation outcomes? Evidence from the Arusha region, Tanzania. Sex Reprod Health Matters. 2020;28(1):1723321. https://doi.org/10.1080/26410397.2020.1723321.
16. Shiferaw Yideta Z, Mekonen L, Seifu W, Shine S. Contraceptive discontinuation, method switching and associated factors among reproductive age women in Jimma town, Southwest Ethiopia, 2013. Fam Med Med Sci Res. 2017;06(01):6–11. https://doi.org/10.4172/2327-4972.1000213.

Table 5 Multivariable analysis for factors associated with contraceptive discontinuation at 3, 6 and 12 months postpartum

	Discontinued		
	3 months OR (95% CI)	**6 months OR (95% CI)**	**12 months OR (95% CI)**
Characteristics			
Number of months since birth to FP use	1.026[0.967,1.088]	1.027[0.965,1.093]	1.001[0.927,1.080]
ANC visit (4-visits vs. < 4)	0.649 [0.408,1.031]*	0.733[0.453,1.188]	0.974[0.542,1.749]
Postnatal attendance7days (Yes)	0.825[0.468,1.455]	0.666[0.362,1.222]	0.679[0.310,1.488]
Age years (reference = 16–19)			
20–24	0.358[0.060,2.125]	0.773[0.185,3.236]	2.041[0.224,18.636]
25–29	0.379[0.062,2.301]	1.053[0.243,4.561]	3.854[0.418,35.509]
30–34	0.31[0.048,2.012]	0.663[0.140,3.132]	1.937[0.190,19.784]
35–39	0.239[0.036,1.593]	0.51[0.101,2.581]	1.961[0.185,20.790]
40–44	0.164[0.019,1.422]	0.356[0.049,2.587]	1.681[0.096,29.540]
Education level (reference = none)			
Primary	0.667[0.237,1.875]	0.728[0.239,2.214]	0.811[0.179,3.672]
Secondary	0.768[0.260,2.265]	0.689[0.214,2.221]	1.017[0.210,4.928]
Higher education	0.715[0.190,2.695]	0.505[0.117,2.172]	0.849[0.127,5.677]
Number of living children	0.813[0.628,1.053]	0.824[0.633,1.073]	0.766[0.546,1.075]
Desire to get pregnant	0.782[0.453,1.351]	0.590[0.329,1.058]	0.657[0.303,1.425]
Received FP counselling during their ANC or PNC	1.037[0.650,1.656]	0.936[0.565,1.551]	0.973[0.527,1.797]
Support from the husband/partner for contraceptive use	0.79[0.498,1.255]	0.771[0.478,1.246]	0.725[0.401,1.309]
Wealth index (reference = poorest)			
Poorer	1.012[0.441,2.320]	1.049[0.465,2.367]	1.765[0.710,4.390]
Medium	1.039[0.539,2.005]	0.891[0.455,1.743]	1.52[0.684,3.378]
Richer	1.043[0.597,1.820]	0.751[0.422,1.336]	0.591[0.288,1.213]
Richest	1.149[0.484,2.726]	1.281[0.535,3.062]	1.262[0.448,3.555]
Method discontinued (reference = injectables)			
Implants	0.092[0.049,0.172]***	0.136[0.069,0.269]***	0.212[0.097,0.464]***
Pills	0.538[0.291,0.995]**	0.499[0.254,0.980]**	0.230[0.069,0.767]**
Condom	0.603[0.225,1.617]	0.799[0.281,2.269]	0.62[0.142,2.712]
Rhythm	0.386[0.215,0.693]***	0.617[0.339,1.121]	1.127[0.581,2.186]
Other	0.595[0.220,1.606]	0.547[0.181,1.656]	1.03[0.241,4.397]
Cons	13.695[1.607,116.692]**	4.295[0.646,28.575]	0.398[0.020,7.732]

***$p < 0.001$; **$p < 0.05$

17. Adal TG. Early discontinuation of long acting reversible contraceptives among married and in union women : a systematic review and meta-analysis. Ann Med Health Sci Res. 2017;7(1):113–8.
18. Do Nascimento Chofakian CB, et al. Contraceptive discontinuation: frequency and associated factors among undergraduate women in Brazil. Reprod Health. 2019;16(1):1–12. https://doi.org/10.1186/s12978-019-0783-9.
19. Samosir, O. B., Kiting, A. S. and Aninditya, F. (2019) 'Determinants of contraceptive discontinuation in Indonesia: further analysis of the 2017 Demographic and Health Survey.'DHS Working Papers, (159), ix-pp. Available at: https://dhsprogram.com/pubs/pdf/WP159/WP159.pdf.
20. MoHCDGEC, et al. Tanzania demographic and health survey 2015/16 final report. In: Tanzania Demographic and Health Survey and Malaria Indicator Survey (TDHS-MIS); 2016. p. 2015–6.
21. Keogh, S. C. et al. (2011) 'Dynamics of postpartum contraceptive use, and their relationship to antenatal intentions, in northern Tanzania'.
22. Elewonibi B, Sato R, Manongi R, Msuya S, Shah I, Canning D. The distance-quality trade-off in women's choice of family planning provider in North Eastern Tanzania. BMJ Glob Health. 2020;5(2):e002149. https://doi.org/10.1136/bmjgh-2019-002149.
23. Eliason, et al. Postpartum fertility behaviours and contraceptive use among women in rural Ghana. Contracept Reprod Med. 2018;3(1):1–12. https://doi.org/10.1186/s40834-018-0066-9.
24. Puri M, Henderson JT, Harper CC, Blum M, Joshi D, Rocca CH. Contraceptive discontinuation and pregnancy postabortion in Nepal: a longitudinal cohort study. Contraception. 2015;91(4):301–7. https://doi.org/10.1016/j.contraception.2014.12.011 Elsevier Inc.
25. Bradley SEK, Schwandt HM, Khan S. Levels, Trends, and Reasons for Contraceptive Discontinuation. DHS Analytical Studies No. 20. Calverton: ICF Macro; 2009.
26. Cohen R, Sheeder J, Arango N, Teal SB, Tocce K. Twelve-month contraceptive continuation and repeat pregnancy among young mothers choosing postdelivery contraceptive implants or postplacental intrauterine devices. Contraception. 2016;93(2):178–83. https://doi.org/10.1016/j.contraception.2015.10.001 Elsevier Inc.

8

Factors associated with modern contraceptive use among women with no fertility intention in sub-Saharan Africa: Evidence from cross-sectional surveys of 29 countries

Bright Opoku Ahinkorah[1], Eugene Budu[2], Richard Gyan Aboagye[3], Ebenezer Agbaglo[4], Francis Arthur-Holmes[5], Collins Adu[6], Anita Gracious Archer[7], Yaa Boahemaa Gyasi Aderoju[8] and Abdul-Aziz Seidu[2,9*]

Abstract

Background: In sub-Saharan Africa, the majority of women of reproductive age who want to avoid pregnancy do not use any method of contraception. This study sought to determine the factors associated with modern contraceptive use among women with no fertility intention in sub-Saharan Africa.

Methods: This study used data from the Demographic and Health Surveys of 29 countries in sub-Saharan Africa. A total of 87,554 women aged 15–49 with no fertility intention and who had completed information on all the variables of interest were considered in this study. Using a multilevel logistic regression analysis, four models were used to examine the individual and contextual factors associated with modern contraceptive use. The results were presented as adjusted odds ratios (aOR), with their respective confidence intervals (CIs). Statistical significance was set at p< 0.05.

(Continued on next page)

* Correspondence: abdul-aziz.seidu@stu.ucc.edu.gh
[2]Department of Population and Health, University of Cape Coast, Cape Coast, Ghana
[9]College of Public Health, Medical and Veterinary Services, James Cook University, Townsville, Australia

(Continued from previous page)

Results: The prevalence of modern contraceptive use was 29.6%. With the individual-level factors, women aged 45–49 had lower odds of using modern contraceptives (aOR = 0.33, 95% CI = 0.28, 0.39). Women who had their first sex at age 15–19 (aOR = 1.12, 95% CI = 1.07, 1.17), those with higher education (aOR = 1.93, 95% CI = 1.75, 2.13), and women who were exposed to newspaper (aOR = 1.15, 95% CI = 1.10, 1.20) and radio (aOR = 1.21, 95% CI = 1.17, 1.26) had higher odds of modern contraceptive use. In terms of the contextual factors, women living in urban areas (aOR = 1.06, 95% CI = 1.02, 1.11), women in the richest wealth quintile (aOR = 1.55, 95% CI = 1.43, 1.67), and those in communities with medium literacy level (aOR = 1.11, 95% CI = 1.06, 1.16) and medium community socio-economic status (aOR = 1.17, 95% CI = 1.10, 1.23) had higher odds of modern contraceptive use. Across the geographic regions in sub-Saharan Africa, women in Southern Africa had higher odds of modern contraceptive use (aOR = 5.29, 95% CI = 4.86, 5.76).

Conclusion: There is a relatively low prevalence of modern contraceptive use among women with no fertility intention in sub-Saharan Africa, with cross-country variations. Women's age, age at first sex, level of education, mass media exposure, place of residence, community literacy level and community socio-economic status were found to be associated with modern contraceptive use. It is, therefore, important for policy makers to consider these factors when designing and implementing programmes or policies to increase contraceptive use among women who have no intention to give birth. Also, policymakers and other key stakeholders should intensify mass education programmes to address disparities in modern contraceptive use among women.

Keywords: Fertility intention, modern contraceptives, sub-Saharan Africa, Women, Women's health

Background

To achieve target 3.7 of the Sustainable Development Goal (SDG) 3 which emphasizes that by 2030 the world should ensure universal access to sexual and reproductive healthcare services, utilization of modern contraceptive is key [1]. Report indicates that modern contraception prevented about 308 million unintended pregnancies in 2017 [2]. An additional 67 million unintended pregnancies could be averted if the needs for modern contraceptives are met [2]. Provision of modern contraception to women who want to avoid pregnancy could cause a reduction in maternal deaths from 308, 000 to 84,000 and newborn mortality from 2.7 million to 538,000 per year respectively [3]. These reductions in unintended pregnancies, and maternal and newborn mortalities can lead to the attainment of the target 3.1 and 3.2 of the SDG 3 which seek to reduce the global maternal mortality ratio to less than 70 per 100,000 live births and end all preventable deaths under 5 years of age by 2030 respectively [1].

Currently, about 1.9 billion women of reproductive age are living in the world. Of this number, 1.1 billion women need family planning [2, 4]. Only 842 million used modern contraceptives in 2019 [2, 4]. However, about 190 million women of reproductive age worldwide who want to avoid pregnancy do not use any contraceptive method, up from 156 million in 2000 [5]. In low-and middle-income countries, 214 million women who wanted to avoid pregnancy in 2019 were not using any method of contraception [2].

In sub-Saharan Africa (SSA), the majority of women of reproductive age who want to avoid pregnancy do not use any method of contraception [6]. Data from the United Nations Department of Economic and Social Affairs and Population Division [5] show that more than 20% of unmet need for family planning were in 15 countries in SSA. A study also reveals that 51 million women of reproductive age had an unmet need for modern contraceptive methods [4]. However, disparities exist in modern contraceptive utilization among women of reproductive age in SSA.

Evidence suggests that the prevalence of modern contraceptive usage among women of reproductive age in 2019 was high in both Estwatini and Namibia (both reporting 52%) and low in Sudan (4%) [5]. Among Ethiopian women, the prevalence of contraceptive use was 51.1% [7]. Also, Gebrecherkos et al. [8] found a 41.8% prevalence of unmet need for modern contraception of which 31.8 and 10% represented the unmet need for spacing and limiting of birth respectively among women of reproductive age in Ethiopia. In Ghana, Wulifa et al. [9] found that 14.98% of the women had an unmet need for modern contraceptives. In Botswana, Letamo and Navaneetham [10] found the unmet need for family planning was reported to be 9.6% among married women, 6.7% for spacing, and 2.9% for limiting. Despite the existing data on unmet needs for family planning, there is still a paucity of data on the magnitude of modern contraception among fecund women or women of reproductive age who do not have the desire to conceive a child in SSA.

Previous studies have suggested that cultural and religious myths and misconceptions undermine modern contraception [9, 11]. Other studies have highlighted that couple related factors (such as partner discussion, approval, and spousal decision making) [10, 12, 13], sociodemographic characteristics (age, educational status, religion, etc.) [10, 14], parity, exposure to mass media [14], knowledge on modern contraceptive methods [15], and fear of side effects [16] are associated with the utilization of modern contraceptives.

Although studies have recognized the importance of modern methods of contraception, few studies have been conducted to determine the factors associated with its utilization among women who have no intention to give birth to another child. This study sought to determine the factors associated with modern contraceptive use among women with no fertility intention in SSA. The findings from this study will provide evidence to inform decision-makers and stakeholders involved in family planning to improve women's access to sexual and reproductive health services, specifically, modern contraceptives in SSA.

Methods

Study design

Data for this study were obtained from the Demographic and Health Surveys (DHS) of 29 countries in SSA. For the purpose of the study, the women's recode files, which contain data on women aged 15–49 were used. The DHS is a nationally representative survey that is conducted in over 85 low- and middle-income countries and focuses on important men, maternal, and child health markers such as contraceptive use [17]. The survey employs a two-stage stratified sampling technique, which makes the data nationally representative. The study by Aliaga and Ruilin [18] provides details of the sampling process. A total of 87,544 women aged 15–49 who had no intention to give birth and had complete information on all the variables of interest in this study were considered. In this study, women with no fertility intention were those who responded "want no more," to the DHS question "would you like to have a (another) child with your husband/partner, or would you prefer not to have any more children with him?" We relied on the 'Strengthening the Reporting of Observational Studies in Epidemiology' (STROBE) statement in writing the manuscript [19]. The dataset is freely available for download at: https://dhsprogram.com/data/available-datasets.cfm.

Variables studied

Outcome variable

The outcome variable for the study was current use of modern contraceptives among women with no fertility intention. We focused on women with no fertility intention as we expected that those category of women would be more likely to use contraceptives to prevent pregnancy. Hence, understanding the use of modern contraceptives among this cohort of women and the factors that drive them to use modern contraceptives is very crucial to reducing unwanted pregnancies and abortions. The variable, modern contraceptives, was derived from a question that elicited the types of contraceptives women with no fertility intention were using during the survey. Responses to this question were coded as "no method", "folkloric method", "traditional method" and "modern method". The modern methods included female sterilization, male sterilization, intrauterine device (IUD), injectables, and implants (Norplant). The modern methods also included contraceptive pill, condoms, emergency contraception, standard day method (SDM), vaginal methods (foam, jelly, suppository), and lactational amenorrhea method (LAM). Country-specific modern methods and other modern contraceptive methods (including cervical cap, contraceptive sponge, and others)which were mentioned by respondents were also regarded as modern contraceptives. Periodic abstinence (rhythm, calendar method), withdrawal (coitus interruptus) and country-specific traditional methods which are proven effectivewere considered as traditional methods. Locally described methods and spiritual methods (such as herbs, amulets, gris-gris, etc.) which are effective but not proven were the folkloric methods [17, 20, 21]. The existing DHS variable on contraceptive use did not include women who were pregnant, those who were infecund, and those who had never had sex. In this study, women using modern methods were coded as '1' while those who were not using any methods, those using traditional methods, and those using folkloric methods were recoded as '0'.

Independent variable

Sixteen independent variables were considered in this study based on their significant associations with modern contraceptive use in previous studies [14, 22–24]. These variables have been broadly grouped into individual-level variables and contextual-level variables. The individual-level variables were age (15–19, 20–24, 25–29, 30–34, 35–39, 40–44 and 45–49 years), marital status (never married, married, cohabiting, widowed and divorced), religion (Christianity, Islam, traditional and no religion), employment status (not working and working), age at first sex (less than 15 years, 15–19 years and 20 years and above), parity (no birth, one birth, two births, three births, four or more births), level of education (no education, primary, secondary and higher), exposure to newspaper (no and yes), exposure to radio (no and yes), and exposure to television (no and yes).

The contextual-level variables were place of residence (urban and rural), wealth index (poorest, poorer, middle, richer and richest), community-level literacy-proportion of women who can read and write (low, medium and

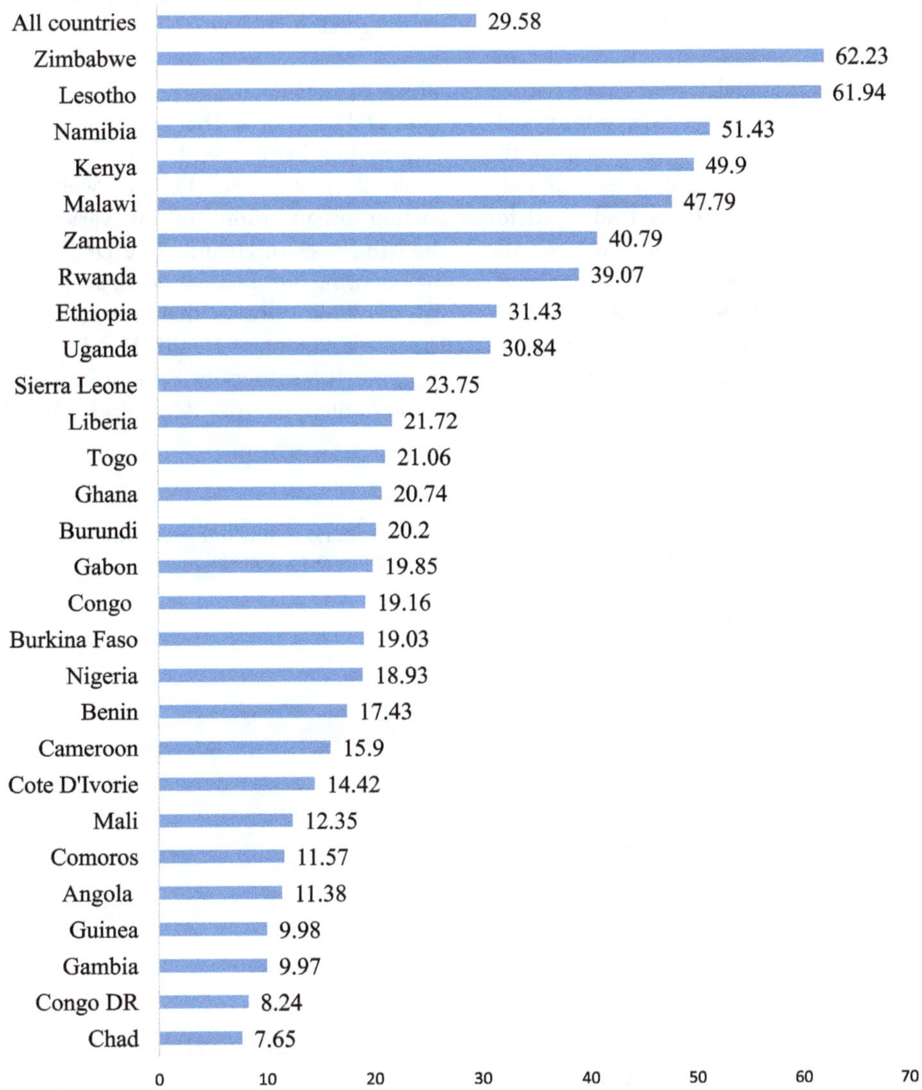

Fig. 1 Prevalence of modern contraceptive use among women with no fertility intention in sub-Saharan Africa

high), community-level socio-economic status - the proportion of women in the richest household quintile (low, medium and high), community knowledge of modern contraceptive method (low, medium and high), and sub-region (West, East, Central and Southern). The countries in West Africa were Burkina Faso, Benin, Cote d'Ivoire, Ghana, Gambia, Guinea, Mali, Nigeria, Sierra Leone, Senegal, and Togo. Burundi, Cameroon, Ethiopia, Gabon, Kenya, Comoros, Malawi, Rwanda, Uganda, Zambia, and Zimbabwe were in East Africa. Angola, Congo DR, Congo, Liberia, and Chad were in Central Africa whiles Lesotho, and Namibia were in Southern Africa [25].

Statistical analyses

The data were analysed with Stata version 16.0. The analysis was conducted in three steps. The first step was the graphical representation of the prevalence of modern contraceptive use among women with no fertility intention in SSA. The second step was a bivariate analysis that calculated the proportion of modern contraceptive use across the explanatory variables with their *p*-values derived from a chi-square test of independence. To check for high correlation among the explanatory variables, a test for multicollinearity was carried out using the variance inflation factor (VIF) and the results showed no evidence of high collinearity (Mean VIF = 1.44, Maximum VIF = 2.15, and Minimum VIF = 1.04). All the variables that showed statistical significance from the Table 2 were moved to the third step of the analysis. In the third step of the analysis, a multilevel logistic regression analysis comprising fixed effects and random effects was fitted. The results of the fixed effects of the model were presented as adjusted odds ratio (aOR) while the random effects were assessed with Intra-Cluster

Correlation (ICC). Model comparison was done using the log-likelihood ratio (LLR) and Akaike's Information Criterion (AIC) tests. Four models were fitted in examining the individualand contextual-level factors associated with modern contraceptive use. The four models comprised an empty model (Model 0) which shows the variations in the use of modern contraceptives in the absence of any explanatory variable. Model I adjusted for the individual-level variables, Model II adjusted for the contextual-level variables and Model III adjusted for all the explanatory variables. Results were presented as adjusted odds ratios (aOR) at 95% Confidence Interval. All frequency distributions were weighted (v005/1000000) while the survey command (SVY) in Stata was used to adjust for the complex sampling structure of the data in the regression analyses.

Ethical approval

The DHS reports that the DHS surveys have been reviewed and approved by Inner City Fund (ICF) Institutional Review Board (IRB) as well as Ethics Boards of partner organisations of the various countries such as the Ministries of Health. The DHS follows the standards for ensuring the protection of respondents' privacy. ICF International ensures that the survey complies with the U.S. Department of Health and Human Services' regulations for the respect of human subjects. This was a secondary analysis of data and therefore no further

Table 1 Description of the study sample

Country	Year of survey	Women aged 15–49 years	Women with no fertlity intention who had information on contraceptive use	Women with complete cases
Angola	2015–16	14,379	339	339
Burkina Faso	2010	17,087	3419	3417
Benin	2018	15,928	3178	3176
Burundi	2016–17	17,269	5790	5787
Congo DR	2013–14	18,827	3368	3366
Congo	2011–12	10,819	1458	1457
Cote D'Ivorie	2011–12	10,060	1365	1364
Cameroon	2018	15,426	2928	2926
Ethiopia	2016	15,683	4718	4715
Gabon	2012	8422	1392	1391
Ghana	2014	9396	2264	2263
Gambia	2013	10,233	1071	1071
Guinea	2012	10,874	1485	1484
Kenya	2014	31,079	5318	5314
Comoros	2012	5329	620	620
Liberia	2013	9239	2001	2000
Lesotho	2014	6621	3439	1716
Mali	2018	10,424	1715	1714
Malawi	2015–16	24,562	8237	8232
Nigeria	2018	41,821	6931	6926
Namibia	2013	10,018	2788	2786
Rwanda	2014–15	13,497	4644	4641
Sierra Leone	2013	16,658	1663	1662
Senegal	2010–11	15,688	2266	2265
Chad	2014–15	17,719	1753	1752
Togo	2013–14	9480	2220	2219
Uganda	2016	18,506	5483	5479
Zambia	2018	13,683	4165	3978
Zimbabwe	2015	9955	3496	3494
Total			89,517	87,554

Table 2 Distribution of modern contraceptive use by individual and contextual-level variables

Variables	Weighted N	Weighted %	Modern contraceptive	p-values
Age				< 0.001
15–19	2164	2.5	15.6	
20–24	4600	5.3	35.0	
25–29	9619	11.0	38.2	
30–34	15,430	17.6	37.9	
35–39	19,635	22.4	34.4	
40–44	19,234	22.0	27.0	
45–49	16,852	19.3	14.8	
Marital status				< 0.001
Never married	5209	6.0	27.4	
Married	57,118	65.2	32.2	
Cohabiting	10,331	11.8	29.4	
Widowed	3607	7.2	13.4	
Divorced	8590	9.8	25.4	
Religion				< 0.001
Christianity	64,891	74.1	33.9	
Islam	19,161	21.9	16.9	
Traditional	1914	2.2	15.0	
No religion	1588	1.8	23.7	
Employment status				0.004
Not working	17,988	20.5	29.0	
Working	69,566	79.5	29.7	
Age at first sex				< 0.001
Less than 15	18,149	20.7	23.9	
15–19 years	54,679	62.5	31.1	
20 years and above	14,726	16.8	31.0	
Parity				< 0.001
No birth	1933	2.2	8.1	
One birth	3867	4.4	25.5	
Two births	8502	9.7	38.6	
Three births	12,988	14.8	36.4	
Four or more births	60,264	68.8	27.8	
Level of education				< 0.001
No education	30,977	35.4	17.6	
Primary	92,933	37.6	34.7	
Secondary	20,324	23.2	37.5	
Higher	3302	3.8	41.8	
Exposure to newspaper				< 0.001
No	71,687	81.9	26.9	
Yes	15,867	18.1	41.8	
Exposure to radio				< 0.001
No	34,741	39.7	24.9	
Yes	51,813	60.3	32.7	

Table 2 Distribution of modern contraceptive use by individual and contextual-level variables *(Continued)*

Variables	Weighted N	Weighted %	Modern contraceptive	p-values
Exposure to television				< 0.001
No	54,414	62.1	27.5	
Yes	33,140	37.9	33.0	
Residence				< 0.001
Urban	30,434	34.8	32.4	
Rural	57,120	65.2	28.1	
Wealth index				
Poorest	16,062	18.4	22.1	< 0.001
Poorer	17,170	19.6	26.7	
Middle	17,582	20.1	29.4	
Richer	18,341	20.9	32.1	
Richest	18,399	21.0	36.5	
Community literacy level				< 0.001
Low	33,855	38.7	24.5	
Medium	29,145	33.4	35.9	
High	24,554	28.0	29.1	
Community socioeconomic status				< 0.001
Low	47,293	54.0	25.4	
Medium	10,087	11.5	36.0	
High	30,174	34.5	34.0	
Community knowledge of modern contraceptive method				< 0.001
Low	81,646	93.3	30.9	
Medium	5908	6.7	11.9	
Sub-region				< 0.001
West Africa	27,561	31.5	17.7	
East Africa	46,577	53.2	37.3	
Central Africa	8914	10.2	13.1	
Southern Africa	4502	5.1	55.4	

NB: p-values obtained from chi-square test

approval was required since the data is available in the public domain. Further information about the DHS data usage and ethical standards are available at http://goo.gl/ny8T6X (Table 1).

Results

Prevalence of modern contraceptive use among women with no fertility intention in sub-Saharan Africa

Figure 1 shows the prevalence of modern contraceptive use among women with no fertility intention in 29 sub-Saharan African countries. The overall prevalence of modern contraceptive use among women with no fertility intention in the 29 sub-Saharan African countries considered in this study was 29.6%. In terms of country-based analysis, Zimbabwe (62.2%) had the highest prevalence of modern contraceptive use while Chad (7.7%) had the lowest prevalence.

Distribution of modern contraceptive use by individual- and contextual-level variables

Table 2 shows the distribution of modern contraceptive use among women with no fertility intention by individual and contextual variables. With the individual-level factors, the highest prevalence of modern contraceptive use was found among women aged 25–29 (38.2%), married women (32.2%), Christians (33.9%), working women (29.7%), those who had their first sex when they were 15–19 years (31.1%), women with two births (38.6%), those with higher level of education (41.8%), and women with exposure to newspaper (41.8%), radio (32.7%), and television (33%). In terms of the contextual-level factors, the highest prevalence of modern contraceptive use was found among women in urban areas (32.4%), those in the richest wealth quintile (36.5%), women in communities with medium community literacy levels (35.9%),

Table 3 Mixed-effects results on the predictors of modern contraceptive use among women with no fertility intention in sub-Saharan Africa

Variables	Model 0	Model I aOR(95%CI)	Model II aOR(95%CI)	Model III aOR(95%CI)
Age				
15–19		1		1
20–24		1.20* (1.04–1.40)		1.03 (0.88–1.20)
25–29		1.26** (1.08–1.46)		0.95 (0.81–1.17)
30–34		1.26** (1.08–1.47)		0.92 (0.78–1.08)
35–39		1.13 (0.74–1.32)		0.86 (0.73–1.01)
40–44		0.86 (0.74–1.01)		0.66*** (0.56–0.78)
45–49		0.43*** (0.37–0.50)		0.33*** (0.28–0.39)
Marital status				
Married		1		1
Not married		0.72*** (0.66–0.77)		0.59*** (0.55–0.65)
Cohabiting		0.61*** (0.58–0.64)		0.73*** (0.69–0.76)
Widowed		0.34*** (0.31–0.37)		0.31*** (0.28–0.33)
Divorced		0.56*** (0.53–0.60)		0.55*** (0.52–0.59)
Religion				
Christianity		1		1
Islam		0.53*** (0.50–0.55)		0.60*** (0.57–0.63)
Traditional		0.51*** (0.44–0.57)		0.78*** (0.69–0.89)
No religion		0.72*** (0.64–0.81)		0.81*** (0.75–0.91)
Employment status				
Working		1		1
Not working		1.00 (0.96–1.04)		0.89*** (0.85–0.93)
Age at first sex				
Less than 15		1		1
15–19		1.23*** (1.18–1.28)		1.12*** (1.07–1.17)
20+		1.15*** (1.09–1.22)		0.96 (0.91–1.02)
Parity				
No birth		1		1
One birth		3.41*** (2.81–4.14)		3.66*** (3.00–4.48)
Two births		6.13*** (5.03–7.47)		7.59*** (6.18–9.32)
Three births		6.30*** (5.16–7.70)		8.85*** (7.19–10.90)
Four or more births		5.55*** (4.54–6.77)		8.78*** (7.13–10.82)
Education				
No education		1		1
Primary		1.96*** (1.88–2.05)		1.56*** (1.49–1.63)
Secondary		2.05*** (1.95–2.16)		1.75*** (1.65–1.85)
Higher		2.23*** (2.03–2.45)		1.93*** (1.75–2.13)
Exposure to newspaper				
No		1		1
Yes		1.40*** (1.34–1.46)		1.15*** (1.10–1.20)
Exposure to radio				
No		1		1
Yes		1.31*** (1.26–1.35)		1.21*** (1.17–1.26)

Table 3 Mixed-effects results on the predictors of modern contraceptive use among women with no fertility intention in sub-Saharan Africa *(Continued)*

Variables	Model 0	Model I aOR(95%CI)	Model II aOR(95%CI)	Model III aOR(95%CI)
Exposure to television				
No		1		1
Yes		0.97 (0.93–1.01)		0.98 (0.94–1.02)
Residence				
Rural			1	1
Urban			1.05* (1.01–1.10)	1.06** (1.02–1.11)
Wealth index				
Poorest			1	1
Poorer			1.36*** (1.39–1.43)	1.26*** (1.19–1.33)
Middle			1.53*** (1.45–1.61)	1.34*** (1.27–1.41)
Richer			1.70*** (1.61–1.80)	1.44*** (1.35–1.52)
Richest			1.99*** (1.86–2.13)	1.55*** (1.43–1.67)
Community literacy level				
Low			1	1
Medium			1.27*** (1.23–1.32)	1.11*** (1.06–1.16)
High			1.12*** (1.07–1.17)	0.95 (0.90–1.00)
Community socioeconomic status				
Low			1	1
Medium			1.14*** (1.08–1.20)	1.17*** (1.10–1.23)
High			1.06* (1.01–1.12)	1.13*** (1.07–1.19)
Community knowledge of modern contraceptive method				
Low			1	1
Medium			0.77*** (0.70–0.84)	0.81*** (0.74–0.89)
Sub-region				
West Africa			1	1
East Africa			2.62*** (2.52–2.72)	2.16*** (2.07–2.27)
Central Africa			0.66*** (0.62–0.72)	0.57*** (0.52–0.62)
Southern Africa			5.08*** (5.08–5.85)	5.29*** (4.86–5.76)
Random effect result				
PSU variance (95% CI)	0.03 (0.02–0.04)	0.02 (0.02–0.03)	0.02 (0.02–0.03)	0.02 (0.01–0.03)
ICC	0.009398	0.0073918	0.0066778	0.0059027
LR Test	Chi-square = 93.90, $p < 0.0001$	Chi-square = 60.28, p < 0.0001	Chi-square = 52.94, p < 0.0001	Chi-square = 39.24, p < 0.0001
Wald chi-square	Reference	8014.01***	6928.45***	11,041.57***
Model fitness				
Log-likelihood	−52,079.447	−47,165.892	−48.68.293	−44,895.43
AIC	104,162.9	94,387.78	96,166.59	89,872.86
N	87,554	87,554	87,554	87,554
Number of clusters	1605	1605	1605	1605

Exponentiated coefficients; 95% confidence intervals in brackets
* $p < 0.05$, ** $p < 0.01$, *** $p < 0.001$,
1 = Reference category; ICC = Intra-Class Correlation; AIC = Akaike's Information Criterion;
Model 0 = The null model, a baseline model without any determinant variable
Model I = Individual-level variables
Model II = Contextual-level variables
Model III = The final model adjusted for individual- and contextual-level variables

and socio-economic status (36.0%), those in communities with low knowledge of modern contraceptives (30.9%), and those who lived in Southern Africa (55.4%). The chi-square test results showed statistically significant associations between all the individual and contextual variables and modern contraceptive use.

Factors associated with modern contraceptive use among women with no fertility intention in sub-Saharan Africa

Measures of association (fixed effects)

Table 3 shows the results of the multilevel logistic regression analyses on the association between modern contraceptive use among women with no fertility intention and the individual- and contextual-level variables. With the individual-level factors, women aged 45–49 had lower odds of using modern contraceptive (aOR = 0.33, 95% CI = 0.28, 0.39) compared to those aged 15–19. Compared to married women, women who were never married, cohabiting, widowed or divorced were less likely to use modern contraceptives. The odds of modern contraceptive use decreased among Muslims, Traditionalists, and women with no religion compared to Christians. Women who were not working were less likely to use modern contraceptives compared to those who were working (aOR = 0.89, 95% CI = 0.85, 0.93). Compared to women who had their first sex at the age below 15, those who had their first sex at age 15–19 were more likely to use modern contraceptives (aOR = 1.12, 95% CI = 1.07,1.17). Women with four or more births were more likely to use modern contraceptives compared to those with no birth (aOR = 8.79, 95% CI = 7.13, 10.82). The likelihood of modern contraceptive use also increased with the level of education with the highest likelihood among those with higher education compared to those with no formal education (aOR = 1.93, 95% CI = 1.75, 2.13). Women who were exposed to newspaper (aOR = 1.15, 95% CI = 1.10, 1.20) and radio (aOR = 1.21, 95% CI = 1.17, 1.26) had higher odds of modern contraceptive use compared to those who were not.

In terms of contextual factors, women in communities with medium knowledge of modern contraceptive method (aOR = 0.81, 95% CI = 0.75, 0.89) were less likely to use modern contraceptives. Conversely, women in urban areas (aOR = 1.06, 95% CI = 1.02, 1.11), women with richest wealth quintile (aOR = 1.55, 95% CI = 1.43,1.67), those in communities with medium literacy level (aOR = 1.11, 95% CI = 1.06, 1.16) and medium community socio-economic status (aOR = 1.17, 95% CI = 1.10, 1.23) had higher odds of modern contraceptive use. Across the geographic regions in SSA, Southern Africa had higher odds of modern contraceptive use (aOR = 5.29, 95% CI = 4.86, 5.76) compared to those in West Africa.

Measures of variation (random effects)

The results of the random effects on the association between modern contraceptive use among women with no fertility intention and the individual and contextual variables show variations in all the models. In Model 0, the clustering of the primary sampling units (PSUs) accounted for significant variations in the odds of modern contraceptive use ($\sigma 2 = 0.03$, 95% CI 0.02–0.04). Model 0 showed that 0.9% of the total variation in modern contraceptive use was attributed to the variance between clusters (ICC = 0.0093). The between-cluster variance was slightly smaller (ICC = 0.0079) in Model I (with individual-level factors only). From Model I, the ICC decreased in Model II (contextual level only model) (ICC = 0.0072). It then increased in Model III (ICC = 0.0067) where all the independent variables (both individual and contextual variables) were considered. This indicates that differences in the clustering of the PSUs account for the variations in modern contraceptive use. The highest log- likelihood (– 44,895.43) and the lowest AIC (89,872.86) were used to determine the best fit model (Table 3).

Discussion

In this study, we investigated the prevalence and correlates of modern contraceptive use among women with no fertility intention in SSA. We found the overall prevalence of modern contraceptive use among the selected women to be 29.6%. This low prevalence suggests that the use of modern contraceptives for fertility prevention is still a problem among women in SSA. In terms of country-based analysis, Zimbabwe (62.2%) had the highest prevalence of modern contraceptive use followed by Lesotho (7.7%). Chad (7.7%) had the lowest prevalence of modern contraceptive use. This finding agrees with that of Yaya et al. (2018), who reported low contraceptive use in several sub-Saharan African countries, including Chad. However, Chikandiwa et al. [26] reported higher use of modern contraception among Zimbabwean women than Kenyan women. In explaining this finding, a study in Zimbabwe showed that over the years, the post-independence Zimbabwean government had encouraged women to use contraceptives, hence resulting in high prevalance of contraceptives among Zimbabwean women [27]. Women aged 45–49 had lower odds of using modern contraceptives compared to those aged 15–19. This finding resonates with that of Adebowale et al. [28]. The lower contraceptive use might be because women aged 15–19 are still in school and as a result might not want to have children to interrupt their academic activities [28]. Another reason could be that younger women (age 15–19) are highly sexually active and had to use modern contraceptives to prevent unwanted pregnancies [29]. Relatedly, women who were never married, cohabiting women, widows, and divorcees were less likely to use modern contraceptives compared to married women. The reason could be that women with no births and those with few births were sexually active and fertile, which demanded that they used more contraceptives to prevent pregnancies. On the other hand, widowed women and divorcees might not be in any sexual relationship, therefore resulting in their low use of modern contraceptives.

With mass media exposure, women who were exposed to newspaper and radio had higher odds of modern contraceptive use, compared to those who were not. This finding highlights the role of mass media in spreading information regarding family planning. Previous studies in Ethiopia [30] and Nigeria [31], as well as Burkina Faso and Senegal [32] have reported the effectiveness of mass media messages in promoting contraceptive use. Ownership of a radio and exposure to family planning radio messages independently encourage women to use modern methods of contraception [33]. This findings therefore suggest the need for sub-Saharan African countries to use mass media as a channel to spread information regarding the use of modern contraceptives to women. This has a capacity to increase contraceptive use among women with no fertility intention.

The odds of modern contraceptive use decreased among Muslims, Traditionalists and women with no religion compared to Christians. A negative relationship between Muslim women and family planning use has been reported by previous studies [34, 35]. Our finding agrees with previous studies conducted in Ethiopia [36, 37], Nigeria [28, 34, 35] and Ghana [38]. The reason for this might be that religious resistance for contraceptive uptake may be more pronounced in Islam than other religions [7, 39]. A study by Hani et al. [40] revealed a strong opposition by husband to the use of contraceptive. This was found as a reason for non-use of contraceptives among Muslim women. As Hani et al. [40] suggested, participation of husband in counseling and involvement of religious leaders in decisions on contraceptive use could improve its use among Muslim women.

Consistent with previous studies in Ethiopia [37], Malawi [41], and Ghana [42], this study recorded lower odds of modern contraceptives use among women who were not working. In most sub-Saharan African countries, contraceptive access is not completely free. At health facilities, levies are charged. Apart from this, distance from family planning clinics is considered as far for most women, particularly those from rural communities. Even in urban areas, family planning clinics are not evenly situated. Transportation cost becomes a barrier to utilization of family planning services [28]. Women need some level of financial autonomy to be able to purchase and use modern contraceptives. Whereas working women may be able to cater for the cost involved in using modern contraceptives, their counterparts who are not working may not [37, 41, 42]. Women who are engaged in occupations that disallow frequent maternity leaves might cause them to use contraceptives.

Moreover, we recorded lower odds of modern contraceptives use among women living in rural areas, and those with medium community knowledge of modern contraceptive method. Similarly, Adebowale et al. [28] reported lower use of modern contraceptives among women with no fertility intention in rural areas in Nigeria. As noted by Asresie et al. [7], inadequate access to family planning service is one of the predominant reasons for the non-use of contraceptives. Thus, the lower use of modern contraceptives among inhabitants of rural areas may be attributed to poor access or unavailability of health facilities in rural areas. Other reasons for low use of modern contraceptives in rural areas could be poor spousal communication, sociocultural norms (especially the husband's role as the primary decision-maker), fear of side-effects and a lack of knowledge [43]. This finding highlights the need for development of programs to increase contraceptive use among women with no fertility intention while taking into consideration the rural-urban disparities.

Finally, we found level of education and community literacy to be significantly associated with the use of modern contraceptives among the study participants. As Nyarko [42] emphasized, well-educated people have contraceptive advantages in two ways. First, their level of education can provide them with accurate knowledge about contraception, contraceptive methods and their benefits. Second, their period of education may encourage them to use modern contraceptive methods to avoid getting pregnant while in school. In terms of community literacy, our study agrees with the findings of Ahinkorah [22], who reported low use of modern contraceptives use among women living in communities with low literacy in SSA. Our study also showed that women in the richest wealth quintile and those in communities with middle socioeconomic status recorded higher odds of modern contraceptives utilization. The use of contraceptives comes with its associated financial burden. While richest women may be in the position to skip any financial hurdles to the use of modern contraceptives, poor women may not [21, 22].

Strengths and limitations

The main strength of this study lies in the use of nationally representative data of each of the countries represented in the study. With this, the findings are generalizable to all women in the countries studied. Another strength lies in the use of sophisticated data collection methods, with experienced field assistants, which generated a higher response rate. We also employed higher order statistical tools for the analysis, which ensured rigorous analysis of the data. Despite these strengths, the study has some limitations that need to be acknowledged. First, with the cross-sectional research approach adopted, we cannot make causal inferences among the studied variables. Also, given the retrospective nature of reporting that characterizes demographic data, the data are likely to be subjected to recall biases. Relatedly, issues of social desirability bias may also be present.

Conclusion

There is a relatively low prevalence of modern contraceptive use among women with no fertility intention in sub-Saharan Africa, with cross-country variations. Women's age, age at first sex, level of education, mass media exposure, religion, employment status, place of residence, community literacy level and community socio-economic status were found to be associated with modern contraceptive use.. It is, therefore, important for policy makers policies to consider these factors when designing and implementing programmes or policies take to increase contraceptive use among women who have no intention to give birth. Also, policymakers and other key stakeholders should intensify mass education programmes to address disparities in modern contraceptive use among women. Such education programmes should target both rural and urban communities to increase women's knowledge and use of modern contraceptives.

Abbreviations

aOR: Adjusted Odds Ratio; CI: Confidence Interval; GDHS: Ghana Demographic and Health Survey; DHS: Demographic and Health Survey; PHC: Population and Housing Census; NHIS: National Health Insurance Scheme

Acknowledgements

We acknowledge Measure DHS for providing us with the data.

Authors' contributions

BOA, EB and AS conceived the study. BOA, EB and AS analysed the data. FA-H intepreted the results. BOA, EB, RA,EA,FA-H,CA,AGA,YBGA and AS drafted the manuscript. All authors reviewed and approved the final version of the manuscript.

Authors' information

School of Public Health, Faculty of Health, University of Technology Sydney, Sydney, Australia (BOA), Department of Population and Health, University of Cape Coast, Cape Coast, Ghana (EB, AS), School of Public Health, University of Health and Allied Sciences, Ho, Ghana (RA), Department of English, University of Cape Coast, Cape Coast, Ghana (EA), Department of Sociology and Social Policy, Lingnan University, 8 Castle Peak Road, Tuen Mun, Hong Kong (FA-H), Department of Health Promotion, Education and Disability Studies, Kwame Nkrumah University of Science and Technology, Kumasi, Ghana (CA); School of Nursing and Midwifery, University of Health and Allied Sciences, Ho, Ghana (AGA), Department of Adult Health Nursing, School of Nursing and Midwifery, University of Cape Coast, Cape Coast, Ghana (YBGA), College of Public Health, Medical and Veterinary Services, James Cook University, Australia (AS).

Author details

[1]School of Public Health, Faculty of Health, University of Technology Sydney, Sydney, Australia. [2]Department of Population and Health, University of Cape Coast, Cape Coast, Ghana. [3]School of Public Health, University of Health and Allied Sciences, Ho, Ghana. [4]Department of English, University of Cape Coast, Cape Coast, Ghana. [5]Department of Sociology and Social Policy, Lingnan University, 8 Castle Peak Road, Tuen Mun, Hong Kong. [6]Department of Health Promotion, Education and Disability Studies, Kwame Nkrumah University of Science and Technology, Kumasi, Ghana. [7]School of Nursing and Midwifery, University of Health and Allied Sciences, Ho, Ghana. [8]Department of Adult Health Nursing, School of Nursing and Midwifery, University of Cape Coast, Cape Coast, Ghana. [9]College of Public Health, Medical and Veterinary Services, James Cook University, Townsville, Australia.

References

1. World Health Organization. World Health Statistics 2018: monitoring health for the SDGs, Sustainable Development Goals: World Health Organization; 2018.
2. World Health Organization. WHO recommendations on self-care interventions: Self-administration of injectable contraception (No. WHO/SRH/20.9): World Health Organization; 2020.
3. Darroch JE, Sully E, Biddlecom A. Adding it up: investing in contraception and maternal and newborn health, 2017—supplementary tables. New York, NY: The Guttmacher Institute; 2017.
4. Kantorová V, Wheldon MC, Ueffing P, Dasgupta AN. Estimating progress towards meeting women's contraceptive needs in 185 countries: A Bayesian hierarchical modelling study. PLoS Med. 2020;17(2):e1003026.
5. United Nations, Department of Economic and Social Affairs, Population Division. Family Planning and the 2030 Agenda for Sustainable Development: Data Booklet. (ST/ESA/SER.A/429). 2019.
6. United Nations, Department of Economic, & Social Affairs, Population Division. Contraceptive Use by Method 2019: Data Booklet (ST/ESA/SER.A/435). 2019.
7. Asresie MB, Fekadu GA, Dagnew GW. Contraceptive use among women with no fertility intention in Ethiopia. PLoS One. 2020;15(6):e0234474. https://doi.org/10.1371/journal.pone.0234474.
8. Gebrecherkos K, Gebremariam B, Gebeyehu A, Siyum H, Kahsay G, Abay M. Unmet need for modern contraception and associated factors among reproductive age group women in Eritrean refugee camps, Tigray, North Ethiopia: a cross-sectional study. BMC Res Notes. 2018;11(1):851. https://doi.org/10.1186/s13104-018-3956-7.
9. Wulifan JK, Mazalale J, Kambala C, Angko W, Asante J, Kpinpuo S, et al. Prevalence and determinants of unmet need for family planning among married women in Ghana-a multinomial logistic regression analysis of the GDHS, 2014. Contracept Reprod Med. 2019;4(1):2.
10. Letamo G, Navaneetham K. Levels, trends and reasons for unmet need for family planning among married women in Botswana: a cross-sectional study. BMJ Open. 2015;5(3):1–11.
11. Gueye A, Speizer IS, Corroon M, Okigbo CC. Belief in family planning myths at the individual and community levels and modern contraceptive use in urban Africa. Int Perspect Sex Reprod Health. 2015;41(4):191.
12. Islam AZ. Factors affecting modern contraceptive use among fecund young women in Bangladesh: does couples' joint participation in household decision making matter? Reprod Health. 2018;15(1):112. https://doi.org/10.1186/s12978-018-0558-8.
13. Belda SS, Haile MT, Melku AT, Tololu AK. Modern contraceptive utilization and associated factors among married pastoralist women in Bale eco-region, Bale Zone, South East Ethiopia. BMC Health Serv Res. 2017;17(1):194.
14. Debebe S, Limenih MA, Biadgo B. Modern contraceptive methods utilization and associated factors among reproductive aged women in rural Dembia District, Northwest Ethiopia: Community based cross-sectional study. Int J Reprod BioMed. 2017;15(6):367.
15. Eliason S, Awoonor-Williams JK, Eliason C, Novignon J, Nonvignon J, Aikins M. Determinants of modern family planning use among women of reproductive age in the Nkwanta district of Ghana: a case–control study. Reprod Health. 2014;11(1):65.
16. Ochako R, Mbondo M, Aloo S, Kaimenyi S, Thompson R, Temmerman M, et al. Barriers to modern contraceptive methods uptake among young women in Kenya: a qualitative study. BMC Public Health. 2015;15(1):1–9.

17. Corsi DJ, Neuman M, Finlay JE, Subramanian SV. Demographic and health surveys: a profile. Int J Epidemiol. 2012;41(6):1602–13.
18. Aliaga A, Ruilin R. Cluster optimal sample size for demographic and health surveys. In: 7th International Conference on Teaching Statistics–ICOTS, vol. 7; 2006. p. 2–7.
19. Von Elm E, Altman DG, Egger M, Pocock SJ, Gøtzsche PC, Vandenbroucke JP. The strengthening the reporting of observational studies in epidemiology (STROBE) statement: guidelines for reporting observational studies. Ann Intern Med. 2007;147(8):573–7. https://doi.org/10.7326/0003-4819-147-8-200710160-00010.
20. Aviisah PA, Dery S, Atsu BK, Yawson A, Alotaibi RM, Rezk HR, et al. Modern contraceptive use among women of reproductive age in Ghana: Analysis of the 2003–2014 Ghana Demographic and Health Surveys. BMC Womens Health. 2018;18(1):141.
21. Ahinkorah BO, Seidu AA, Appiah F, Budu E, Adu C, Aderoju YBG, et al. Individual and community-level factors associated with modern contraceptive use among adolescent girls and young women in Mali: a mixed effects multilevel analysis of the 2018 Mali demographic and health survey. Contracept Reprod Med. 2020;5(1):1–12.
22. Ahinkorah BO. Predictors of modern contraceptive use among adolescent girls and young women in sub-Saharan Africa: a mixed effects multilevel analysis of data from 29 demographic and health surveys. Contracept Reprod Med. 2020;5(1):1–12.
23. Ejembi CL, Dahiru T, Aliyu AA. DHS working papers; 2015.
24. Lasong J, Zhang Y, Gebremedhin SA, Opoku S, Abaidoo CS, Mkandawire T, et al. Determinants of modern contraceptive use among married women of reproductive age: a cross-sectional study in rural Zambia. BMJ Open. 2020;10(3):e030980. https://doi.org/10.1136/bmjopen-2019-030980.
25. United Nations 1999, Standard country or area codes for statistics use, 1999 (Revision 4), viewed May 23 2020, https://unstats.un.org/unsd/publications/catalogue?selectID=109. Accessed 23 Nov 2020.
26. Chikandiwa A, Burgess E, Otwombe K, Chimoyi L. Use of contraceptives, high risk births and under-five mortality in Sub Saharan Africa: evidence from Kenyan (2014) and Zimbabwean (2011) demographic health surveys. BMC Womens Health. 2018;18(1):173.
27. Mturi A, Joshua K. Falling fertility and increase in use of uontraception in Zimbabwe. Afr J Reprod Health. 2011;15(2):31–44.
28. Adebowale SA, Adeoye IA, Palamuleni ME. Contraceptive use among Nigerian women with no fertility intention: interaction amid potential causative factors. Afr Popul Stud. 2013;27(2):127–39. https://doi.org/10.11564/27-2-435.
29. Ba DM, Ssentongo P, Agbese E, Kjerulff KH. Prevalence and predictors of contraceptive use among women of reproductive age in 17 sub-Saharan African countries: a large population-based study. Sexual Reprod Healthcare. 2019;21:26–32. https://doi.org/10.1016/j.srhc.2019.06.002.
30. Ahmed M, Seid A. Association between exposure to mass media family planning messages and utilization of modern contraceptive among urban and rural youth women in Ethiopia. Int J Women's Health. 2020;12:719–29. https://doi.org/10.2147/IJWH.S266755.
31. Measurement L, Team EPN. Evaluation of the Nigerian urban reproductive health initiative (NURHI) program. Stud Fam Plan. 2017;48:253–68.
32. Jacobs J, Marino M, Edelman A, Jensen J, Darney B. Mass media exposure and modern contraceptive use among married west African adolescents. Eur J Contracept Reprod Health Care. 2017;22(6):439–49. https://doi.org/10.1080/13625187.2017.1409889.
33. Islam MM, Hasan AS. Mass media exposure and its impact on family planning in Bangladesh. J Biosoc Sci. 2020;32(4):513–26.
34. Avong NH. Relationship between religion and use of modern contraceptives among the Atyap in Kaduna state, Nigeria. Res Humanit Soc Sci. 2012;2(8):82–9.
35. Viswan SP, Ravindran TS, Kandala NB, Petzold MG, Fonn S. Sexual autonomy and contraceptive use among women in Nigeria: findings from the demographic and health survey data. Int J Women's Health. 2017;9:581–90. https://doi.org/10.2147/IJWH.S133760.
36. Musa A, Assefa N, Weldegebreal F, Mitiku H, Teklemariam Z. Factor associated with experience of modern contraceptive use before pregnancy among women who gave birth in Kersa HDSS, Ethiopia. BMC Public Health. 2016;16(1):614. https://doi.org/10.1186/s12889-016-3292-6.
37. Lakew Y, Reda AA, Tamene H, Benedict S, Deribe K. Geographical variation and factors influencing modern contraceptive use among married women in Ethiopia: evidence from a national population based survey. Reprod Health. 2013;10(1):52. 24067083 https://doi.org/10.1186/1742-4755-10-52.
38. Crissman HP, Adanu RM, Harlow SD. Women's sexual empowerment and contraceptive use in Ghana. Stud Fam Plan. 2012;43(3):201–12. https://doi.org/10.1111/j.1728-4465.2012.00318.x PMID: 23185863.
39. Alsaleem MA, et al. Contraceptive use as limiters and spacers among women of reproductive age in southwestern, Saudi Arabia. Saudi Med J. 2018;39(11):1109. https://doi.org/10.15537/smj.2018.11.22817 PMID: 30397710.
40. Hani RA, Peleg R, Freud T, Treister-Goltzman Y. Knowledge, attitudes and contraceptive use among Muslim Bedouin women in southern Israel. Health Soc Care Commun. 2020;1(2):1–8.
41. Palamuleni ME. Socio-economic and demographic factors affecting contraceptive use in Malawi. Afr J Reprod Health. 2013;17(3):91–104. 24069771.
42. Nyarko SH. Spatial variations and socioeconomic determinants of modern contraceptive use in Ghana: a Bayesian multilevel analysis. PLoS One. 2020;15(3):e0230139. https://doi.org/10.1371/journal.pone.0230139.
43. Muanda MF, Ndongo GP, Messina LJ, Bertrand JT. Barriers to modern contraceptive use in rural areas in DRC. Cult Health Sex. 2017;19(9):1011–23.

9

Predictors of modern contraceptive use among adolescent girls and young women in sub-Saharan Africa: A mixed effects multilevel analysis of data from 29 demographic and health surveys

Bright Opoku Ahinkorah

Abstract

Background: The use of modern contraceptives among adolescent girls and young women (AGYW) in sub-Saharan Africa (SSA) remains an issue that needs urgent attention. This present study assesses the individual and contextual factors associated with modern contraceptive use among AGYW in SSA.

Methods: Data for this study was obtained from the latest Demographic and Health Surveys (DHS) conducted between January 2010 and December 2018 across 29 countries in SSA. Data were analysed with Stata version 14.2 by employing both Pearson's chi-square test of independence and a multilevel binary logistic regression. The selection of variables for the multilevel models was based on their statistical significance at the chi-square test at a $p < 0.05$. Model fitness for the multilevel models was checked using the log likelihood ratios and Akaike's Information Criterion (AIC) and the results were presented using adjusted odds ratios (aOR) at 95% confidence interval (CI).

Results: It was found that 24.7% of AGYW in SSA use modern contraceptives. In terms of the individual level factors, the study showed that AGYW aged 15–19 [aOR = 0.86, CI = 0.83–0.90], those who were married [aOR = 0.83, CI = 0.79–0.87], Muslims [aOR = 0.59, CI = 0.57–0.62], working [aOR = 0.92, CI = 0.89–0.95], those who had no child [aOR = 0.44, CI = 0.42–0.47], those who had no exposure to newspaper/magazine [aOR = 0.44, CI = 0.63–0.71] and radio [aOR = 0.82, CI = 0.78–0.86] had lower odds of using modern contraceptives. Conversely, the use of modern contraceptives was high among AGYW whose age at first sex was 15–19 years [aOR = 1.20, CI = 1.12–1.28]. With the contextual factors, the odds of using modern contraceptives was low among AGYW who lived in rural areas [aOR = 0.89, CI = 0.85–0.93] and in communities with low literacy level [aOR = 0.73, CI = 0.70–0.77] and low socio-economic status [aOR = 0.69, CI = 0.65–0.73].

Conclusion: Several individual and contextual factors are associated with modern contraceptive use among AGYW in SSA. Therefore, Governments in the various countries considered in this study should intensify mass education on the use of modern contraceptives. This education should be more centered on AGYW who are in socio-economically disadvantaged communities, those who are not married, Muslims, those with high parity and high fertility preferences and those who are working.

Keywords: Utilization of modern contraceptives, Adolescent girls, Young women, Sub-Saharan Africa, Reproductive health

Correspondence: brightahinkorah@gmail.com
School of Public Health, Faculty of Health, University of Technology Sydney, Sydney, Australia

Background

The sexual and reproductive health (SRH) of adolescent girls and young women (AGYW) aged 15–24 forms a key component of the global burden of sexual ill health [1]. This is because neglecting SRH of AGYW has detrimental effect on their transition to adulthood [2]. The SRH of AGYW has become critical because it has been estimated that 16 million girls aged 15–19 give birth each year, and this constitutes about 11% of all births worldwide and 95% of these births occur in low-and middle-income countries (LMICs), including sub-Saharan Africa (SSA) [3]. Other studies have indicated that most of these births result from unintended pregnancies and in SSA, 44% of these unintended pregnancies occur among AGYW [4, 5]. This unquestionably accounts for the high unsafe abortion rates among AGYW in SSA [6]. Apart from these SRH challenges, AGYW in SSA also face risk of exposure to HIV and other sexually transmitted infections (STIs) [1].

As part of efforts to deal with the SRH challenges of AGYW, the United Nations in 2015 developed the Sustainable Development Goals and Goal 3.7 focuses on ensuring universal access to sexual and reproductive health-care services, including family planning, information and education, and the integration of reproductive health into national strategies and programmes by 2030 [7]. The achievement of this Goal, especially for AGYW who often go through a lot of SRH challenges depends on the access, consistent and effective use of modern contraceptives [8, 9].

However, studies have indicated that the use of modern contraceptives among AGYW in SSA remains an issue that needs urgent attention [10–12]. Globally, it is estimated that over 220 million women in LMICs have an unmet need for contraception [13]. Although the prevalence of unmet need for contraception among AGYW in SSA is unknown, approximately 25% of women in the subregion (i.e. about 47 million) have unmet need for contraception [14], with a majority of them being AGYW [15–17].

Theoretically, the use of modern contraceptives among AGYW can be understood within the theoretical underpinning of the Health Belief Model which provides explanations to the likelihood of using modern contraceptives among AGYW from the point of perceived risks [18]. In this regard, AGYW who consider themselves as being at risk of unintended pregnancies and STIs may be more likely to use modern contraceptives compared to those who consider themselves not to be at risk. In the absence of risk perception, studies have shown that despite the desire of AGYW to use contraceptives, a majority of them have challenges with access to contraceptive services [15–17]. These challenges can be understood within the context of Anderson and Newmans' Health Care Utilisation Model which proposes that the use of a service, which includes modern contraceptives is influenced by predisposing factors such as demographics, health beliefs and social structures; enabling factors which include the availability of health personnel and facilities, waiting time and health insurance subscription and need for care factors which focuses on factors which are people's perception and evaluation of their health that serve as motivation to use a service [19].

Based on these theoretical underpinnings, it can be affirmedthat individual and contextual factors play a key role in the use of modern contraceptives among AGYW. However, studies on modern contraceptives use among AGYW in SSA have often focused on individual level factors such as age, marital status, religion, ethnicity, level of education, wealth status and occupation [17, 20–23]. Apart from their focus on individual level factors, most of these studies examined the predictors of contraceptive use (which includes traditional methods) instead of looking at modern contraceptives which have been considered the most effective of all contraceptive methods [24–26]. Again, studies on predictors of contraceptives among AGYW in SSA have been done in specific countries like Congo [20], Ghana [23] Malawi [21], South Africa [17] and Tanzania [22]. Although a recent study explored the predictors of modern contraceptive use among young women in LMICs, which included countries in SSA, the major focus of the authors was on community level factors that influence modern contraceptive use [27]. One of the gaps in this study which the current study seeks to fill is the lack of understanding of the interaction between individual and contextual-level factors in influencing the use of modern contraceptives of among AGYW. Again, Mutumba, Wekesa [27] used data from the 2008 to 2016 Demographic and Health Surveys (DHS). However, the current study considers current DHS data from 2010 and 2018 since variations in contraceptive accessibility and usage may have happened in the last few years. Using a multilevel modelling approach, this present study assesses the individual and contextual factors associated with modern contraceptive use among AGYW in SSA. Findings from this study will help to formulate useful interventions and strategies in addressing the use of modern contraceptive among AGYW in the sub-region.

Methods

Data source

Data for this study was obtained from the latest DHS conducted between January 2010 and December 2018 across 29 countries in SSA. The survey was designed to collect and provide data on various demographic indicators such as contraceptive use [28]. The details of the methodology employed in the DHS are documented by Corsi, Neuman [29]. In this study, only AGYW (15–24 years) who had ever had sex and had information on the use of contraceptives were considered ($n = 91,083$).

Table 1 Detailed description of the countries, survey years and the sample used in this study

Country	Survey year	Adolescent girls and young women	Sample (N)	Sample (%)
1. Angola	2015–16	6423	4822	5.3
2. Benin	2017–18	6251	4084	4.5
3. Burkina Faso	2010	6592	4319	4.7
4. Burundi	2016–17	7218	2579	2.8
5. Cameroon	2011	6708	4187	4.6
6. Chad	2014–15	6884	3374	3.7
7. Comoros	2012	2282	683	0.8
8. Congo	2011–12	3963	3235	3.6
9. Côte d'Ivoire	2011–12	3984	2814	3.1
10. DR Congo	2013–14	7661	4953	5.4
11. Ethiopia	2016	6401	2625	2.9
12. Gabon	2012	3407	2487	2.7
13. Gambia	2013	4564	1875	2.1
14. Ghana	2014	3327	2046	2.3
15. Guinea	2018	4267	2315	2.5
16. Kenya	2014	11,483	3215	3.5
17. Lesotho	2014	2842	589	0.7
18. Liberia	2013	3499	2921	3.2
19. Malawi	2015–16	10,369	7382	8.1
20. Mali	2018	4116	2649	2.9
21. Namibia	2013	3577	2151	2.4
22. Nigeria	2018	15,267	4740	5.2
23. Rwanda	2014–15	5252	2084	2.3
24. Senegal	2010–11	6773	2433	2.7
25. Sierra Leone	2013	6739	3059	3.4
26. Togo	2013–14	3337	2188	2.4
27. Uganda	2016	8058	5303	5.8
28. Zambia	2018	5799	3832	4.2
29. Zimbabwe	2015	3938	2138	2.4

Table 1 gives detailed description of the countries, survey years and the sample used in this study. The datasets for the DHS are available at http://dhsprogram.com/data/available-datasets.cfm.

Definition of variables

Outcome variable

The outcome variable for the study was 'current modern contraceptive usage'. It was derived from the question, "Are you currently using any type of contraceptive"? Responses to this question were coded as "no method", "folkloric method", "traditional method" and "modern method". Details of the specific contraceptives under each of the methods have been described elsewhere [30]. The existing DHS variable excluded women who were pregnant and those who had never had sex. For the purpose of this study, AGYWwho were using modern methods were coded as '1' whiles those who were not using any methods, those using traditional methods and folkloric methods were recoded as '0' [31, 32].

Independent variables

Fifteen independent variables, grouped into individual and contextual level factors were considered in this study. These variables were not determined a priori; but were selected based on their theoretical relevance and practical significance with usage of modern contraceptives [26, 33–35].

Individual level factors

The individual level factors were age, marital status, religion, employment status, age at first sex, parity, frequency of reading newspaper/magazine, listening to radio and watching television, desire for more children and ideal number of children. Age was coded as '15–19' and '20–24'. Marrital status was recoded into 'never married', 'married', 'cohabiting' and 'widowed/divorced/ separated'. Religion was recoded as 'Christianity', 'Islam' and 'other'. 'Working' and 'not working' were the categories for employment status. Age at first sex was recoded as 'less than 15 years' '15–19 years' and '20–24 years'. Parity was recoded as 'zero birth', 'one birth', 'two births', 'three births', and four or more births'. Frequency of reading newspaper/magazine, listening to radio and watching television were each coded as 'not at all' 'less than once a week' and 'at least once a week'. 'Desire for more children and idela number of children were derived from the questions, "do you desire to have a/another child?" and "what is the ideal number of children you want to have?". For this study, desire for more children was coded as "have another", "undecided" and "no more". Ideal number of children was also coded as "0–3″, "4–5″ and 6+".

Community level factors

Residence, community literacy level (proportion of women who can read and write), community socio-economic status (proportion of women in the richest household quintile) and community knowledge level of modern contraceptive (proportion of women with knowledge on modern contraceptives) were considered as contextual level factors. Residence was coded as 'urban' and 'rural'. Community literacy level, community socio-economic status and community knowledge level of modern contraceptives were each coded as 'low', 'middle' and 'high'.

Statistical analyses

The data were analysed with Stata version 14.2 for windows following a three-step analytical approach. The first approach involved the use of percentages to describe the prevalence of modern contraceptive use among AGYW in SSA. This was followed by the distribution of modern contraceptive use across the individual and contextual level factors. Statistical significance of the association between each of the factors and modern contraceptive use was measured using Pearson's chi-square test of independence [χ^2] at a p-value of less than 0.05 (see Table 1). Finally, a two-level multilevel binary logistic regression analysis was carried out to examine the association between modern contraceptive use and the individual and contextual factors. The use of a multilevel binary logistic regression in this study was to cater for the different levels at which sampling was done for the DHS (individual, household and cluster levels). The two-level modelling in this study implies that women were nested within households and households were nested within clusters. Clusters were considered as random effects to cater for the unexplained variability at the contextual level [36]. Only variables that showed statistically significant associations with modern contraceptive utilization at the chi-square test were included in the multilevel binary logistic regression models.

In terms of the modelling, four models, comprising the empty model (model 0), model 1 model 2 and model 3 were fitted. Model 0 showed the variance in modern contraceptive use attributed to the clustering of the primary sampling units (PSUs) without the explanatory variables. Model 1 and model 2 contained the individual and contextual level factors respectively while model 3 contained all the individual and contextual level factors. The Stata command "melogit" was used in fitting these models. Model comparison was done using the log likelihood and Akaike's Information Criterion (AIC) tests. The lowest AIC (90,917.38) and highest log likelihood (−45, 426.69) were used to determine the best fit model (see Table 2). Odds ratio and associated 95% confidence intervals (CIs) were presented for all the models apart from model 0 (see Table 2). To check for high correlation among the explanatory variables, a test for multicollinearity was carried out using the variance inflation factor (VIF) and the results showed no evidence of high collinearity (Mean VIF = 1.35, Maximum VIF = 1.86, and Minimum VIF = 1.06). Sample weight (v005/1,000,000) and SVY command were used to correct for over and under-sampling and the complex survey design and generalizability of the findings respectively. The findings were presented using the Strengthening Reporting of Observational studies in Epidemiology (STROBE) reporting guidelines [37].

Ethical approval

Ethical clearance were obtained from the Ethics Committee of ORC Macro Inc. as well as Ethics Boards of partner organisations of the various countries such as the Ministries of Health. The DHS follows the standards for ensuring the protection of respondents' privacy. Inner City Fund (ICF) International ensured that the survey complies with the U.S. Department of Health and Human Services regulations for the respect of human subjects. This was a secondary analyses of data and therefore no further approval was required since the data is available in the public domain. Further information about the DHS data usage and ethical standards are available at http://goo.gl/ny8T6X.

Results

Figure 1 displays the results on the prevalence of modern contraceptive use among AGYW in SSA. It was found that 24.7% of AGYW in the 29 countries in SSA considered in this study use modern contraception. Lesotho recorded the highest prevalence of modern contraceptive use among AGYW (59.2%) while Chad had the lowest prevalence of 5.1%.

Table 2 Distribution of modern contraceptive use across individual and contextual factors of adolescent girls and young women in sub-Saharan Africa

Variables	Weighted N	Weighted %	Modern contraceptive use	χ2 (*p*-value)
Age				365.7 (< 0.001)
15–19	33,197	36.4	21.1	
20–24	57,886	63.6	26.8	
Marital status				476.9 (< 0.001)
Never married	33,359	36.6	28.5	
Married	38,564	42.3	21.3	
Cohabiting	14,012	15.4	24.6	
Widowed/divorced/separated	5148	5.7	25.7	
Religion				8.2 (< 0.001)
Christianity	60,928	66.9	29.1	
Islam	25,992	28.5	15.0	
Other	4162	4.6	20.5	
Employment status				45.3 (< 0.001)
Not working	37,956	41.7	26.2	
Working	53,127	58.3	23.6	
Age at first sex				281.8 (< 0.001)
Less than 15 years	19,252	21.1	20.1	
15–19 years	65,236	71.6	25.9	
20–24 years	6595	7.2	26.2	
Parity				371.0 (< 0.001)
No birth	33,799	37.1	22.3	
One birth	31,748	34.9	27.0	
Two births	16,884	18.5	27.6	
Three births	6577	7.2	21.7	
Four or more births	2074	2.3	14.7	
Frequency of reading newspaper/magazine				7.9 (< 0.001)
Not at all	70,291	77.2	21.4	
Less than once a week	10,880	12.0	35.4	
At least once a week	9912	10.9	36.5	
Frequency of listening to radio				698.1 (< 0.001)
Not at all	36,24	40.1	20.5	
Less than once a week	17,828	19.6	26.0	
At least once a week	36,731	40.3	28.3	
Frequency of watching television				640.2 (< 0.001)
Not at all	48,953	53.8	21.6	
Less than once a week	11,640	12.8	25.9	
At least once a week	30,490	33.5	29.3	
Desire for more children				263.2 (< 0.001)
Have another	81,348	89.3	24.4	
Undecided	3668	4.0	20.1	
No more	6067	6.7	31.7	
Ideal number of children				12.5 (< 0.001)
0–3	28,448	31.2	33.7	

Table 2 Distribution of modern contraceptive use across individual and contextual factors of adolescent girls and young women in sub-Saharan Africa *(Continued)*

Variables	Weighted N	Weighted %	Modern contraceptive use	χ2 (*p*-value)
4–5	41,582	45.7	25.6	
6+	21,052	23.1	10.8	
Place of residence				969.0 (< 0.001)
Urban	37,290	40.9	30.0	
Rural	53,793	59.1	21.0	
Community literacy level				3.3 (< 0.001)
Low	29,156	32.0	18.1	
Moderate	33,323	36.6	27.0	
High	28,603	31.4	28.8	
Community socio-economic status				7.3 (< 0.001)
Low	50,072	55.0	19.9	
Moderate	7563	8.3	30.7	
High	33,448	36.7	30.5	
Community knowledge of modern method				6.0 (< 0.001)
Low	72,827	78.0	27.1	
Moderate	16,786	18.4	15.6	
High	1470	1.6	9.5	

Source: Demographic and Health Surveys

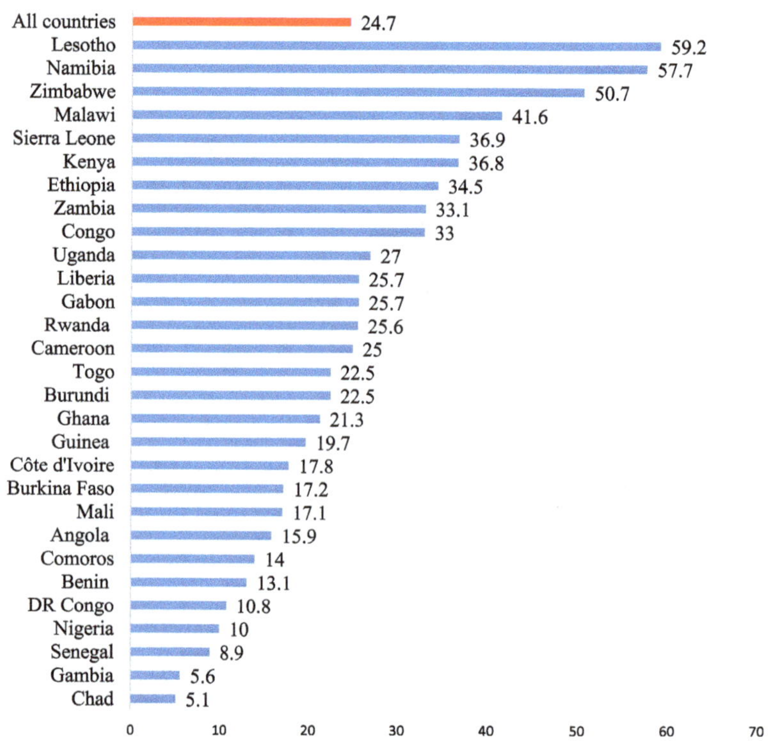

Fig. 1 Prevalence of modern contraceptive usage among adolescent girls and young women in SSA. Source: Demographic and Health Surveys

Distribution of modern contraceptive use across the individual and contextual level factors

Table 2 shows results on the distribution of modern contraceptive use across the individual and contextual level factors of AGYW in SSA. The results indicate that the use of modern contraceptives was high among AGYW aged 20–24 (26.8%), those who had never married (28.5%), Christians (29.1%), those who were not working (26.2%), those who had their first sex between 20 and 24 years (26.2%), those with two births (27.6%) and those who read newspaper/magazine, listened to radio or watched television at least once a week. A greater proportion of AGYW also used modern contraceptives if they desired to have no more children (31.7%), had 0–3 as their ideal number of children (33.7%), lived in urban areas (30%), lived in communities with high literacy (28.8%), moderate socio-economic status (30.7%) and low knowledge of modern methods (27.1%). The chi-square test results also revealed all the individual and contextual factors had statistically significant associations with modern contraceptive usage.

Association between individual and contextual level factors and modern contraceptive use among AGYW in SSA

In terms of the individual level factors, the study showed that AGYW aged 15–19 were less likely to use modern contraceptives [aOR = 0.86, CI = 0.83–0.90] compared with those aged 20–24. AGYW who were either married [aOR = 0.83, CI = 0.79–0.87], cohabiting [aOR = 0.69, CI = 0.66–0.73], or widowed/divorced/separated [aOR = 0.77, CI = 0.72–0.83] had lower odds of using modern contraceptives, compared with those who had never married. The likelihood of modern contraceptive use was also low among Muslims [aOR = 0.59, CI = 0.57–0.62] and AGYW who belonged to 'other' religions [aOR = 0.68, CI = 0.62–0.74] compared to Christians. AGYW who were working [aOR = 0.92, CI = 0.89–0.95], those who had no child [aOR = 0.44, CI = 0.42–0.47], those who had no exposure to newspaper/magazine [aOR = 0.44, CI = 0.63–0.71] and radio [aOR = 0.82, CI = 0.78–0.86] had lower odds of using modern contraceptives. The likelihood of modern contraceptive use among AGYW reduced among those who were not decided on their desire for more children [aOR = 0.72, CI = 0.65–0.80] and those whose ideal number of children was 6+ [aOR = 0.38, CI = 0.35–0.40]. Conversely, the use of modern contraceptives was high among AGYW whose age at first sex was 15–19 years [aOR = 1.20, CI = 1.12–1.28] compared to those whose first sex happened between the ages of 20–24. With the contextual factors, the odds of using modern contraceptives was low among AGYW who lived in rural areas [aOR = 0.89, CI = 0.85–0.93], communities with low literacy level [aOR = 0.73, CI = 0.70–0.77], low socio-economic status [aOR = 0.69, CI = 0.65–0.73] and high knowledge of modern contraceptives [aOR = 0.33, CI = 0.27–0.41] compared to those who lived in urban areas, communities with high literacy level, high socio-economic status and low knowledge on modern contraceptives (see Table 3).

Discussion

This study assessed the individual and contextual level correlates of modern contraceptive use among AGYW in SSA. It was found that 24.7% of AGYW in SSA use modern contraceptives. Age, marital status, religion, employment status, parity, exposure to mass media, desire for more children, ideal number of children and age at first sex were identified as individual level predictors of modern contraceptive use among AGYW in SSA. In terms of the contextual level factors, place of residence, community literacy level, community socio-economic status and community knowledge of modern contraceptives had associations with the utilization of modern contraceptives among AGYW in SSA.

In this study, the use of modern contraceptives was low among AGYW in SSA. In line with this finding, Mutumba, Wekesa [27] also found a low prevalence of 17.8% of modern contraceptive use among young women in LMICs. AGYW in chad had the lowest prevalence of modern contraceptive use. In a recent study on contraceptive use among adolescents and adult women in LMICs, Li, Patton [38] identified Chad as one of the countries with a low contraceptive prevalence. AGYW in Chad are less likely to use modern contraceptives because in Chad, national guidelines authorized only doctors based in hospitals to provide modern contraceptives such as IUDs and implants. Again, few providers in the country have been given the training to provide contraceptive services. This often results in the lack of skills and confidence to deliver these services [39]. The cost of modern contraceptive services has also been considered as a barrier to the use of modern contraceptives, especially among AGYW in Chad [39].

This study showed that AGYW aged 15–19 were less likely to use modern contraceptives compared with those aged 20–24. This finding corroborates the findings obtained in previous studies [20, 21]. The possible reason for this finding is that AGYW aged 20–24 are assumed to have a better understanding of the consequences of engaging in sexual acts without contraception compared to those aged 15–19 [21]. AGYW aged 15–19 may also have challenges accessing family planning services either because they have no knowledge on where to obtain contraception or cannot afford the services [40, 41]. Relatedly, this study identified a high usage of modern contraceptives among AGYW who had

Table 3 Mixed effects results on individual and contextual factors associated with modern contraceptive use among adolescent girls and young women in sub-Saharan Africa

Variables	Model 0 aOR[95%CI]	Model 1 aOR[95%CI]	Model 2 aOR[95%CI]	Model 3 aOR[95%CI]
Age				
15–19		0.82*** (0.79–0.86)		0.86*** (0.83–0.90)
20–24		1		1
Marital status				
Not married		1		1
Married		0.80*** (0.76–0.83)		0.83*** (0.79–0.87)
Cohabiting		0.68*** (0.65–0.72)		0.69*** (0.66–0.73)
Widowed/separated/divorced		0.78*** (0.72–0.84)		0.77*** (0.72–0.83)
Religion				
Christianity		1		1
Islam		0.58*** (0.55–0.60)		0.59*** (0.57–0.62)
Other		0.69*** (0.63–0.75)		0.68*** (0.62–0.74)
Employment status				
Not working		1		1
Working		0.89*** (0.86–0.92)		0.92*** (0.89–0.95)
Age at first sex				
Less than 15 years		0.99 (0.91–1.06)		1.03 (0.95–1.11)
15–19 years		1.18*** (1.11–1.26)		1.20*** (1.12–1.28)
20–24 years		1		1
Parity				
Zero birth		0.48*** (0.45–0.50)		0.44*** (0.42–0.47)
One birth		0.78*** (0.75–0.82)		0.76*** (0.72–0.80)
Two births		1		1
Three births		0.92* (0.85–0.98)		0.94 (0.87–1.01)
Four or more births		0.85** (0.75–0.96)		0.88 (0.77–1.00)
Frequency of reading newspaper/magazine				
Not at all		0.65*** (0.61–1.82)		0.67*** (0.63–0.71)
Less than once a week		1.02 (0.96–1.08)		0.98 (0.91–1.04)
At least once a week		1		1
Frequency of listening to radio				
Not at all		0.80*** (0.77–0.83)		0.82*** (0.78–0.86)
Less than once a week		1.00 (0.95–1.04)		0.99 (0.95–1.04)
At least once a week		1		1
Frequency of watching television				
Not at all		0.85*** (0.81–0.88)		0.97 (0.93–1.01)
Less than once a week		0.92** (0.88.0.97)		1.00 (0.95–1.06)
At least once a week		1		1
Desire for more children				
Have another		1.10** (1.03–1.17)		1.08* (1.01–1.15)
Undecided		0.70*** (0.63–0.77)		0.72*** (0.65–0.80)
No more		1		1
Ideal number of children				
0–3		1		1

Table 3 Mixed effects results on individual and contextual factors associated with modern contraceptive use among adolescent girls and young women in sub-Saharan Africa *(Continued)*

Variables	Model 0 aOR[95%CI]	Model 1 aOR[95%CI]	Model 2 aOR[95%CI]	Model 3 aOR[95%CI]
4–5		0.73*** (0.70–0.75)		0.78*** (0.75–0.81)
6+		0.31*** (0.29–0.32)		0.38*** (0.35–0.40)
Place of Residence				
Urban			1	1
Rural			0.83*** (0.79–0.86)	0.89*** (0.85–0.93)
Community literacy level				
Low			0.63*** (0.60–0.66)	0.73*** (0.70–0.77)
Moderate			0.98 (0.94–1.02)	0.95* (0.92–0.99)
High			1	1
Community socio-economic status				
Low			0.66*** (0.63–0.70)	0.69*** (0.65–0.73)
Moderate			1	1
High			0.96 (0.91–1.02)	0.90*** (0.84–0.95)
Community knowledge of modern method				
Low			1	1
Moderate			0.43*** (0.40–0.44)	0.53*** (0.51–0.56)
High			0.24*** (0.19–0.29)	0.33*** (0.27–0.41)
Random effect result				
PSU variance (95% CI)	0.03 (0.02–0.04)	0.02 (0.01–0.03)	0.03 (0.01–0.04)	0.02 (0.01–0.03)
ICC	0.008	0.006	0.007	0.006
LR Test	$\chi 2 = 91.46$, $p < 0.001$	$\chi 2 = 47.41$, $p < 0.001$	$\chi 2 = 68.69$, $p < 0.001$	$\chi 2 = 45.92$, $p < 0.001$
Wald chi-square	Reference	6019.62***	3323.50***	7015.95***
Model fitness				
Log-likelihood	−49,667.17	−46,122.51	−47,848.36	−45,426.69
AIC	99,338.16	92,295.02	95,714.72	90,917.38
N	91,083	91,083	91,083	91,083

Source: Demographic and Health Surveys
1 Reference category, *PSU* Primary Sampling Unit, *ICC* Intra-Class Correlation, *LR Test* Likelihood ratio Test, *AIC* Akaike's Information Criterion
*$p < 0.05$, **$p < 0.01$, ***$p < 0.001$

their first sex between the ages of 15–19 and those who had never married. The possible reason for these findings is the link between marital status and modern contraceptive use. Studies have explained that AGYW who have never married are more likely to use modern contraceptives to prevent unintended pregnancies [42, 43] while those who are married are confronted with pressure to have a child soon after marriage which expose them to pregnancy even if they had the intention to delay pregnancy [44]. This is true, especially among those whose age at first sex occurs below 20 years as this is more likely to occur outside wedlock [45, 46]. The findings are also in line with the theoretical underpinning of the Health Belief Model which explains that AGYW who consider themselves as being at risk of unintended pregnancies and STIs may be more likely to use modern contraceptives compared to those who consider themselves not to be at risk [18].

Muslim AGYW and those who belonged to 'other' religions were less likely to use modern contraceptives compared to Christians. This finding is supported by the findings of other studies [47–49]. This may be attributed to differences in religious teachings regarding the use of contraceptives for fertility control [47]. As found in this study, in religions where high parity is desired and fertility preferences are high, there is low likelihood of the use of modern contraceptives. Specifically for Muslim AGYW, a study by Abdi, Okal [50] in two Muslim communities in Kenya showed that Muslim women tend to have high desire for more children due to the belief that children are a blessing from God. Thus, to receive more of the blessings God has in stock for them in the form of children, they will be less likely to use modern contraceptives. This finding could be true especially when previous studies have found high prevalence of child marriage among Muslims and other religious adherents compared to Christians [51, 52]. Despite this finding, there is the need for future qualitative research to explore further on why Christian AGYW are more likely to use modern contraceptives compared to Muslims and AGYW who belong to 'other' religion. In the meantime, there is the need to formulate and disseminate particular culturally appropriate messages targeting sexually active AGYW on the importance of modern contraceptive use in line with their religious beliefs and practices.

In this study, AGYW who lived in socio-economically disadvantaged communities (rural areas, communities with low literacy level and low socio-economic status) were less likely to use modern contraceptives compared to those who lived in socio-economically advantaged communities. This finding is in agreement with the findings of previous studies [53, 54]. This finding could be attributed to economic empowerment that gives AGYW in socio-economically advantaged communities more economic power to access modern contraceptives as the barriers in terms of cost are catered for [55–57]. Theoretically, AGYW who are in socio-economically disadvantaged communities might not have the perceived behavioural control to utilise modern contraceptives when they are financially not viable to purchase these modern contraceptives [58]. Despite the role of advantaged socio-economic status on the use of modern contraceptives, AGYW who were working had lower odds of using modern contraceptives compared to those who were not working. The possible reason for this finding could be that the majority of non-working AGYW may be in school and hence may consider the use of contraceptives as a means of preventing pregnancy and delaying fertility. Similar findings were obtained in Nigeria [36] and Ghana [59].

Non-exposure to media (radio and newspaper/magazine) decreased the odds of modern contraceptive use among AGYW in this study. This finding relates to the findings of studies in other SSA countries like Ghana [23], Mali [60], Nigeria [61, 62] and Senegal [63]. It can be affirmed that access to mass media is likely to lead to exposure to family planning messages which can bring about change in AGYW's negative attitude with respect to contraception [61]. Relatedly, Sharma, Ghimire [64] also observed that women who are exposed to family planning messages through health facilities, radio, and television have a greater likelihood to use modern contraceptives in Nepal. However, AGYW who lived in communities with high knowledge on modern contraceptives were less likely to use modern contraceptives. Further research is needed to understand this counter-intuitive finding.

Strengths and limitations

The use of nationally representative and current datasets in this study and the focus on AGYW in SSA is a major strength in this study. Again, the large sample size, the use of rigorous statistical analysis that considers both individual and contextual level factors associated with modern contraceptive use and the use of validated instruments in the DHS strengthen the validity of findings from the dataset. However, the use of cross-sectional design in the surveys makes it impossible to establish causality with respect to the findings. There is also the possibility of response bias since the issue on contraceptive use may lead to provision of social desirable responses and AGYW may also find it challenging to recall previous events on the use of modern contraception. The differences in survey years can also affect the comparability of the findings since modernization may play a role in the prevalence of modern contraceptives use in more current surveys compared to older ones.

Conclusion

Modern contraceptive use among the AGYW in SSA remains low and this can result in high rates of unwanted or mistimed pregnancies and risk of contracting STIs including HIV/AIDS. Therefore, Governments in the various countries considered in this study through their policy makers should put in measures that will halt barriers to access and use of modern contraceptives whilst intensifying mass education on modern contraceptive methods. This education should be more centered on AGYW who are in socio-economically disadvantaged communities, those who are not married, Muslims, those with high parity and high fertility preferences and those who are working. Further studies is essential to unearth the reasons why AGYW who live in communities with high knowledge on modern contraceptives are less likely to use modern contraceptives.

Abbreviations

AGYW: Adolescent girls and young women; AIC: Akaike's Information Criterion; aOR: Adjusted odds ratios; DHS: Demographic and Health Survey; ICC: Intra-Class Correlation; LR Test: Likelihood ratio Test; PSU: Primary Sampling Unit; SRH: Sexual and reproductive health; SSA: Sub-Saharan Africa

Acknowledgements

The author thanks the MEASURE DHS project for their support and for free access to the original data.

Author's contributions

BOA contributed to the study design and conceptualization. BOA reviewed the literature and performed the analysis. BOA provided technical support and critically reviewed the manuscript for its intellectual content. BOA had final responsibility to submit for publication. The author read and amended drafts of the paper and approved the final version.

References

1. Morris JL, Rushwan H. Adolescent sexual and reproductive health: the global challenges. Int J Gynecol Obstet. 2015;131:S40–S2.
2. Patton GC, Sawyer SM, Santelli JS, Ross DA, Afifi R, Allen NB, et al. Our future: a lancet commission on adolescent health and wellbeing. Lancet. 2016;387(10036):2423–78.
3. Adolescent pregnancy. Fact sheet No. 364 [Internet]. 2014 [cited Accessed July 4, 2020]. Available from: http://www.who.int/mediacentre/factsheets/fs364/en/.
4. Ameyaw EK, Budu E, Sambah F, Baatiema L, Appiah F, Seidu A-A, et al. Prevalence and determinants of unintended pregnancy in sub-Saharan Africa: a multi-country analysis of demographic and health surveys. PLoS One. 2019;14(8).
5. Geda YF. Determinants of teenage pregnancy in Ethiopia: a case–control study, 2019. Curr Med Issues. 2019;17(4):112.
6. Fertility among very young adolescents. [Internet]. Population Division, United Nations Department of Economic and Social Affairs. 2019.
7. United Nations. Sustainable development goals. New York: United Nations; 2015.
8. Darroch JE. Trends in contraceptive use. Contraception. 2013;87(3):259–63.
9. Darroch JE, Singh S. Trends in contraceptive need and use in developing countries in 2003, 2008, and 2012: an analysis of national surveys. Lancet. 2013;381(9879):1756–62.
10. Tsui AO, Brown W, Li Q. Contraceptive practice in sub-Saharan Africa. Popul Dev Rev. 2017;43(Suppl Suppl 1):166.
11. Behrman JA, Wright KQ, Grant MJ, Soler-Hampejsek E. Trends in modern contraceptive use among young adult women in sub-Saharan Africa 1990 to 2014. Stud Fam Plan. 2018;49(4):319–44.
12. Radovich E, Dennis ML, Wong KLM, Ali M, Lynch CA, Cleland J, et al. Who meets the contraceptive needs of young women in sub-Saharan Africa? J Adolesc Health. 2018;62(3):273–80.
13. Singh S, Darroch JE. Adding it up: costs and benefits of contraceptive services. New York: Guttmacher Institute and UNFPA; 2012. p. 1269–86.
14. Darroch JE, Sedgh G, Ball H. Contraceptive technologies: responding to women's needs. New York: Guttmacher Institute. 2011;201(1).
15. Ochako R, Mbondo M, Aloo S, Kaimenyi S, Thompson R, Temmerman M, et al. Barriers to modern contraceptive methods uptake among young women in Kenya: a qualitative study. BMC Public Health. 2015;15(1):118.
16. Durowade KA, Omokanye LO, Elegbede OE, Adetokunbo S, Olomofe CO, Ajiboye AD, et al. Barriers to contraceptive uptake among women of reproductive age in a semi-Urban Community of Ekiti state, Southwest Nigeria. Ethiop J Health Sci. 2017;27(2):121–8.
17. Makola L, Mlangeni L, Mabaso M, Chibi B, Sokhela Z, Silimfe Z, et al. Predictors of contraceptive use among adolescent girls and young women (AGYW) aged 15 to 24 years in South Africa: results from the 2012 national population-based household survey. BMC Womens Health. 2019;19(1):158.
18. Rosenthal DA, Hall C, Moore SM. AIDS, adolescents, and sexual risk taking: a test of the health belief model. Aust Psychol. 1992;27(3):166–71.
19. Azfredrick EC. Using Anderson's model of health service utilization to examine use of services by adolescent girls in South-Eastern Nigeria. Int J Adolesc Youth. 2016;21(4):523–9.
20. Casey SE, Gallagher MC, Kakesa J, Kalyanpur A, Muselemu J-B, Rafanoharana RV, et al. Contraceptive use among adolescent and young women in North and South Kivu, Democratic Republic of the Congo: a cross-sectional population-based survey. PLoS Med. 2020;17(3):e1003086.
21. Mandiwa C, Namondwe B, Makwinja A, Zamawe C. Factors associated with contraceptive use among young women in Malawi: analysis of the 2015–16 Malawi demographic and health survey data. Contracept Reprod Med. 2018;3(1):1–8.
22. Nsanya MK, Atchison CJ, Bottomley C, Doyle AM, Kapiga SH. Modern contraceptive use among sexually active women aged 15–19 years in North-Western Tanzania: results from the adolescent 360 (A360) baseline survey. BMJ Open. 2019;9(8):e030485.
23. Appiah F, Seidu A-A, Ahinkorah BO, Baatiema L, Ameyaw EK. Trends and determinants of contraceptive use among female adolescents in Ghana: analysis of 2003–2014 demographic and health surveys. SSM-Population Health. 2020;10:100554.
24. Abiye AA, Fekede B, Jemberie AM, Molla BA, Tolla BK, Tefera BS, et al. Modern contraceptive use and associated factors among reproductive age group women in three Peri-Urban Communities in Central Ethiopia. J Drug Deliv Ther. 2019;9(6-s):93–102.
25. Ajayi AI, Adeniyi OV, Akpan W. Use of traditional and modern contraceptives among childbearing women: findings from a mixed methods study in two southwestern Nigerian states. BMC Public Health. 2018;18(1):604.
26. Debebe S, Limenih MA, Biadgo B. Modern contraceptive methods utilization and associated factors among reproductive aged women in rural Dembia District, Northwest Ethiopia: community based cross-sectional study. Int J Reprod BioMed. 2017;15(6):367.
27. Mutumba M, Wekesa E, Stephenson R. Community influences on modern contraceptive use among young women in low and middle-income countries: a cross-sectional multi-country analysis. BMC Public Health. 2018;18(1):430.
28. Fabic MS, Choi Y, Bird S. A systematic review of demographic and health surveys: data availability and utilization for research. Bull World Health Organ. 2012;90:604–12.
29. Corsi DJ, Neuman M, Finlay JE, Subramanian SV. Demographic and health surveys: a profile. Int J Epidemiol. 2012;41(6):1602–13.
30. Ahinkorah BO, Hagan JEJ, Seidu A-A, Sambah F, Adoboi F, Schack T. Female adolescents' reproductive health decisionmaking capacity and contraceptive use in subSaharan Africa: what does the future hold? PLoS One. 2020;15(7):1–20.
31. Namasivayam A, Lovell S, Namutamba S, Schluter PJ. Predictors of modern contraceptive use among women and men in Uganda: a population-level analysis. BMJ Open. 2020;10(2):e034675.
32. Yussuf MH, Elewonibi BR, Rwabilimbo MM, Mboya IB, Mahande MJ. Trends and predictors of changes in modern contraceptive use among women aged 15–49 years in Tanzania from 2004–2016: evidence from Tanzania demographic and health surveys. PLoS One. 2020;15(6):e0234980.
33. Aviisah PA, Dery S, Atsu BK, Yawson A, Alotaibi RM, Rezk HR, et al. Modern contraceptive use among women of reproductive age in Ghana: analysis of the 2003–2014 Ghana demographic and health surveys. BMC Womens Health. 2018;18(1):141.
34. Lasong J, Zhang Y, Gebremedhin SA, Opoku S, Abaidoo CS, Mkandawire T, et al. Determinants of modern contraceptive use among married women of reproductive age: a cross-sectional study in rural Zambia. BMJ Open. 2020;10(3):e030980.
35. Ejembi CL, Dahiru T, Aliyu AA. DHS working papers; 2015.
36. Solanke BL, Oyinlola FF, Oyeleye OJ, Ilesanmi BB. Maternal and community factors associated with unmet contraceptive need among childbearing women in Northern Nigeria. Contracept Reprod Med. 2019;4(1):11.
37. Von Elm E, Altman DG, Egger M, Pocock SJ, Gøtzsche PC, Vandenbroucke JP, et al. The strengthening the reporting of observational studies in epidemiology (STROBE) statement: guidelines for reporting observational studies. Int J Surg. 2014;12(12):1495–9.
38. Li Z, Patton G, Sabet F, Zhou Z, Subramanian SV, Lu C. Contraceptive use in adolescent girls and adult women in low-and middle-income countries. JAMA Netw Open. 2020;3(2):e1921437-e.
39. Rattan J, Noznesky E, Curry DW, Galavotti C, Hwang S, Rodriguez M. Rapid contraceptive uptake and changing method mix with high use of long-acting reversible contraceptives in crisis-affected populations in Chad and the Democratic Republic of the Congo. Glob Health Sci Pract. 2016;4(Supplement 2):S5–S20.
40. Binu W, Marama T, Gerbaba M, Sinaga M. Sexual and reproductive health services utilization and associated factors among secondary school students in Nekemte town, Ethiopia. Reprod Health. 2018;15(1):64.
41. Tamang L, Raynes-Greenow C, McGeechan K, Black K. Factors associated with contraceptive use among sexually active Nepalese youths in the Kathmandu Valley. Contracept Reprod Med. 2017;2(1):13.
42. Grindlay K, Dako-Gyeke P, Ngo TD, Eva G, Gobah L, Reiger ST, et al. Contraceptive use and unintended pregnancy among young women and men in Accra, Ghana. PLoS One. 2018;13(8):e0201663.
43. Ahinkorah BO, Seidu A-A, Appiah F, Baatiema L, Sambah F, Budu E, et al. What has reproductive health decision-making capacity got to do with unintended pregnancy? Evidence from the 2014 Ghana demographic and health survey. PLoS One. 2019;14(10):e0223389.
44. UNFPA. Girlhood, not motherhood: preventing adolescent pregnancy. In: Fund UNP, editor. New York 2015.
45. Cremin I, Mushati P, Hallett T, Mupambireyi Z, Nyamukapa C, Garnett GP, et al. Measuring trends in age at first sex and age at marriage in Manicaland, Zimbabwe. Sex Transm Infect. 2009;85(Suppl 1):i34–40.
46. Żaba B, Isingo R, Wringe A, Marston M, Slaymaker E, Urassa M. Influence of timing of sexual debut and first marriage on sexual behaviour in later life: findings from four survey rounds in the Kisesa cohort in northern Tanzania. Sex Transm Infect. 2009;85(Suppl 1):i20–i6.
47. Obasohan PE. Religion, ethnicity and contraceptive use among reproductive age women in Nigeria. Int J MCH AIDS. 2015;3(1):63.
48. Adedini SA, Babalola S, Ibeawuchi C, Omotoso O, Akiode A, Odeku M. Role of religious leaders in promoting contraceptive use in Nigeria: evidence from the Nigerian urban reproductive health initiative. Glob Health Sci Pract. 2018;6(3):500–14.
49. Tigabu S, Demelew T, Seid A, Sime B, Manyazewal T. Socioeconomic and religious differentials in contraceptive uptake in western Ethiopia: a mixed-methods phenomenological study. BMC Womens Health. 2018;18(1):1–10.
50. Abdi B, Okal J, Serour G, Temmerman M. "Children are a blessing from god"–a qualitative study exploring the socio-cultural factors influencing contraceptive use in two Muslim communities in Kenya. Reprod Health. 2020;17:1–11.

51. Yaya S, Odusina EK, Bishwajit G. Prevalence of child marriage and its impact on fertility outcomes in 34 sub-Saharan African countries. BMC Int Health Hum Rights. 2019;19(1):33.
52. Odusina EK, Bishwajit G, Yaya S. Prevalence of child marriage and its impact on fertility outcomes in 34 sub-Saharan African countries. J Adolesc Health. 2013;52:552–8.
53. Adebowale SA, Adedini SA, Ibisomi LD, Palamuleni ME. Differential effect of wealth quintile on modern contraceptive use and fertility: evidence from Malawian women. BMC Womens Health. 2014;14(1):40.
54. Rutaremwa G, Kabagenyi A, Wandera SO, Jhamba T, Akiror E, Nviiri HL. Predictors of modern contraceptive use during the postpartum period among women in Uganda: a population-based cross sectional study. BMC Public Health. 2015;15(1):262.
55. Aremu O. The influence of socioeconomic status on women's preferences for modern contraceptive providers in Nigeria: a multilevel choice modeling. Patient Preference Adherence. 2013;7:1213.
56. Abekah-Nkrumah G, Abor PA. Socioeconomic determinants of use of reproductive health services in Ghana. Heal Econ Rev. 2016;6(1):9.
57. Lamidi EO. State variations in women's socioeconomic status and use of modern contraceptives in Nigeria. PLoS One. 2015;10(8):e0135172.
58. Ajzen I. The theory of planned behavior. Organ Behav Hum Decis Process. 1991;50(2):179–211.
59. Guure C, Maya ET, Dery S, Vrom B-C, Alotaibi RM, Rezk HR, et al. Factors influencing unmet need for family planning among Ghanaian married/ union women: a multinomial mixed effects logistic regression modelling approach. Arch Public Health. 2019;77(1):11.
60. Zamawe COF, Banda M, Dube AN. The impact of a community driven mass media campaign on the utilisation of maternal health care services in rural Malawi. BMC Pregnancy Childbirth. 2016;16(1):21.
61. Ajaero CK, Odimegwu C, Ajaero ID, Nwachukwu CA. Access to mass media messages, and use of family planning in Nigeria: a spatio-demographic analysis from the 2013 DHS. BMC Public Health. 2016;16(1):427.
62. Bajoga UA, Atagame KL, Okigbo CC. Media influence on sexual activity and contraceptive use: a cross sectional survey among young women in urban Nigeria. Afr J Reprod Health. 2015;19(3):100–10.
63. Jacobs J, Marino M, Edelman A, Jensen J, Darney B. Mass media exposure and modern contraceptive use among married West African adolescents. Eur J Contracept Reprod Health Care. 2017;22(6):439–49.
64. Sharma SK, Ghimire DR, Pratap N. Ethnic differentials of the impact of family planning program on contraceptive use in Nepal. Demogr Res. 2011;25: 837–68.

10

Contraceptive method use, discontinuation and failure rates among women aged 15–49 years: Evidence from selected low income settings in Kumasi, Ghana

Ayaga A. Bawah[1*], Ryoko Sato[2], Patrick Asuming[1], Elizabeth G. Henry[2], Caesar Agula[1], Charles Agyei-Asabere[1], David Canning[2] and Iqbal Shah[2]

Abstract

Background: This paper provides estimates of contraceptive discontinuation and failure rates in a poor urban setting in Ghana. Contraceptive use is for the purposes of preventing unintended or mistimed pregnancies. Unfortunately, evidence abounds in many parts of the world where there is considerable levels of contraceptive failure and high levels of discontinuation resulting in unintended pregnancies.

Methods: We estimated discontinuation rates during a 12-month period since starting use by applying single and multiple decrement life table methods to the contraceptive calendar data collected in a survey of women in reproductive age of 15–49 years.

Results: Modern contraceptive method use was estimated to be 13.7% at the time of the survey. The results show that contraceptive method discontinuation vary markedly by type of contraceptive method but are high for almost all methods, except for implants (23.7%). Discontinuation rate for emergency contraception was estimated at 88.5%, withdrawal 87.6%, and male condom use 80.9%. However, discontinuation rates were moderately high for rhythm (63.6%), pills (65.6%) and injectables (56%). In terms of failure rates, overall contraceptive failure for all methods was estimated at 7.9%. The factors significantly associated with method failure include being within age bracket 40–44 years (OR = 0.3, $p < 0.05$), having secondary/higher education (OR = 0.4, $p < 0.01$), belonging to the richest household wealth scale (OR = 3.3, $p < 0.01$), currently in union with a partner (OR = 2.2, $p < 0.01$), and using contraceptive methods such as rhythm (OR = 5.6, $p < 0.01$) and withdrawal (OR = 3.7, $p < 0.01$). On the flip side, the odds for method discontinuation were significantly higher for women in their 20s and mid 30s, formerly in union (OR = 1.9, $p < 0.05$) and use of withdrawal method (OR = 1.4, $p < 0.05$) and lower for women formerly in union (OR = 0.4, $p < 0.01$) and use of implants (OR = 0.2, $p < 0.01$) and injectables (OR = 0.6, $p < 0.01$).

Conclusion: While contraceptives use is low, both discontinuation and failure rates are high and variable among different methods. Failure and discontinuation rates are lowest for long-acting methods such as implants while higher failure rates are more prevalent among women who rely on withdrawal and the rhythm methods.

Keywords: Contraceptives, Method failure, Discontinuation, Kumasi, Ghana

* Correspondence: aabawah@ug.edu.gh
[1]University of Ghana, Legon, Accra, Ghana

Background

Family planning and contraceptive use remain an effective intervention for addressing women's reproductive health needs and particularly, preventing unintended and/or, mistimed pregnancies. Indeed, one of the major fertility regulation interventions that received international attention and donor support, particularly in developing countries was the introduction of large-scale family planning programs [1]. Contraceptive use is mainly for the purposes of preventing unintended or mistimed pregnancies [2–4]. Singh, Sedgh and Hussain [4] reported that 40% of an estimated 213 million worldwide pregnancies that occurred in 2012 were unintended. While these rates vary across regions and countries, the highest unintended pregnancy rates are found in Middle and Eastern Africa [4]. High rates of unintended pregnancies are also observed in West Africa where it was reported that 26% of the 17.6 million pregnancies were unintended [4]. In Ghana, about 37% of all pregnancies are also unintended, with 23% being mistimed and 14% being unwanted pregnancies [5, 6].

Unintended pregnancies are a major public health problem which affects both individuals and the society at large. Problems arising out of unintended pregnancies range from health, through emotional and psychosocial problems, as well as economic and in many cases, such pregnancies mark the termination of the educational careers for many girls and women and deprive them of work opportunities, particularly in developing countries.

It is often assumed that women who are using contraceptives are protected from getting pregnant. However, some of the unintended pregnancies happened while the women were reported to be using contraceptives. For instance, in 2008 Kost et al. reported that as much of 12.4% women in the United States of America who were using reversible methods in 2002 had experienced a contraceptive failure after 12 months of initiation of use [7]. Trussell found slightly higher rates (14.9%) using the same dataset [8]. Using data from 43 countries Polis et al. [9] found 12-month failure rate varied across subregions and by method. Overall failure rates were lowest for long-acting reversible methods; for example 0.6% for implants, 1.4% for IUD and 1.7% for injectables and highest for traditional methods such as withdrawal or period abstinence (13.9%). More recent results from a paper by Bradley et al. [10] show similar patterns of failure with respect to method, although more generally their rates are higher than those reported by Polis et al. in 2016. For instance, Bradley et al. estimate failure rate for implants as 0.03 (per 100 episodes), that for IUD as 1.2, and approximately 2.0 for injectables. Failure rates are higher for pills (6.3%), condom (8.6% and periodic abstinence 19.0% [10]. What this suggests is that contraceptive failure or user-failure resulting from incorrect or inconsistent method use prevent women from realizing their reproductive intentions.

As noted above, some of unintended pregnancies are a result of contraceptive method failure, which is also one of the reported reasons for method discontinuation. Other often cited reasons for discontinuation are side effects or health concerns and desire to become pregnant or no further need for using a method [3]. Analysis by Ali, Cleland and Shah using data from 60 Demographic and Health Surveys also show that discontinuation rates and reasons for discontinuation, vary by method [3].

The demographic impact of contraceptive use depends not only on its prevalence but also on the duration and effectiveness of use. As desired family size declines and contraceptive prevalence rises, contraceptive effectiveness becomes an increasingly important determinant of fertility [11]. For example, if desired fertility is six births per woman, an increase in contraceptive effectiveness from 85 to 90% would result in a decline in total fertility of about 0.20 births. In contrast, if desired fertility is two births per woman, then the same increase in contraceptive effectiveness would reduce the total fertility rate by more than one birth [12].

In addition to the demographic impact, the analysis of contraceptive discontinuation, and in particular, contraceptive method failure, is important because it can inform efforts to improve service delivery in various ways. For instance, the rate at which women discontinue the use of a method due to reported side effects may signal the need for improved counseling, and that information about the method needs to be communicated much more effectively [13–15]. High levels of discontinuation due to access or availability problems suggest that supply and/or distribution mechanisms need examination. Combined with knowledge of the modes of delivery for different methods, discontinuation rates can help identify the inadequacies of particular types of service delivery and the potential effects of contemplated changes in modes.

This paper reports on estimates of contraceptive method use, discontinuation and contraceptive method failure rates and their determinants in an urban poor setting in the city of Kumasi in southern Ghana. Kumasi was one of two cities in Ghana where Willows International, in partnership with government of Ghana and four other organizations, implemented the *Reducing Maternal Mortality and Morbidity (R3M)* program that aimed to improve access to family planning and safe abortion services [16]. The interventions implemented included a package of reproductive health information programs that focused on provision of reproductive health information and home-based family planning counseling and referral services for women who desire to adopt family planning. Women identified as being at high risk of unintended pregnancy as well as other reproductive health problems were referred to selected health facilities for services.

Methods

Study setting and sampling procedure

This paper is based on data collected in four communities in the Kumasi metropolis as part of a retrospective, cross-sectional survey by Willows Impact Evaluation (WIE) study to evaluate the impact of the Willows program. Data were collected in Willows intervention areas: Asawase-Aboabo and Sepe-Buokrom communities and comparison areas: Angloga and Sepe-Timpom communities. These communities share similar socio-economic, demographic and ethnic mix characteristics and usually vulnerable to the exigencies of urbanization such as floods and cholera and often disproportionately limited in terms of access to health care.

WIE study employed a multi-level cluster sampling procedure for a representative sample. In the first level, 200 clusters (100 each for intervention and comparison areas) were randomly sampled from sub-divisions of Enumeration Area (EA) maps obtained from the Ghana Statistical Service (GSS). A complete listing of all women aged 15–49 years in the sampled clusters was done. In the second level, about 20 households with at least a woman within the age band 15–19 years were randomly sampled from each sampled cluster. In the last level, where there were more women within the age bracket 15–49 years in a household, one was randomly selected.

Data collection and tools used

A population-based survey was implemented during the period January–July 2018. Data collected included indicators of contraceptive use and method preferences, indices of unmet need, discontinuation and whether or not women got pregnant while using a method. These data were collected using an electronic version of a paper questionnaire with both standard direct survey questions and the use of a retrospective contraceptive calendar covering reproductive events during the 5 years prior to the survey, based on the Demographic and Health Survey (DHS). CommCare version 2.40.1, an electronic data capture system, was used for programming of the paper questionnaire into an electronic version for data collection [17]. CommCare allows for the capture and storage of data in real-time, with features to program inbuilt checks to prevent inconsistent and common errors from getting into the data. It also offers the ability to monitor and control the experiences of data collectors in the field and ensures that interviewers follow strict protocol which helps to reduce errors that commonly get into the data when using manual or paper-based data collection techniques. This paper draws on these data to estimate contraceptive use, discontinuation and failure rates, among all sexually active women who were using contraceptives during the period.

Measures

Three status indicators of contraceptive use dynamics permit the estimation of contraceptive failure and discontinuation rates. These include getting pregnant while using a method of contraception, timing in switching from one method to another or abandoning the use completely. Contraceptive failure is estimated by calculating the number of observations with reported pregnancy while on a method relative to all who were using the method, while discontinuation rates are estimated as those who stop using a method for whatever reason and duration. Discontinuing the use of a method may or may not be followed by method switching. Method switching occurs when a woman switches from the use of a contraceptive method to another method. Women who switch from one method to another are considered to have discontinued the previous method. The unit of analysis is an episode of contraceptive use, which begins at the point in the reproductive calendar when a woman reports initiating use of a contraceptive method and ends when she reports discontinuing that method [9].

The estimation procedure is based on all women who reported that they were sexually active and had used a method of contraceptive at some point during the period as captured in the contraceptive calendar. The period covered by the contraceptive calendar is 5 years preceding the survey. An individual woman may contribute more than one episode to the calculation during the period. Women who reported that they discontinued the use of any method during the period because they became pregnant while using the method are captured as method failure. This permits the identification of episodes of use and discontinuation.

The analysis is restricted to episodes within the last 5 years preceding the survey using data from the contraceptive calendar. For periods of use between births occurring within the 5 years it is possible to calculate periods of starting dates taking into consideration reported duration of use and nine-month gestational period for more recent births [18].

The study considered the use of methods such as sterilization, intrauterine device (IUD), injectables, implants, pills and male/female condom, emergency contraceptive (EC), lactational amenorrhea as modern methods, consistent with the 2017 Ghana Maternal Health Survey [19]. Withdrawal and calendar/rhythm/periodic abstinence were considered as traditional methods.

Measurements for explanatory variables used in the regression models were: age (1. 15–19 years, 2. 20–24 years, 3. 25–29 years, 4. 30–34 years, 35–39 years and 40+ years), religion (1. Catholic, 2. Methodist/Anglican/ Presbyterian, 3. Pentecostal, 4. other Christians, 5. Moslem and 6. other/no religion), educational level (1. none, 2. primary and 3. secondary/higher), household wealth index (1. poorest, 2. poorer, 3. middle, 4. richer and 5. richest), marital status (1. single, 2. currently in union with a partner and 3. formerly in a union with a partner), contraceptive method (1. male condom, 2. rhythm, 3. withdrawal, 4. injection, 5. pill and 6. implant) and knowledge of family planning methods. Women who used EC were dropped from the regression analysis because it is meant for emergency situations and expected to be discontinued after use. These variables were selected based on previous literature [20–22] and other possible reasons that could affect the dependent variables.

Method of analysis

Discontinuation rates are estimated using single and multiple decrement life table procedures as implemented in the DHS programme [23]. It calculates the probabilities of discontinuation for specific methods in the absence of competing reasons for discontinuation. The procedure calculates percentage of episodes discontinued within 12 months by reason for discontinuation, by method.

To estimate the determinants of both discontinuation and failure rates, we used logistic regression methods, dichotomizing each into occurrence or non-occurrence of the event (*discontinuation* vs *continuation* and *failure* vs *non-failure*). In the first regression model, occurrence of method failure was coded "1" whereas non-failure coded "0". For the second model, occurrence of method discontinuation was coded "1" and continuous use coded "0". Covariates of the models with probability values less than or equal to 5% were considered significant. The pseudo-R^2 and the f-statistics were used to examine goodness of fit and the overall significance of the models, respectively. Multicollinearity was also checked to ensure that the regressors were not correlated. Moreover, STATA 14.2 which was used for the analysis automatically checks for multicollinearity and often deletes variables that are correlated.

Results

Background characteristics of women

A sample of 4230 women in urban-poor settings of Kumasi, Ghana consented to participate in the study and had completed interviews. Of the 4230 women, data of 4220 women after cleaning were used for the analysis. Table 1 provides information on the background characteristic of respondents. Majority of the respondents are less than 30 years of age, with the highest concentration in the age group 25–29 (≈21%). With respect to education, 74.2% of the women had at least some education whereas 25.8% had not had any formal education. However, 26.6% of the women had attained secondary or higher education whereas 47.6% had attained only primary education.

In terms of household wealth of the respondents, about 7.7% of them are categorized as being in the poorest category while 5.3% are in the richest category. The greater proportion of them are either in the medium or richer categories. Majority (37.2%) of the respondents are in the middle category.

With regards to marital status, 39.2% of the respondents were reported to be single, whereas 51.5% were said to be in a union with a partner at the time of the survey. About 9.3% of the respondents reported that they were formerly in a union with a partner. With respect to religious affiliation, most of the respondents professed as being Christians (56.5%) with majority of the Christians being Pentecostal (30.0%). However, a large proportion of them also reported as being Moslem 42.2% and a small minority of 21.3% indicating no religion.

In terms of knowledge of contraceptive methods, respondents had knowledge of an average of 8.6 methods out of a total of 13.

Method mix for women

Figure 1 shows method mix for women. The results show a broad mix of various contraceptive methods that women in this area use for fertility regulation. Overall, modern contraceptive prevalence rate in this population was estimated to be 13.7% at the time of the survey. However, as Fig. 1 suggests, women in these communities use both modern and non-modern methods of contraceptives for purposes of fertility regulation. The majority of contraceptive users use calendar/rhythm method which is a traditional method (26.4%), followed by implants (14.1%), then injectables (11.9%). Other modern methods that women use include male condom (9.1%), emergency contraception (7.3%), female sterilization (4.5%), IUD (3.2) and lactational amenorrhea method (LAM) (4.6%). Another traditional method commonly used was the withdrawal method which is reported to be 8.1%. A few of the women (1.6%) also reported using Primolut N-tablet (commonly referred to as N-tablet in Ghana). The N-tablet contains norethisterone and is often used as a pre- or post-coital tablet by women to prevent pregnancy.

Method discontinuation and method failure by type of FP

The first part of Table 2 reports results for 12-months discontinuation rates for women by method and reasons

Table 1 Distribution of women, by background characteristics

Background characteristics	Case [Percent] (*N* = 4220)
Age (years)	
15–19	556 [13.2%]
20–24	730 [17.3%]
25–29	869 [20.6%]
30–34	700 [16.6%]
35–39	610 [14.4%]
40–44	402 [9.5%]
45–49	353 [8.4%]
Education	
None	1089 [25.8%]
Primary	2008 [47.6%]
Secondary or higher	1123 [26.6%]
Household Wealth Index	
Poorest	323 [7.7%]
Poorer	829 [19.6%]
Medium	11,571 [37.2%]
Richer	1230 [29.2%]
Richest	267 [6.3%]
Marital Status	
Currently in union with a partner	1656 [39.2%]
Formerly in union with a partner	2173 [51.5%]
Currently in union with a partner	391 [9.3%]
Religion	
Catholic	237 [5.6%]
Anglican/Methodist/Presbyterian	371 [8.8%]
Pentecostal	1265 [30.0%]
Other Christian	511 [12.1%]
Moslem	1780 [42.2%]
Other/No religion	56 [1.3%]
	Mean [Std. Dev.]
Number of contraceptive methods known (0–13)	8.6 [2.0]

for discontinuing use of particular methods. The first part of the table represents episodes of use. Rates vary markedly by method but are overall high for almost all methods, except for implants (23.7%). As expected, the rates were very high for EC (88.5%), withdrawal (87.6%) and male condom use (80.9%). The rates were however moderately high for rhythm (63.6%), pills (65.6%) and injectables (56%).

In terms of reasons for discontinuation of specific methods, the most frequently cited reason for discontinuing the use of implants is side effects/health concerns. The methods mostly discontinued by women due to method failure are the rhythm method (6.6%) and withdrawal (7.7%). Interestingly, the most cited reason for discontinuation for most of the methods is either infrequent sex, opposition from husband or some fatalistic reason.

The second part of Table 2 presents results of contraceptive failure rates. The overall contraceptive failure rate is 7.9%, with rhythm and withdrawal methods recording the highest failure rates. It is important to note the difference between the failure rate for all methods reported in the two divides of Table 2. The first part of Table 2 include all episodes whereas the second part include episodes that discontinued which accounts for differences in the denominators.

Associated factors of method failure and discontinuation

Table 3 presents logistic regression results showing the determinants of method failure and method discontinuation. The regression for the determinants of method failure is based on those who discontinued use because of method failure relative to all users while that for discontinuation is based on all discontinued events i.e. all who discontinued for whatever reason.

For failure, the significant determinants are age of woman, education, household wealth scale, marital status, and contraceptive method type. Similarly, apart from education, the rest of the other variables mentioned above are also significantly associated with discontinuation. For instance, women who have secondary or higher levels of education are 0.4 times as unlikely to experience method failure relative to those without education. Also, women within the age band 40–44 years have lower odds (OR = 0.3, $p = 0.05$) for method failure compared with women aged 15–19 years. Surprisingly, women who are better off on the household wealth scale are more likely to experience method failure relative to those in the poorest class, controlling for the type of method used. For example, those in the richest wealth scale are 3.3 times as likely to experience method failure juxtaposed with those in the poorest wealth quintile, and this statistically significant at 1%. Women who are currently in union with a partner (OR = 2.2, $p < 0.01$) are more likely to experience method failure relative to those not married. Unsurprisingly, the likelihood of method failure is higher among methods considered less effective (rhythm and withdrawal) compared with condom.

With regards to method discontinuation, age is significantly associated with method discontinuation. Women within the age band 20–29 years have higher odds of discontinuation relative to younger women (16–19). For instance, comparing with aged 15–19 years, women within the age group 25–29 years are 2.4 times as likely to discontinue the use of a method. Further, results show that women within the richer (OR = 0.7, $p < 0.05$) and richest (OR = 0.5, $p < 0.05$) wealth scales have lower odds

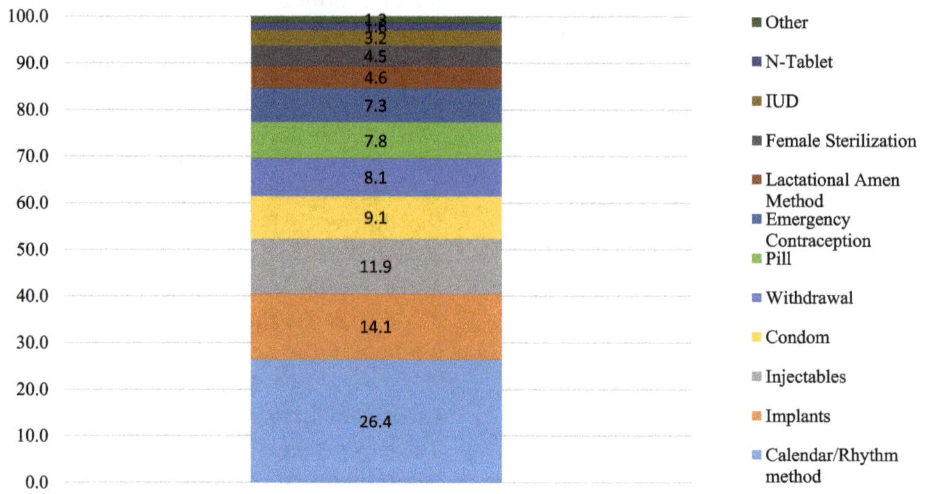

Fig. 1 Method Mix for Women 16–49 in Kumasi, Ghana 2018

relative to their counterparts in the poorest wealth scale. Unlike method failure, women who reported currently being in union with a partner (OR = 0.4, $p < 0.01$) are less likely to discontinue use of a method relative to women who are single. On a flip side, those formerly in union are about 2 times as likely to discontinue use of a method compared with single women. The likelihood of method discontinuation is also lower for the use of rhythm (OR = 0.6, $p < 0.01$), injectable (OR = 0.6, $p < 0.01$) and implant ((OR = 0.2, $p < 0.01$) and higher for withdrawal (OR = 1.4, $p < 0.05$).

Figure 2 shows the reproductive statuses of women 3 months following discontinuation of a method for any reason. Majority of women who reportedly discontinued a method as a result of failure remained pregnant (57%) 3 months following the discontinuation. About 9.1% of the women who reported method failure as the reason for discontinuation terminated the pregnancy. The remaining 16% of the women who reported no method

Table 2 Method discontinuation and failure rates by type of FP

Contraceptive method	Reasons for discontinuation (%)									Prevalence of Method Failure by type of FP		
	Method failure	Desire to become pregnant	Other fertility related reasons (infrequent sex, husband oppose, fatalistic)	Side effects or health concerns	Wanted more effective method	Other method related	Other/ DK	All reasons	Number	Number of episodes	Number of failures (failure rate (%))	% of total failures
Rhythm	6.6	5.5	36.6	0.0	10.3	1.0	3.5	63.6	964	740	106 (14.3)	45.5
Emergency Contraception	4.0	3.0	55.6	12.7	2.8	4.2	6.2	88.5	620	560	27 (4.8)	11.6
Withdrawal	7.7	7.3	45.7	0.3	19.8	1.7	5.1	87.6	619	550	50 (9.1)	21.5
Male condom	2.1	5.6	50.1	1.8	7.0	7.0	7.4	80.9	532	454	11 (2.4)	4.7
Injectables	2.5	9.4	8.7	25.7	0.9	3.1	5.8	56.0	360	258	12 (4.7)	5.2
Pills	5.7	8.1	19.3	20.3	4.0	4.3	4.1	65.6	343	273	25 (9.2)	10.7
Implants	0.5	2.5	2.1	16.6	0.0	0.0	2.0	23.7	228	104	2 (1.9_	0.9
All methods/ Total	4.8	5.8	36.9	7.8	8.1	3.0	5.0	71.4	3666	2939	233 (7.9)	100.00

Table 3 Logistic regression of associated factors to Method Failure / Discontinuation

Indicator Variable	Method Failure				Discontinuation			
Age Category	**Odds ratio**	***P*-value**	**95%-CI**		**Odds ratio**	**P-value**	**95%-CI**	
RC (15–19)								
20–24	0.54	0.19	0.22	1.35	1.89	0.00	1.23	2.92
25–29	0.96	0.93	0.39	2.39	2.44	0.00	1.55	3.84
30–34	0.71	0.48	0.27	1.88	1.67	0.03	1.05	2.67
35–39	0.69	0.48	0.24	1.94	1.59	0.06	0.97	2.61
40–44	0.29	0.05	0.08	1.00	1.65	0.08	0.93	2.92
45–49	0.11	0.05	0.01	1.02	1.72	0.18	0.76	3.87
Religion								
RC (Catholic)								
Anglican/Methodist/Presbyterian	1.70	0.23	0.71	4.09	1.05	0.84	0.64	1.72
Pentecostal	1.42	0.36	0.66	3.06	1.33	0.16	0.89	2.00
Other Christian	1.55	0.32	0.65	3.69	0.75	0.21	0.49	1.18
Muslim	1.08	0.83	0.50	2.34	1.48	0.05	0.99	2.22
Other/No religion	0.86	0.86	0.15	5.01	1.33	0.50	0.58	3.03
Education								
RC (No Education)								
Primary	0.71	0.16	0.44	1.15	1.08	0.55	0.84	1.38
Secondary or higher	0.44	0.00	0.24	0.80	1.18	0.28	0.88	1.61
Household wealth index								
RC (Poorest)								
Poorer	1.61	0.24	0.72	3.60	0.45	0.00	0.31	0.65
Medium	2.00	0.05	1.00	4.03	0.66	0.02	0.46	0.94
Richer	1.72	0.15	0.82	3.60	0.69	0.04	0.48	0.99
Richest	3.32	0.00	1.36	8.10	0.51	0.01	0.30	0.88
Marital Status								
RC (Single)								
Currently in union with a partner	2.18	0.00	1.40	3.40	0.45	0.00	0.34	0.58
Formerly in union with a partner	0.94	0.88	0.41	2.17	1.95	0.02	1.10	3.46
Contraceptive method								
RC (Condom)								
Rhythm	5.63	0.00	2.88	11.00	0.65	0.00	0.47	0.88
Emergency Contraception#	.				.			
Withdrawal	3.71	0.00	1.84	7.47	1.43	0.04	1.01	2.02
Injection	1.12	0.80	0.43	2.93	0.58	0.00	0.41	0.83
Pill	2.85	0.00	1.30	6.28	0.90	0.59	0.62	1.31
Implant	0.39	0.24	0.08	1.92	0.19	0.00	0.13	0.28
Knowledge of number of FP methods	1.10	0.17	0.96	1.27	1.03	0.46	0.95	1.10
Constant	0.00	0.00	0.00	0.03	3.85	0.00	1.71	8.65
	Number of obs. = 2378; Wald Chi2(25) = 115.3; Prob > Chi2 = 0.00; Pseudo R2 = 0.12; Log pseudolikelihood = –625.7				*Number of obs. = 3043; Wald Chi2(25) = 288.75; Prob > Chi2 = 0.00; Pseudo R2 = 0.10; Log pseudolikelihood = –1428.6*			

#_Emergency contraceptive was dropped from the regression analysis because it is meant for emergency situations and expected to be discontinued after use

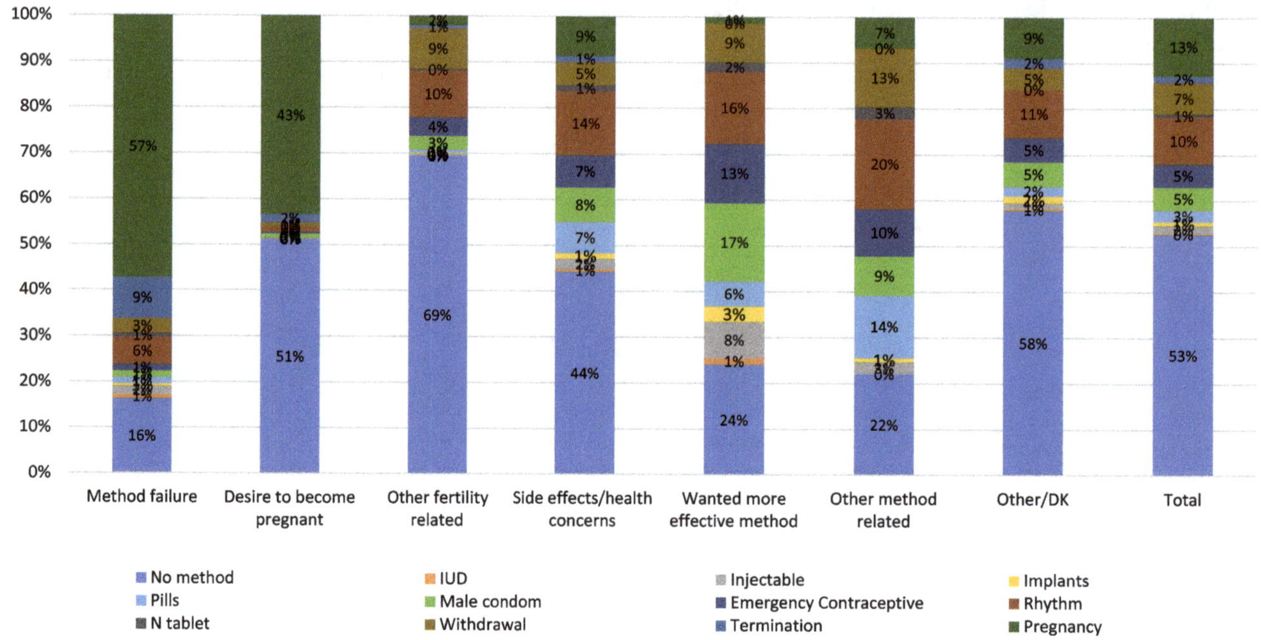

Fig. 2 Events after Discontinuation (in 3 months)

are likely to still be pregnant since they reported a method failure.

For those who desired to become pregnant, the 51% of them did not use a method following discontinuation. Indeed, about 43% of these women became pregnant 3 months following their discontinuation of the method.

Discussion

Contraceptive use, discontinuation and failure rates in low-income urban settings

Modern use of contraceptives in low-income urban settings in Southern Ghana is extremely low, about half the national average (25%) [19]. While contraceptives use is low, discontinuation rates are quite high and variable among different methods. Discontinuation rates are lowest for long-acting methods such as implants while failure rates are more prevalent among women who rely on withdrawal and the rhythm methods.

It is not surprising that the rhythm and withdrawal methods have relatively high failure rates because they are entirely under user control with high risk of inconsistent and incorrect use. On the other hand, as expected, failure rates are lowest among implant users. Surprisingly, we find relatively high rates of failure among women who use injectables and oral pills which are considered as relatively more effective compared to condoms or emergency contraceptives, though all depend on user's correct use to be effective.

With such low use of contraceptives and high discontinuation and failure rates, it is likely that women in these communities will be predisposed to various reproductive health challenges particularly those related to unwanted and mistimed pregnancies, as observed in other parts of Africa and elsewhere in the developing world. Indeed, research published in 2019 [5] using data from the 2014 Ghana Demographic and Health Survey showed that 40% of pregnancies were unintended. Our own data used for this paper show that 33.9% of the women reported that their last pregnancy was not intended.

Determinants of method failure and discontinuation

Contraceptive method failure is one of the reasons for contraceptive discontinuation. Results suggest that women who use methods such as rhythm, withdrawal and pills are more likely to experience method failure. This is interesting because these methods are often unreliable because of the difficulty in their administration and operationalization. Indeed, Polis et al. have shown that the rhythm and withdrawal methods have the lowest success rates. Results also suggests that the chances of women in their 40s and older to have had experienced method failure is low. Most women beyond 40s are either about entering to, or already in their menopausal ages and would have minimal chances of conception. It is therefore unclear whether the lower odd for method failure is as a result of their fertility chances or other factors such as experience in the proper use of methods overtime. Women with tertiary or higher formal education are associated with lower odds of method failure. This outcome is expected because these women often tend to have more knowledge of contraceptive methods and are more inclined to use effective or modern methods which have less risk of failure. In fact, a plethora of studies in Ghana (e.g., [24–26]) have shown that higher education is associated with the use of effective contraceptive methods. Further, women who reported currently in union with a partner have higher odds of method failure relative to those who are single. It is likely to be the case that single women will take extra care to use more effective methods because they may not want to get pregnant.

Regarding factors associated with method discontinuation and not related to failure, we found that women in their 20s were more likely to discontinue use in low-income settings of Ghana. This outcome contrast with findings for the whole country [22]. Modey and colleagues, using data from the Ghana Demographic Health Survey, 2008 showed that age was not a predictor of method discontinuation. However, our finding is expected because younger aged women are associated with highest levels of fertility. In other words, women in these groups are more likely to have begun active childbearing and so are more likely to discontinue use if they were previously using any contraceptives.

This study is limited in a few ways. The population surveyed is not representative of the entire population of the Kumasi metropolis. The communities selected for this study are low income communities, predominantly of migrant populations and extremely poor with low educational attainment. Secondly, calendar method by which these data are collected is likely to introduce recall biases because of the retrospective interviewing that is associated with the calendar method.

Also, using episodes of use as the main unit of analysis is not straightforward because one could potentially have several episodes of use within the period in consideration.

Conclusion

Our results highlight the profound program challenges in maintaining contraceptive uptake because of high failure and discontinuation rates in this urban poor setting. The combination of low contraceptive use with high discontinuation and low switching to more effective methods require urgent attention of policy makers and program managers to address the gaps in the provision of counselling and provision of services. The implications of the high discontinuation and or, failure rates suggest that women must be counselled properly on the various methods of contraceptive, their effectiveness and side effects to enable women make appropriate choices to reduce high rates of discontinuation and failure.

Abbreviations

DHS: Demographic and Health Survey; EA: Enumeration Area; EC: Emergency Contraceptive; GHS: Ghana Health Service; GSS: Ghana Statistical Service; IUD: Intrauterine Device; LAM: Lactational Amenorrhea Method; R3M: Reducing Maternal Mortality and Morbidity; WIE: Willows Impact Evaluation

Acknowledgements

We acknowledge the administrative supports from the Regional Institute for Population Studies, University of Ghana and Department of Global Health and Population, Harvard T.H. Chan School of Public Health.

Authors' contributions

AAB conceived idea, guided data analysis and prepared full first draft of the manuscript. RS conducted the statistical analysis. PA supported with analysis. EGH supported analysis and writing. CA reviewed first draft and supported revisions of subsequent drafts. CAA supported data management. DC reviewed and helped with revisions. IS reviewed the entire manuscript and helped with revisions of the text. The author(s) read and approved the final manuscript.

Author details

[1]University of Ghana, Legon, Accra, Ghana. [2]TH Chan School of Public Health, Harvard University, Boston, USA.

References

1. Bongaarts J, Cleland J, Townsend JW, Bertrand JT, Gupta MD. Family planning programs for the 21st century: Rationale and design. New York: The Population Council; 2012.
2. Cleland A, Ali MM. Reproductive consequences of contraceptive failure in 19 developing countries. Obstetrics Gynaecol. 2004;104(2):314–20. https://doi.org/10.1097/01.AOG.0000134789.73663.fd.
3. Ali MM, Cleland J, Shah IH. Causes and Consequences of Contraceptive Discontinuation: Evidence from 60 Demographic and Health Surveys. Geneva: World Health Organization; 2012. http://www.who.int/reproductivehealth/publications/family_planning/9789241504058/en/
4. Sedgh G, Singh S, Hussain R. Intended and unintended pregnancies worldwide in 2012 and recent trends. Stud Fam Plan. 2014;45(3):301–14.
5. Nyarko SH. Unintended pregnancy among pregnant women in Ghana: prevalence and predictors. J Pregnancy. 2019; https://doi.org/10.1155/2019/2920491.
6. GSS, GHS and Macro International. Proceedings of the GSS, GHS and Macro International, Calverton, Md, USA. Ghana Statistical Service. 2007.
7. Kost K, Singh S, Vaughan B, Trussell J, Bankole A. Estimates of contraceptive failure from the 2002 National Survey of family growth. Contraception. 2008; 77(1):10–21.
8. Trussell J. Estimates of contraceptive failure from the 1995 National Survey of family growth. Contraception. 2008;78:85.
9. Polis, CB, Bradley, SEK, Bankole, A, Onda, T, Croft, T, Singh, S. Contraceptive failure rates in the developing world: an analysis of demographic and health survey data in 43 countries 2016. https://www.guttmacher.org/report/contraceptive-failure-rates-in-developing-world
10. Bradley S, Polis CB, Bankole A, Croft T. Global contraceptive failure rates: who is Most at risk? Stud Fam Plan. 2019;50(1):3–24 https://doi.org/10.1111/sifp.12085.
11. Wang D, Diamond I. The impact on fertility of contraceptive failure in China in the 1980s. J Biosoc Sci. 1995;27:277–84.
12. Bongaarts, J and Rodríguez, J. A new method for estimating contraceptive failure rates. In Measuring the Dynamics of Contraceptive Use. New York: United Nations 1991. 52–64.
13. Datey S, Gaur LN, Saxena BN. Vaginal bleeding patterns of women using different contraceptive methods (implants, injectables, IUDs, oral pills) - an Indian experience. Contraception. 1995;51:155–65.
14. Petta C, Amatya AR, Farr G, Chi I-c. An analysis of the personal reasons for discontinuing IUD use. Contraception. 1994;50:339–47.
15. Amatya R, Akhter H, McMahan J, Williamson N, Gates D, Ahmed Y. The effect of husband counseling on NORPLANT® contraceptive acceptability in Bangladesh. Contraception. 1994;50:263–73.
16. Sundaram AJF, Bankole A, Singh S. Factors associated with abortion-seeking and obtaining a safe abortion in Ghana. Stud Family Planning. 2012;43(4): 273–86.
17. Dimagi Inc. CommCare (version 2.40.1) [Mobile application software]. (2018).

18. Ali M, Cleland J. Contraceptive discontinuation in six developing countries: a cause-specific analysis author(s): Mohammed Ali and John Cleland source. Int Fam Plan Perspect. 1995;21(3):92–7.
19. Ghana Statistical Service (GSS), Ghana Health Service (GHS), and ICF. Ghana Maternal Health Survey 2017. Accra, Ghana: GSS, GHS, and ICF; 2018.
20. Sato R, Elewonibi B, Msuya S, Manongi R, Canning D, Shah I. Why do women discontinue contraception and what are the post-discontinuation outcomes? Evidence from the Arusha region, Tanzania. Sexual Reproductive Health Matters. 2020;28(1):172–321.
21. Yideta Z, Mekonen L, Seifu W, Shine S. Contraceptive discontinuation, method switching and associated factors among reproductive age women in Jimma town, Southwest Ethiopia, 2013. Fam Med Med Sci Res. 2017; 6(213):2.
22. Modey EJ, Aryeetey R, Adanu R. Contraceptive discontinuation and switching among Ghanaian women: evidence from the Ghana demographic and health survey, 2008. Afr J Reprod Health. 2014;18(1):84–92.
23. Croft, Trevor N., Aileen M. J. Marshall, Courtney K. Allen, et al. Guide to DHS Statistics. Rockville: ICF. 2018.
24. Nyarko SH. Spatial variations and socioeconomic determinants of modern contraceptive use in Ghana: a Bayesian multilevel analysis. PLoS One. 2020; 15(3):e0230139.
25. Aviisah PA, Dery S, Atsu BK, Yawson A, Alotaibi RM, Rezk HR, Guure C. Modern contraceptive use among women of reproductive age in Ghana: analysis of the 2003–2014 Ghana demographic and health surveys. BMC Womens Health. 2018;18(1):141.
26. Eliason S, Awoonor-Williams JK, Eliason C, Novignon J, Nonvignon J, Aikins M. Determinants of modern family planning use among women of reproductive age in the Nkwanta district of Ghana: a case–control study. Reprod Health. 2014;11(1):65.

11

Contraceptive prevalence rate and associated factors among reproductive age women in four emerging regions of Ethiopia

Delayehu Bekele[1], Feiruz Surur[1], Balkachew Nigatu[1], Alula Teklu[2], Tewodros Getinet[3], Munir Kassa[4], Merhawi Gebremedhin[5], Berhe Gebremichael[5*] and Yonas Abesha[6]

Abstract

Background: Ethiopia is the second most populous country in Africa, known for its high fertility and low contraceptive use. The magnitude of contraceptive use in the emerging regions of the country is below the national average. However, there is a paucity of evidence regarding the reasons for low contraceptive use in these regions. Therefore, this study aimed to assess contraceptive use and associated factors in the emerging regions of Ethiopia.

Methods: For the quantitative part, a community based cross-sectional study was conducted among 2891 reproductive age women who were selected by multistage sampling technique. Data were collected face to face using an open data kit software, and STATA version 14 was used for data analysis. Frequencies, percentages, summary measures and tables were used to summarize and present the data. Bivariable and multivariable logistic regression analyses were performed to identify factors associated with contraceptive use, by computing odds ratio with 95% confidence interval. Level of significance was considered at p-value < 0.05. For the qualitative part, phenomenological study was conducted among 252 health care workers and community members who were selected purposely. The data were collected by focused group discussions, in-depth interviews and key informant interviews. The data were audio-recorded in the local languages, and then translated to English verbatim. NVivo version 11 was used to analyze the data through a thematic analysis method.

Results: The overall contraceptive prevalence rate was 22.2%; with 11.7, 38.6, 25.5 and 8.8% for Afar, Benshangul Gumuz, Gambela and Somali Regions, respectively. Age, religion, education, marital status, family size, ideal children, knowledge and attitude were significantly associated with contraceptive use. Additionally, the qualitative study identified three themes as barriers to contraceptive use: individual, health care system and sociocultural factors.

Conclusions: Contraceptive prevalence rate was low in this study compared to the national average. Age, religion, education, marital status, family size, ideal children, knowledge and attitude were significantly associated with contraceptive use. From the qualitative aspect, individual, health care system and sociocultural factors were identified as barriers to contraceptive use. Therefore, the emerging regions of Ethiopia need special focus in increasing contraceptive use through behavioral influence/change.

Keywords: Contraceptive prevalence rate, Emerging regions, Ethiopia, Reproductive age women

* Correspondence: berhegere09@gmail.com
[5]School of Public Health, Haramaya University, Harar, Ethiopia

Introduction

Ethiopia is a low income country with poor health service coverage, including family planning (FP), particularly in the emerging regions [1]. The Ethiopian government has made a massive expansion of health facilities and trained human support capacity [2]. Accordingly, contraceptive prevalence rate (CPR) of the country has increased from 8% in 2000 to 41.4% in 2019 [3]. However, there was a significant regional variation in CPR among the emerging regions, with 3% in Somali Region and 38.5% in Benishangul Gumuz (BG) Region. Different factors such as age, education, family size, spousal communication on FP, number of live children, spousal approval on FP, ideal number of desired children, residence, religion, knowledge, and attitudes influence the uptake in contraceptive use [4–7].

Ethiopia has set an ambitious plan to improve primary health care services. To this effect, the Federal Ministry of Health (FMoH) has developed a health sector transformation plan (HSTP), with due emphasis given to FP. Accordingly, CPR was expected to reach 55% by 2020 [8]. However, 41.4% of married women were using modern contraceptive at national level, as of the Ethiopian Mini Demographic and Health Survey of 2019 [3]. Meanwhile, rapid expansion of health facilities/institutions and FP services task shifting to the lower levels, including health posts, has been made progressively since the last decade [2, 9]. Health post and health centers are the front line for FP services delivery and about 16,559 health posts and 3982 health centers are providing contraceptives in the nation [2], granting 90% access to FP [10].

Despite promising changes in the country, both community surveys and facility reports show that contraceptive use in the emerging regions is far below the national goal. The FMoH reported that contraceptive acceptance rate was very low in emerging regions [11]. In contrast, emerging regions are known to be highly polygamous (19 to 29%) in addition to high ideal desire of children (4.5–10.5) [12], with poor access to FP services [13]. To the level of our knowledge, there is no large-scale study done in the emerging regions with depth analysis. In response to this, a large scale study, with quantitative and qualitative approaches, was done to assess the overall contraceptive use and its associated factors among reproductive age women in the four emerging regions of Ethiopia.

Materials and methods

Study area and period

The study was conducted in the emerging regions of Ethiopia from 01 to 30 June 2017. According to the Ethiopian government, BG, Gambela, Afar and Somali are considered as emerging regions. Afar and Somali are pastoral regions while BG and Gambela are agrarian regions. According to 2014 population projection, the total population for Afar, BG, Gambela and Somali were 1, 678,000 (755,000 females), 976,000 (481,000 females), 396,000 (189,000 females), and 5,307,000 (2,420,000 females), respectively [14].

The health service delivery of Ethiopia has been restructured into a three-tier system. The first tier, the primary health care unit (PHCU), is composed of a health center (HC), satellite health posts (HP), and a primary hospital. While the second and third tiers are general hospitals and specialized hospitals, respectively. Family planning (FP) is provided extensively at the PHCU. According to the current approach, one woreda, with an average population of 100,000, needs to have one primary hospital, four HCs, and 20–33 HPs. So far, about 380 HCs and 1998 HPs are found in the four emerging regions, and the regions are characterized by a low health care provider to population ratio [2].

Study design and population

A community based cross-sectional study design was applied for the quantitative study while phenomenological study design/approach was used for the qualitative one. For the quantitative data, reproductive age women (15–49 years old) were the study population; whereas health professionals working at different levels and community inhabitants, including community and religious leaders were the study population for the qualitative study. Individuals with serious medical or mental health problems and known infertile women were excluded from the study.

Sample size determination and sampling procedure

Considering the sociocultural differences among the regions, the sample size was estimated independently for each emerging region. Since there was no similar literature showing the proportion of contraceptive use in the same context, we used $p = 50\%$ that provides the maximum sample size. Single population proportion formula was used by considering confidence level = 95%, margin of error = 1%, design effect = 2 and 10% for anticipated non-response. Mathematically, $\boldsymbol{n_h} = (\boldsymbol{z^2})\ (\boldsymbol{p})\ (\boldsymbol{1\text{-}p})\ (\boldsymbol{d})\ (\boldsymbol{r})\ /\ (\boldsymbol{c})\ (\mathbf{a})\ (\boldsymbol{e^2})$, where n_h = sample size in terms of number of households to be selected, z = level of confidence, p = proportion, d = design effect, r = multiplier to account for the anticipated rate of non-response, c = proportion of total population contributed by the target population of the survey, a = average household size, and e^2 = *margin* of error. Based on the formula, the final sample size was fixed at a total of 2929 women (i.e. 683, 805, 678 and 753 women for Afar, BG, Somali and Gambela Regions, respectively).

Regarding the sampling procedure, all woredas of each emerging region were listed (*woreda is the second smallest administrative unit in Ethiopia*). Accordingly, there were 30, 20, 53 and 13 woredas in Afar, BG, Somali and Gambela Regions, respectively. In the first stage, 20% of the total woredas were selected from each region by lottery method (i.e. 6, 4, 10 and 3 woredas for Afar, BG, Somali and Gambela Regions, respectively). Then, five kebeles (*kebele is the smallest administrative unit in Ethiopia*) were randomly selected from each woreda. In the third stage, two enumeration areas were randomly selected from each kebele. One enumeration area is expected to have an average of 80 households. Fresh households which were not documented in the lists received from woreda/kebele files were recorded by the research team and included in the sampling process. Finally, a systematic random sampling was used to select the actual participants of the study (i.e. the reproductive age women). Sampling intervals of 7, 4, 12 and 3 were calculated for Afar, BG, Somali and Gambela Regions, respectively, by dividing the total household list to the expected sample per enumeration areas. Lottery method was used to select the first household from the interval for each region. In case a household has two or more eligible women, one of them was selected using lottery method for interview.

For the qualitative part, a total of 252 individuals participated who were selected purposely; it included 15 focused group discussions (FGDs) ($n = 120$), 80 in-depth interviews (IDIs) ($n = 80$) and 52 key informant interviews (KIIs) ($n = 52$). Four FGDs were conducted in each region, except for Afar Region which were three FGDs. In addition, 20 IDIs and 13 KIIs were conducted in each region. The study participants for the FGDs were selected separately for male and female groups. Accordingly, eight of the FGDs were female groups and the remaining seven were male groups. The participants in the FGDs were community members, including community (clan) and religious leaders. The number of participants per FGD ranges from 6 to 12 individuals, and all discussions were conducted for duration of one to 2 h. On the other hand, 20 IDIs and 13 KIIs were conducted in each region. The participants for the IDIs were reproductive age women, and the participants for the KIIs were health care workers, and regional and woreda FP services coordinators. Each interview took duration of 30 min to an hour.

Data collection methods

For the quantitative study, a questionnaire was adapted from different prior literature and formatted to best respond to research questions. The questionnaire includes questions on socio-demography, reproductive history, and FP knowledge, attitude and utilization. The questions were developed and constructed by the investigators after reviewing different previous literature. Repeated discussions were conducted among the investigators during the development of the questionnaire. Each question was critically assessed in these group discussions to align with the research questions and objectives. Then, first draft of the questionnaire was reviewed by the FMoH technical team of expert, and their feedback was incorporated. The questionnaire was initially prepared in English, and was later translated into three local languages (Amharic, Somali, and Afar languages) by language experts for the purpose of data collection.

Data collectors and supervisors, who were native local languages speakers and health related professionals, were recruited and deployed to the data collection process. A survey operation guideline (SOG) was developed, and four-day training was provided by the investigators to assist field staffs. Most of the data collectors and supervisors were recruited from the respective regions; the training was conducted in each region separately. Data were collected face to face by the mobile application, open data kit (ODK). The overall data collection was supervised by the investigators centrally. The investigators had routine communications with the data collectors, supervisors and data manager through field visits, phone calls and social media communications. Supervisors were closely following and supporting the data collectors at the field sites and were communicating with the investigators regarding the data collection process on daily basis. Since the data were collected using ODK, the data collectors submit their data to central server and communicate with the investigators, supervisors, and data manager for any support they want during the field work. If connection was absent, the data collectors were able to save the data and continue data collection after reconnecting to an internet source. The data were submitted to and stored in a central data storage system (server) and the data manager at the central office routinely monitored the incoming data, notifying field staff and investigators if any potential errors occurred.

For the qualitative part, the study used FGD, IDI and KII guides to collect the data. The guiding questions were developed and assessed critically by the investigators and FMoH technical team of experts to fit with the research question (i.e. to find out the barriers of contraceptive use). The tool was initially developed in English and translated into the local languages by experts. Then, it was pretested before the actual data collection. Data collectors and supervisors were recruited considering fluency in the local language and previous experience in qualitative data collection/supervision. Four-day training was provided both to the data collectors and supervisors regarding the data collection process. The data collection team for the FGDs had male and female interviewers and collected the data from the male and female groups separately until the saturation of ideas in at least two consecutive FGDs. The collected data from the aforementioned three sources (i.e. from FGDs, IDIs and KIIs) were audio-recorded.

Operational definition

Emerging regions: In Ethiopia, emerging regions are defined as least developed regions characterized by poor level of infrastructure and services; border and internal (clan) conflicts; strongly traditional in social practices; predominantly rural with small, scattered and nomadic population; dominated by pastoral and agro-pastoral as the basic means of livelihood; gender inequalities; poor capacity of regional and local government systems to deliver basic infrastructures and services [15].

Contraceptive prevalence rate (CPR): is the proportion of reproductive age women who were using at least one modern contraceptive method during the study period; i.e. the proportion of current contraceptive users.

Contraceptive use: is the utilization of at least one modern contraceptive method by reproductive age women.

Current contraceptive users: are reproductive age women who were using at least one modern contraceptive method during the study period.

Data quality control

The questionnaire was translated into the local languages; i.e. Afar, Amharic and Somali languages for data collection and then translated back into English for analysis and reporting. The questionnaire was reviewed and assessed by technical team of experts from FMoH. Before the actual data collection, 5% of the questionnaires were pretested in woredas which were not included in this study. Data collectors and supervisors were trained for 4 days on the data collection process to have a common understanding. The data collectors were closely supervised by the supervisors and investigators. Completeness of each questionnaire was checked by the investigators and data manager on daily basis. To minimize transcription and translation inconsistencies of the qualitative data, the transcribed and translated data were compared to the audio-recorded one by other individuals with similar background and educational level.

Data processing and analysis

The quantitative data were first downloaded from the server as an Excel (.xls) files, and then exported to STATA version 14. Data were checked for completeness, coded, and cleaned before analysis. The characteristics of study participants was described and presented using frequencies, percentages, and summary measures such as mean and standard deviation (SD).

To assess knowledge of the participants, 12 questions related to the types of contraceptive methods were asked. Each question's response was coded as "1" for "yes" and "0" for "no". The internal consistency (α) of the items was checked and found to be 0.87, which indicates an acceptable level of reliability. Then, score was computed for each participant, which ranges from 0 to 12. The score was tested for normality and was found normally distributed. Finally, a composite knowledge variable was created from the score considering mean as a cut-off-point. Participants with a score of mean and above were classified as having "good knowledge", and those with a score of below the mean were categorized as having "poor knowledge".

Similarly, attitude of the participants on contraceptive methods was assessed using 9 attitude related questions. Some questions were in the form of a Likert scale while others were not. Thus, all the questions were re-coded in binary form. The internal consistency (α) of the items was found to be 0.78, indicating acceptable reliability. Just as for the knowledge assessment, attitude score was computed for each participant, ranging from 0 to 9. The score was tested for normality and was normally distributed. Finally, a composite variable was created from the score considering mean as a cut-off-point. Participants with a score of mean and above were classified as having a "favorable attitude" whereas those with a score of below the mean were categorized as having an "unfavorable attitude".

Contraceptive use (the dependent variable) was coded as "0" for non-users and "1" for users. A bivariable logistic regression analysis was performed to assess the association between the dependent variable and each independent variable. Variables with p-value ≤ 0.25 from the bivariable logistic regression analysis had been included in the final multivariable logistic regression analysis model to control for confounding factors. Multicollinearity test was done among the independent variables using variance inflation factor (VIF), and no significant (VIF > 10) collinearity was detected. A model goodness-of-fit was checked by a Hosmer-Lemeshow test and the model was well fitted ($p = 0.43$).

The collected qualitative data were first transcribed in the local languages and translated to English by native speakers of the local languages who had BSc degree in the field of health sciences. Then, the data were exported into NVivo version 11 for analysis and coding was done line by line, segment by segment, and paragraph based. All coded items were categorized into specific themes and sub-themes. Thematic analysis was applied to derive the main themes and sub-themes, and the results are presented by narrative approach.

Results

Socio-demographic characteristics of participants

Twenty-three woredas (Somali = 9, Afar = 6, BG =4, and Gambela = 4) were included in this study. With 99.1%

overall response rate, 643 (22.2%), 794 (27.5%), 752 (26%), and 702 (24.3%) of participants were from Afar, BG, Gambela, and Somali Regions, respectively. Mean age of the participants was 26.8 (± 7.5 SD) years, 2135 (73.8%) were from rural area, and 1525 (52.7%) had no formal education. More than three-fourth (76.5%) of participants were married or in union and 1713 (59.3%) were Muslims. The overall mean family size of the participants' households was 5.9 persons (± 2.8 SD), with the highest mean family size in Somali Region (6.7 ± 3.2 SD) followed by Afar and Gambela Regions (6.1 ± 2.7 SD for each). Regarding occupation, 89.4, 75.9, 58.2, and 75.1% of participants from Afar, BG, Gambela and Somali Regions were daily laborers/farmers, respectively. There was no participant from Afar Region with a monthly household income greater than the median (1000 Ethiopian Birr (ETB)), but participants from BG (55.5%), Gambela (48.8%) and Somali (67.6%) Regions reported monthly income greater than the median (1000 ETB). Six hundred twenty-six (21.6%) of participants had radio, 544 (18.8%) had television, and 1373 (47.5%) had their own cellphone. One-fourth (26.4%) of participants had history of watching/listening/reading TV/radio/newspaper at least once a week (Table 1).

Reproductive characteristics of participants

Self-reported numbers of women who had ever had sexual intercourse was 85.6% (91.7,89.2, 80.2 and 81.6% for Afar, BG, Gambela, Somali Regions, respectively). Mean age of participants at first sex was 17.2 ± 2.8 SD years. Of those, who ever had sex, 71.5, 61, 60.6 and 44.2% participants from Afar, BG, Gambela and Somali, respectively, had sex before turning 18 years old. More than three-fourth (76.5%) had history of pregnancy where the last pregnancies were unwanted for 24.4% of participants. Mean age at first pregnancy was 18.5 (± 2.9 SD) years and average number of live children was 4.2 ± (2.7 SD); average live children was higher for Somali women (4.4 ± 2.8 SD) while lower for BG (3 ± 2.1 SD). More than one-third (69.3%) of the participants had a desire to have additional children in the future. Mean desire of ideal children was 7.5 (± 3.5 SD) with the highest mean ideal children (10.2 ± 3.5SD) in Somali Region and lowest in BG Region (5.5 ± 2.9 SD). About 5.4 and 13.4% of ever pregnant mothers reported a history of stillbirth and abortion, respectively (Table 1).

Knowledge and attitude of women on family planning

The study showed that 2394 (82.8%) of the participants had knowledge of at least one contraceptive method. Only one third (33%) knew six or more (half of the list) contraceptives types. The mean knowledge score of FP was 4.3 (± 3.4 SD) and 1254 (43.4%) of the respondents had good FP knowledge. Good knowledge was higher for BG (62.7%) followed by Gambela (41.1%) women. The most common contraceptive methods among participants were injectables, (72.3%), followed by pills (67.6%), and implants (51.7%). Health Extension Workers (HEWs) were the major source of contraceptive methods for 45.2% of the respondents, with health care providers (28.8%) and friends (24.7%) following as sources for the participants (Table 2).

The mean score for the overall attitude of FP was 4.0 (± 2.5 SD), and attitude mean score was higher among current contraceptive users (6.1 ± 1.8 SD) compared with non-users (4 ± 2.4 SD). More than half (52.3%) of the respondents had a favorable attitude (≥ mean score) towards FP. The mean attitude score of contraceptive use was also differed by location of residence where 4.5 (± 2.4 SD) for urban residents and 3.8 (± 2.5 SD) among rural dwellers. Meanwhile, there was a high regional variation in attitude mean score of contraceptive use with the lowest score in Somali Region (2.4 ± 1.8 SD) and highest score in BG Region (5.8 ± 2SD) (Table 3).

Contraceptive prevalence rate

The overall CPR was 579 (22.2%); it was 11.7, 38.6, 25.5, and 8.8% for Afar, BG, Gambela and Somali Regions, respectively. The contraceptive prevalence rate (CPR) was higher among urban than rural women (28.4% versus 19.9%). Similarly, CPR was higher among Christian than Muslim women (32.3% versus 15%). The contraceptive prevalence rate (CPR) was 12.4, 32.2, 29 and 43.3% for women with no formal education, primary level, secondary level, and above secondary level, respectively. Contraceptive prevalence rate (CPR) was higher among employed than daily laborer/farmer women (41% versus 21.6%). Women with family monthly income above the median (26.8%) had higher CPR than those with less than the median income (18.5%). Besides, women who listen/watch radio/TV at least once per week had higher CPR (34%) compared with those who never listen/watch (18.1%). Women with good knowledge and favorable attitude had CPR of 36.1 and 38.2%, respectively.

Factors associated with contraceptive use

The bivariable logistic regression analysis result showed that large family size, having high number of live children, and desiring high number of ideal children were negatively associated with contraceptive use. Similarly, being from urban area, older age, being married or in union, being Christian, higher education level, having an educated husband, having radio/TV, listening/watching radio/TV, high monthly family income, being employed, and having good knowledge and favorable attitude towards FP were positively associated with contraceptive use ($p < 0.05$) (Table 4).

Table 1 Socio-demographic and reproductive characteristics of reproductive age women in four emerging regions of Ethiopia (in frequencies and percentages), 2017

Background characteristics	Emerging regions				
	Afar ($n = 643$)	BG ($n = 794$)	Gambela ($n = 752$)	Somali ($n = 702$)	Total ($n = 2891$)
Rural residence	468(72.8)	652(82.1)	528(70.2)	487(69.4)	2135(73.8)
Age (in years)					
15–24	222(34.5)	326(41.0)	383(51.0)	260(37.0)	1191(41.2)
25–34	331(51.5)	292(36.8)	271(36.0)	305(43.5)	1199(41.5)
35–49	90(14.0)	176(22.2)	98(13.0)	137(19.5)	501(17.3)
Educational status					
No education	504(78.4)	305(38.4)	219(29.1)	497(70.8)	1525(52.7)
Primary	107(16.6)	318(40.1)	279(37.1)	95(13.5)	799(27.6)
Secondary	17(2.6)	93(11.7)	178(23.7)	72(10.3)	360(12.5)
Above Secondary	15(2.3)	78(9.8)	76(10.1)	38(5.4)	207(7.2)
Partner's education					
No education	414(64.4)	207(26.1)	170(22.6)	359(51.1)	1150(39.8)
Primary	77(12)	238(30)	113(15)	36(5.1)	464(16.1)
Secondary	27(4.2)	97(12.2)	125(16.6)	57(8.1)	306(10.6)
Above Secondary	28(4.4)	94(11.8)	181(24.1)	53(7.5)	356(12.3)
Not Applicable	97(15.1)	158(19.9)	163(21.7)	197(28.1)	615(21.3)
Family monthly income > median(1000 ETB)	0	441(55.5)	366(48.8)	474(67.6)	1281(44.4)
Muslim in religion	622(96.7)	387(48.7)	26(3.5)	678(96.6)	1713(59.3)
Employment status					
Labor work	575(89.4)	603 (75.9)	438 (58)	527(57)	2143(74.1)
Merchant	22(3.4)	50(6.3)	35(4.6)	68(9.7)	175 (6.1)
Employee	21(3.2)	48(6)	74(9.8)	34(4.8)	177(6.12)
Student	25(3.8)	93(11.7)	205(27.3)	73(10.4)	396 (13.7)
Having radio/TV/mobile phone	386(60)	482(60.7)	390(51.8)	432(61.5)	1690(58.5)
Listening Radio/TV at least once a week	183(28.5)	309(38.9)	109(14.5)	161(23)	762(26.4)
Family size					
1–5	292(45.4)	504(63.5)	353(46.9)	271(38.6)	1420(49.1)
6–10	314(48.8)	275(34.6)	358(47.6)	352(50.1)	1299(44.9)
>=11	37(5.8)	15(2)	41(5.4)	79(11.3)	172(6)
Ideal number of children > mean (5 children)	(536(83.4)	401 (50.5)	573(76.2)	666(94.9	2176(75.3)
Ever had sexual intercourse	590(91.7)	708(89.2)	603(80.2)	573(81.6)	2474(85.6)
Mean Age at first sex	16.6(2.3)	16.8(3.1)	17.2(2.8)	18(2.9)	17.2(2.8)
Practice sex before 18 years	363(71.5)	411(61)	368(60.6)	244(44.2)	1386(59.2)
Last pregnancy wanted	353(68.7)	498(78.5)	320(59)	501(96)	1672(75.6)
Total number of pregnancy > = mean (5 children)	233(45.3)	212(33.4)	158(29.2)	281(53.8)	884(40)
Ever face abortion	54(8.4)	110(13.9)	57(7.6)	75(10.7)	296(13.4)
Ever face stillbirth	0	50(7.9)	38(7.1)	32(6.1)	120(5.4)
Having live children > 4	136(26.5)	130(20.5)	75(13.8)	164(31.4)	505(22.8)

Table 2 Knowledge of contraceptive methods (in frequencies and percentages) among reproductive-age women in the four emerging regions of Ethiopia, 2017

Variable	Emerging regions				
	Afar (*n* = 643)	BG (*n* = 794)	Gambella (*n* = 752)	Somali (*n* = 702)	Total (*n* = 2891)
Know at least one contraceptive method	581(90.4)	761(95.8)	538(71.5)	514(73.2)	2394(82.8)
Know male condom	313(48.7)	475(59.8)	397(52.8)	200(28.5)	1385(47.9)
Know pill	462(71.9)	664(83.6)	428(56.9)	400(57.0)	1954(67.6)
Know injectable	506(78.7)	730(91.9)	446(59.3)	407(58.0)	2089(72.3)
Know IUD	95(14.8)	471(59.3)	153(20.3)	96(13.7)	815(28.2)
Know implants	211(32.8)	696(87.7)	336(44.7)	252(35.9)	1495(51.7)
Know tubal ligation	73(11.4)	204(25.7)	132(17.6)	47(6.7)	456(15.8)
Know vasectomy	56(8.7)	97(12.2)	115(15.3)	38(5.4)	306(10.6)
Female condom	77(12.0)	173(21.8)	256(34.0)	71(10.1)	577(20.0)
Know LAM	349(54.3)	244(30.7)	158(21.0)	368(52.4)	1119(38.7)
Know rhythm	230(35.8)	388(48.9)	285(37.9)	224(31.9)	1127(39.0)
Know withdrawal	109(17.0)	171(21.5)	72(9.6)	76(10.8)	428(14.8)
Know emergency contraceptive	141(21.9)	187(23.6)	181(24.1)	122(17.4)	631(21.8)
Good overall knowledge (composite)	222(34.5)	498(62.7)	309(41.1)	225(32.1)	1254(43.4)
Source of contraceptive information					
Friends	170(26)	208(26.2)	174(23.1)	163(23.2)	715(24.7)
School	90(14)	186(23.4)	158(21)	77(11)	511(17.7)
Family	73(11)	95(12.0)	44(5.9)	47(6.7)	259(9)
HEWs	310(48.2)	561(70.7)	276(36.7)	159(22.6)	1306(45.2)
Health care providers	220(34.2)	300(37.8)	124(16.5)	190(27.1)	834(28.8)
Radio	107(16.6)	93(11.7)	4(0.5)	25(3.6)	229(7.9)
Television	62(9.6)	92(11.6)	40(5.3)	63(9)	257(8.9)
Printed-materials	8(1.2)	3(0.4)	0(0.0)	1(0.1)	12(0.4)
Internet/Social Media	8(12)	1(0.1)	4(0.5)	20(2.8)	33(1.1)

In the multivariable logistic regression analysis, being in the age group of 35–49 years, being married, being Christian, primary level or more education, and having good knowledge and favorable attitude towards FP were positive predictors of contraceptive use. Whereas, having large family size and high ideal children were negatively associated with contraceptive use ($p < 0.05$) (Table 4).

In addition to the quantitative result, three themes of barriers of contraceptive use were identified from the qualitative study. These are individual, health care system and sociocultural factors.

The individual factors include four sub-themes: poor FP knowledge, lack of women's decision-making power, fear of side effects, and being busy. Poor FP knowledge was reported by most of the participants as one of the primary bottlenecks to contraceptive use. The participants also responded that fear of side effects was a barrier to use contraceptive methods in the study areas. Moreover, most of the participants agreed that contraceptive use was primarily decided by husbands and this was higher for rural than urban residents. Participants also indicated that there are women who were unable to properly use contraceptive methods due to being busy of domestic workloads.

> *"…..we want to use contraceptive methods, but we fear the side effects such as excessive bleeding and infertility. In addition, men are decision makers and have great role in protecting us from using contraceptives. My husband decides on me regarding every activity done in our life. There are women in our community who have interest to use contraceptives, but refused by their husbands."* ***IDI participant (reproductive age woman), from Afar Region***

The health care system factors include four sub-themes: lack of accessibility to contraceptive methods, low financial support, lack of guiding policy, and low monitoring system. Majority of the respondents concluded that poor transportation access, lack of roads,

Table 3 Attitude of contraceptive methods (in frequency and percentage) among reproductive-age women in the four emerging regions of Ethiopia, 2017

Variable	Emerging regions				
	Afar (*n* = 643)	BG (*n* = 794)	Gambella (*n* = 752)	Somali (*n* = 702)	Total (*n* = 2891)
Discussion with one's partner on FP					
Frequently	29(6.1)	177(28.0)	115(24.1)	35(7.1)	356(17.1)
Sometimes	51(10.7)	239(37.8)	109(22.8)	30(6.0)	429(20.6)
Rarely	78(16.3)	58(9.2)	20(4.2)	36(7.3)	192(9.2)
Never	320(66.9)	159(25.1)	234(49.0)	395(79.6)	1108(53.1)
Discussion with family/relative					
Frequently	14(2.2)	52(6.5)	25(3.3)	6(0.9)	97(3.4)
Sometimes	53(8.2)	220(27.7)	108(14.4)	29(4.1)	410(14.2)
Rarely	68(10.6)	116(14.6)	64(8.5)	70(10.0)	318(11.0)
Never	508(79.0)	406(51.1)	555(73.8)	597 (85.0)	2066(71.5)
Discussion with friends					
Frequently	23(3.6)	66(8.3)	51(6.8)	14(2.0)	154(5.3)
Sometimes	67(10.4)	239(30.1)	180(23.9)	53(7.5)	539(18.6)
Rarely	77(12)	143(18.0)	79(10.5)	73(10.4)	372(12.9)
Never	476(74.0)	346(43.6)	442(58.8)	562(80.1)	1826(63.2)
Contraception has benefit for women					
Yes	264(41.1)	691(87.0)	452(60.1)	323(46.0)	1730(59.8)
No	194(30.2)	45(5.7)	95(12.6)	110(15.70)	444(15.4)
Don't know	185(28.8)	58(7.3)	205(273)	269(38.3)	717(24.8)
Large family size affects economic condition negatively					
Strongly agree	54(8.4)	257(32.4)	163(21.7)	37 (5.3)	511(17.7)
Agree	174(27.1)	417(52.5)	259(34.4)	123(17.5)	973(33.7)
Neutral	52(8.1)	31(3.9)	91(12.1)	51(7.3)	225(7.8)
Disagree	269(41.8)	69(8.7)	178(23.7)	349(49.7)	865(29.9)
Strongly disagree	94(14.6)	20(2.5)	61(8.1)	142(20.2)	317(11.0)
Large family size earns respect by the husband					
Strongly agree	129(20.1)	32(4.0)	78(10.4)	138(19.7)	377(13.0)
Agree	226(35.1)	237(29.8)	144(19.1)	324(46.2)	931(32.2)
Neutral	69(10.7)	77(9.7)	99(13.2)	79(11.3)	324(11.2)
Disagree	182(28.3)	419(52.8)	325(43.2)	119(17.0)	1045(36.1)
Strongly disagree	37(5.8)	29(3.7)	106(14.1)	42(6.0)	214(7.4)
Large family size earns the respect of the community					
Strongly agree	107(16.6)	26(3.3)	75(10.0)	157(22.4)	365(12.6)
Agree	212(33.0)	252(31.7)	164(21.8)	327(46.6)	955(33.0)
Neutral	92(14.3)	87(11.0)	111(14.8)	81(11.5)	371(12.8)
Disagree	183(28.5)	406(51.1)	294(39.1)	105(15.0)	988(34.2)
Strongly disagree	49(7.6)	23(2.9)	108(14.4)	32(4.6)	212(7.3)
Large family size earns respect by a religious leader					
Strongly agree	156(24.3)	18(2.3)	98(13.0)	122(17.4)	394(13.6)
Agree	169(26.3)	253(31.9)	163(21.7)	297(42.3)	882(30.5)
Neutral	120(18.7)	171(21.5)	101(13.4)	122(17.4)	514(17.8)
Disagree	152(23.6)	329(41.4)	248(33.0)	135(19.2)	864(29.9)

Table 3 Attitude of contraceptive methods (in frequency and percentage) among reproductive-age women in the four emerging regions of Ethiopia, 2017 *(Continued)*

Variable	Emerging regions				
	Afar (n = 643)	BG (n = 794)	Gambella (n = 752)	Somali (n = 702)	Total (n = 2891)
Strongly disagree	46(7.2)	23(2.9)	142(18.9)	26(3.7)	237(8.2)
Large family size affects maternal and child health					
Strongly agree	78(12.1)	190(23.9)	125(16.6)	46(6.6)	439(15.2)
Agree	168(26.1)	455(57.3)	263(35.0)	266(37.9)	1152(39.8)
Neutral	79(12.3)	44(5.5)	106(14.1)	88(12.5)	317(11.0)
Disagree	250(38.9)	94(11.8)	198(26.3)	240(34.2)	782(27.0)
Strongly disagree	68(10.6)	11(1.4)	60(8.0)	62(8.8)	201(7.0)
Overall attitude (composite)					
Favorable	214(33.3)	687(86.5)	464(61.7)	146(20.8)	1511(52.3)
Unfavorable	429(66.7)	107(13.5)	288(38.3)	556(79.2)	1380(47.7)

long distances to access health facilities and shortage of available contraceptive methods were the reasons to low contraceptive use. Shortage of funds at the health facility and health administration levels was also indicated as a major reason for low contraceptive use. Health professionals and FP service coordinators indicated that even though they had good plans and strategies regarding FP services, they were unable to implement them due to budget problems. In addition, they pointed out that there were poor monitoring systems and guiding policies on FP for the emerging regions.

> *" ... because of distance and poor road infrastructures, it is difficult to provide FP services; the areas are not accessible to transport, especially during the summer. There are also problems that affect the provision of FP services such as shortage of budget, poor monitoring systems and lack of clear policies and guidelines."* ***KII participant, FP service coordinator from Somali Region***

The sociocultural factors include seven sub-themes: male dominance, desire for large family size, poor attitudes towards FP, a nomadic lifestyle, myths on FP, fear of adultery, and poor FP acceptance. Almost all participants agreed that a woman who wishes to use contraceptive methods should first obtain her husband's approval. Women who use contraceptives without the knowledge of their husbands may face divorce, physical attack, family conflict, polygamy and mistrust. Another factor which was reported as a reason to low contraceptive use was the desirability of a large family. Communities in these emerging regions generally want to have a large family size in order to cope up with inter and intra clan competitions. As a result, clan leaders do not allow their clan members to use contraceptive methods in order to increase clan size.

Participants also reported that there is a belief in the community that modern contraceptive use requires a balanced diet and failure to do so results in negative health outcomes. Thus, women with shortage of food are not recommended taking contraceptives. Another reported misperception was some individuals believe the provision of FP is carried out in order to accomplish government interests, and the community is not yet well convinced on the issues of FP. Some individuals also believe that contraceptive use is perceived as killing the already conceived life and therefore is considered as a sin by the followers of some religions.

> *" ... we need to have children with no gaps and nothing used. Allah feeds for all, including our children. Our community should not use contraceptives. We are Muslims; we do not use contraceptives because our religion does not allow us to do so and utilization is considered as sin."* ***Female FGD participant, from Somali Region***

Another finding from this report indicated that letting a wife use contraceptives is equivalent to letting her commit adultery. There is a belief in the community that if a mother uses contraceptives, she will have large periods of time between births, making her healthy, beautiful, and very attractive to other men. Consequently, she may commit adultery.

> *".....when a woman starts to use contraceptives, she has more time to care herself well and becomes beautiful and attractive. This can lead her to commit adultery which may finally result in divorce and other social problems. Therefore, I do not recommend women to use contraceptive methods."* ***Male FGD participant, from BG Region***

Table 4 Factors associated with current contraceptive use among reproductive age women in four emerging regions of Ethiopia, 2017

Independent variables	Categories	Contraceptive use		COR (95% CI)	AOR (95% CI)
		Yes	No		
Residence	Rural	382	1531	1.00	1.00
	Urban	197	496	1.6(1.3, 1.9)**	1.1 (0.8, 1.6)
Age	15–24	223	658	1.00	1.00
	25–34	234	613	1.1(0.9, 1.3)	1.2 (0.9, 1.8)
	35–49	62	333	0.5(0.4, 0.7) *	1.6(1.1, 2.4)*
Marital status	Single	39	478	1.00	1.00
	Married	519	1423	4.5(3.2, 6.2)**	8.4(5.5, 12.7)**
	Others	21	126	2(1.1, 3.6)*	4.5(2.0, 9.9)**
Family size	1–5	407	874	1.00	1.00
	6–10	167	999	0.4(0.3, 0.4)**	0.65(0.5, 0.8)*
	≥ 11	5	154	0.1(0.03, 0.2)**	0.2(0.1, 0.5)*
Religion	Muslim	228	1290	1.00	1.00
	Non-Muslim	351	737	2.7(2.2, 3.3)**	1.3(1.1, 1.7)*
Level of education	No	168	1192	1.00	1.00
	Primary	235	496	3.4(2.6, 4.2)**	2.1(1.6, 2.8)**
	Secondary	95	233	2.8(2.1, 3.8)**	1.8(1.2, 2.7)*
	Above secondary	81	106	5.4(3.8, 7.5)**	2.1(1.3, 3.4)*
Husband level of education	No	121	891	1.00	1.00
	Primary	165	246	4.9(3.7, 6.4)**	1.4(1.0, 2.1
	Secondary	111	154	5.3(3.8, 7.2)**	1.1(0.7, 1.8)
	Above secondary	126	183	5.1(3.7, 6.8)**	1.1(0.6, 1.9)
Occupation	Farmer	410	1492	1.00	1.00
	Merchant	50	118	1.5(1.1, 2.1)*	1.2(0.7, 2.4)
	Employee	66	95	2.5(1.8, 3.5)**	1.2(0.6, 2.4)
	Student	53	322	0.59(0.4, 0.8)**	1.2(0.60, 2.2)
Household monthly income	< 1000 ETB	266	1175	1.00	1.00
	≥ 1000 ETB	312	850	1.6(1.3, 1.9)**	1.1(0.8, 1.5)
Having TV/Radio	No	419	1688	1.00	1.00
	Yes	160	339	1.9(1.5, 2.4)**	1.1(0.8, 1.6)
Watch/listening TV/radio	No	344	1543	1.00	1.00
	Yes	235	484	2.2(1.8, 2.6)**	1.1(.8, 1.6)
Total number of live children	≤ 4	506	1491	1.00	1.00
	> 4	73	536	0.42(0.3, 0.5)**	0.8(0.5, 1.2)
Number of ideal desired children	1–4	260	394	1.00	1.00
	≥ 5	319	1633	0.3(0.2, 0.4)**	0.8(0.6, 0.9)*
Knowledge on FP	Poor	169	1302	1.00	1.00
	Good	410	725	4.4(3.0, 5.3)**	6.6(4.6, 9.6)**
Attitude towards FP	Unfavorable	54	1176	1.00	1.00
	Favorable	525	851	13.4(10.0, 18.0)**	2.1(1.6, 2.8)**

* = *p*-value < 0.05, ** = *p*-value< 0.001, *CI* Confidence interval, *COR* Crude odds ratio, *AOR* Adjusted odds ratio

Discussion

With the objective to assess the magnitude of current contraceptive use and associated factors, this study revealed that the overall CPR was 22.2%; high variation was observed in CPR among regions (11.7% in Afar, 38.6% in BG, 25.5% in Gambela and 8.8% in Somali). Age, marital status, family size, religion, educational status, ideal desire of children, knowledge and attitude were found statistically significant predictors for current contraceptive use. Additionally, the qualitative finding identified three themes (individual, health care system and sociocultural related factors) as main barriers of contraceptive use.

The overall CPR in this study was lower than study findings from different parts of Ethiopia, which ranges between 38.3% in Mojo (Oromia Region) and 82.6% in Bench Maji (Southern Nations, Nationalities and Peoples Region) [5, 8, 16–20]. Moreover, the prevalence was lower than study reports from Turkey (53%) [21] and Haryana state of India (62%) [22]. These variations may be attributed to the differences in culture, geographic location, religious perspectives, and scope of the study including study setting. Besides, women living in emerging regions have lower access to contraceptive methods and contraceptive acceptance rate [11]. Furthermore, the qualitative aspect of this study identified individual, health care system and sociocultural barriers against contraceptive use, and these barriers might have contributed to the low CPR in this study.

Inter-regional variation was also observed in CPR. The current study showed CPR was 11.7% for Afar Region which is almost similar with the finding of the Ethiopian Mini Demographic and Health Survey of 2019 (12.7%) [3], but higher than another study done in the region (8.5%) [23]. The current CPR of BG Region (38.6%) was similar with the aforementioned national mini survey finding (38.5%), while the CPR of Somali Region (8.8%) was a bit higher than the national mini survey finding (3%). In Gambela Region, CPR was 25.5% which is lower than the national mini survey finding (33.8%). These all discrepancies may be attributed to differences in sample size and scale of the studies.

In this study, urban and rural residence was not stratified; rather it was randomly selected, potentially giving over representation of urban residents which is ideally assumed as high contraceptive users. Pocket study done in the Kebri Beyah of Somali Region showed similar finding with the current study [10]; however, studies done in the Assosa Woreda of BG Region showed significant variation with the current findings [24]. This variation may be related with sample size and residence of study participants.

The participants in the age group of 35–49 years were more likely to use contraceptives compared to those in the age group of 15–24 years. This indicates that women mostly start using contraceptives after they achieve the desired number of children. Women also get more freedom from husband pressure as they get older, hence this may give them an opportunity to use more contraceptives than younger women. This finding was in line with studies done in Dodota Woreda (Oromoia Region of Ethiopia) [7], but contradicts with study done in the town of Arba Minch (Southern Nations, Nationalities and Peoples Region, Ethiopia) [8].

Religion was also found to be an important predictor of contraceptive use that Christians were more likely to use contraceptives compared to Muslims. As insured by the qualitative study, the Muslim religion encourages its followers to have more children, and therefore may see using contraceptives as against this goal.

Married women were more likely to use contraceptives than unmarried ones. Similarly, family size categories of 6–10 and 11 or above were at lower odds of contraceptive use than those with family size of 1–5. Meanwhile, desiring an ideal number of children greater than five was negatively associated with current contraceptive use. This finding contradicts with a research conducted in the town of Modjo, Ethiopia [18], where higher fertility was a significant predictor of contraceptive use; this difference may be attributed to sample size, scope of the study, and sociocultural character of participants. Logically, those with family size less than five are younger than their respective counter parts; as a result, the young could be more educated than the older groups as educational resources are improving with time in developing countries. Moreover, young generations use social media more; hence, they may have better access to FP than older generation. Older generations could also stick highly towards religion and culture. It is also logical that women who desire minimum ideal children can use contraceptives to fulfill their objectives. The impact of different socio-demographic variables like a high level of education, high income, and residence, or low desire of ideal children can indirectly affect the use of contraceptives.

Educational level of participants was identified as a significant factor of contraceptive use in this study. Women with education levels of primary, secondary and above secondary were more likely to use contraceptives than less educated women. Educated women can better understand the advantage of FP use. Women's power of decision-making and personal income also increases with education level which ultimately helps couples to accept contraceptive use easier. Different studies conducted in different part of Ethiopia and other countries have revealed similar finding with this study [7, 8, 17, 18, 23, 25, 26].

Participants who had a good knowledge and favorable attitude on FP were more likely to use contraceptive than their respective counterparts. Even though education and knowledge have not shown any co-linearity, they are interrelated to each other in that mothers may have favorable attitude as a result of education and good knowledge of FP. Having good knowledge is a prerequisite to having a favorable attitude–both good knowledge and favorable attitude are prerequisite to be a FP user provided that an informed choice is an option. This finding was in line with pocket studies conducted in Ethiopia and elsewhere in other countries [4, 8, 20, 23, 26–28]. It is also supported by the qualitative results of this study that poor knowledge, poor attitude and poor acceptance of FP were the barriers to contraceptive use.

Strength and limitations of the study

The strength of the study is it used large sample size, is multi-center (involving four regions) and covered quantitative and qualitative approaches. However, the study might not show the causal relationship since it used cross-sectional design.

Conclusions

Overall, CPR was low (22.2%) in the emerging regions of Ethiopia compared to the national magnitude, which is 41.4%. Age, marital status, family size, religion, education, ideal number of children, and knowledge and attitude toward FP were important predictors for current contraceptive use among women in the emerging regions. High regional variation in CPR was observed. Most of the factors that affect the contraceptive use can be improved through behavioral change. Therefore, FMoH, the respective regional health bureaus, and developmental partners should work on improving mass communication through media outlets, and health education by health extension workers should be further strengthened. Similarly, woreda health offices along with community representatives, religious leaders, and local stakeholders should give more emphasis on disseminating FP related messages; this would ultimately bring positive change through improved FP usage.

Abbreviations

AOR: Adjusted odds ratio; BG: Benshangul gumuz; CI: Confidence interval; COR: Crude odds ratio; CPR: Contraceptive prevalence rate; ETB: Ethiopian birr; FGD: Focused group discussion; FMoH: Federal ministry of health; FP: Family planning; HC: Health center; HP: Health post; IDI: In-depth interview; KII: Key informant interview; ODK: Open data kit; PHCU: Primary health care unit; SD: Standard deviation; SOG: Survey operation guideline; VIF: Variance inflation factor

Acknowledgments

We would like to extend our gratitude to FMOH for providing budget and technical support. Heads of regional health bureau of the four emerging regions, supervisors and data collectors are acknowledged for their unreserved effort. Also, we are grateful to Mr. Asher Maria for his language edition. Lastly but not least, we acknowledge all participants.

Authors' contributions

The study was created and designed by TG, DB, FS, AM, YA, BN, and MK. Detail analysis was done by TG, MG and BG. The manuscript was prepared by MG and BG, and then edited by TG, DB, FS, AM, YA, BN. All the authors provided support throughout the process, read, and approved the final manuscript.

Author details

[1]Department of Obstetrics and Gynecology, Saint Paul's Hospital Millennium Medical College, Addis Ababa, Ethiopia. [2]Research Office, Saint Paul's Hospital Millennium Medical College, Addis Ababa, Ethiopia. [3]Public Health Department, Saint Paul's Hospital Millennium Medical College, Addis Ababa, Ethiopia. [4]Federal Ministry of Health, Ministry's Office, Addis Ababa, Ethiopia. [5]School of Public Health, Haramaya University, Harar, Ethiopia. [6]Private Consultancy Practice, Addis Ababa, Ethiopia.

References

1. AssefaY HPS, Gilks CF, Admassu M, Tesfaye D, WVan D. Primary health care contributions to universal health coverage, Ethiopia. Bull World Health Organ. 2020;98:894–905 Available from: https://www.ncbi.nlm.nih.gov/pmc/articles/PMC7716108/pdf/BLT.19.248328.pdf.
2. Federal Democratic Republic of Ethiopia Ministry of Health. Health Sector Transformation Plan: 2015/16–2019/20. 2015. Available from: https://www.globalfinancingfacility.org/sites/gff_new/files/Ethiopia-health-system-transformation-plan.pdf.
3. Ethiopian Public Health Institute (EPHI) [Ethiopia] and ICF. Ethiopia Mini Demographic and Health Survey 2019: Key indicators. Rockville, Maryland, USA: EPHI and ICF; 2019. Available from: https://dhsprogram.com/pubs/pdf/PR120/PR120.pdf
4. Lwelamira J, Mnyamagola G, Msaki MM. Knowledge, attitude and practice (KAP) towards modern contraceptives among married women of reproductive age in Mpwapwa District, Central Tanzania. Curr Res J Soc Sci. 2012;3:235–45 Available from: http://www.airitilibrary.com/Publication/alDetailedMesh?DocID=20413246-201205-201512250021-201512250021-235-245.
5. Lamaro T, Tadele N. Family planning service utilization and its associated factors among married women in Benchi-Maji Zone, Southwest, Ethiopia: community-based cross-sectional study. Clin Mother Child Health. 2017;14(258). https://doi.org/10.4172/2090-7214.1000258.
6. Aynekulu WT, Buruh G. Measuring fertility intention, family planning utilization and associated factors among married couples in Mekelle City, Tigray, Ethiopia, cross sectional study. Int J Pharm Bio Sci. 2013;6:2278–3997 Available from: http://ijpbsf.com/journal%20data/IJPBSFSept13_1_15_Ethiopia.pdf.
7. Kedir GJ, Legesse TW, Seid Y. Contraceptive utilization among couples and associated factors in Dodota district, Oromia Region, Ethiopia. Biomed J Sci Tech Res. 2018;4(1). https://doi.org/10.26717/BJSTR.2018.04.000986 Available from: https://biomedres.us/pdfs/BJSTR.MS.ID.000986.pdf.
8. Samuel A, Uliso A, Olle B, Dambe D, Nigatu M, Sorato MM. Assessment of modern contraceptive method utilization and associated factors among women of reproductive age group in Arba Minch town, SNNPR, Ethiopia: community based cross-sectional study. Open J Epidemiol. 2017;15(6):367–74.
9. Federal Democratic Republic of Ethiopia Ministry of Health. Health extension program evaluation and improvement document: Amharic version. 2018. Available from: http://repository.iifphc.org/bitstream/handle/123456789/511/HEP%20Optimization_Discussion%20%20document%202010EC.pdf?sequence=1&isAllowed=y.
10. Nigussie AT, Girma D, Tura G. Postpartum family planning utilization and associated factors among women who gave birth in the past 12 months, Kebribeyah town, Somali region, Eastern Ethiopia. J Women's Health Care. 2016;5(6):1–12. https://doi.org/10.4172/2167-0420.1000340.
11. Federal Democratic Republic of Ethiopia Ministry of Health. Health and health related indicators: Version 1, Ethiopian Fiscal Year 2007. 2015. Available from: https://www.dktethiopia.org/sites/default/files/PublicationFiles/Health%20and%20Health%20Related%20Indicator%202008.pdf.
12. Central Statistical Agency (CSA) and ICF. Ethiopia Demographic and Health Survey. Addis Ababa, Ethiopia, and Rockville, Maryland, USA: CSA and ICF; 2016. Available from: https://dhsprogram.com/pubs/pdf/FR328/FR328.pdf

13. Federal Democratic Republic of Ethiopia Ministry of Health. National guideline for family planning services in Ethiopia. 2011. Available from: https://stage.prb.org/wp-content/uploads/2018/05/National-Guideline-for-Family-Planning-Services-in-Ethiopia-2011.pdf.
14. Central Statistical Agency (CSA). Population projections for Ethiopia; 2007-2037. 2013. Available from: https://www.statsethiopia.gov.et/wp-content/uploads/2019/05/ICPS-Population-Projection-2007-2037-produced-in-2012.pdf.
15. Government of Ethiopia Ministry of Federal Affairs. Emerging Regions Development Program (ERDP). 2011. Available from: https://info.undp.org/docs/pdc/Documents/ETH/00047309_Emerging%20Regions%20Development%20Programme%20(00056833).pdf.
16. Yitayal M, Berhane Y, Worku A, Kebede Y. The community-based health extension program significantly improved contraceptive utilization in west gojjam zone, Ethiopia. J Multidisciplinary Healthc. 2014;7:201 Available from: https://www.ncbi.nlm.nih.gov/pmc/articles/PMC4031203/pdf/jmdh-7-201.pdf.
17. Gebremeskel F, Getahun D, Kanko T, Tilahun A, Endrias B, Alamirew B, et al. Prevalence of modern contraceptive utilization and associated factors among women of reproductive age group at Boditi town, Wolayita zone, SNNPR, Ethiopia. Am J Nurs Sci 2017; 6(6): 447–453. Available from: http://www.sciencepublishinggroup.com/journal/paperinfo?journalid=152&doi=https://doi.org/10.11648/j.ajns.20170606.12.
18. Gizaw A, Regassa N. Family planning service utilization in mojo town, Ethiopia: a population based study. J Geogr Reg Planning. 2011;4(6):355–63.
19. Girum T, Shegaze M, Tariku Y. The role of currently married men in family planning and its associated factors in Agaro Town, South West Ethiopia. Ann Med Health Sci Res. 2017;7(6):119–24.
20. Gebremariam A, Addissie A. Modern contraceptive method mix and factors affecting utilization of modern contraceptives among married women in Adigrat town, Tigray, Northern, Ethiopia. Fam Med Med Sci Res. 2014;3(04): 139. https://doi.org/10.4172/2327-4972.1000139.
21. Ayaz S, Efe ŞY. Family planning attitudes of women and affecting factors. J Turk Ger Gynecol Assoc. 2009;10(3):137. Available from: https://www.ncbi.nlm.nih.gov/pmc/articles/PMC3939116/pdf/jtgga-10-3-137.pdf–41.
22. Gupta V, Mohapatra D, Kumar V. Family planning knowledge, attitude, and practices among the currently married women (aged 15–45 years) in an urban area of Rohtak district, Haryana. Int J Med Sci Public Health. 2016;5(4): 627–32. Available from: https://www.ijmsph.com/?mno=199530. https://doi.org/10.5455/ijmsph.2016.12082015100.
23. Alemayehu M, Lemma H, Abrha K, Adama Y, Fisseha G, Yebyo H, Gebeye E., Negash K., Yousuf J., Fantu T., Gebregzabher T., Medhanyie A.A. Family planning use and associated factors among pastoralist community of afar region, eastern Ethiopia. BMC Womens Health 2016; 16(1): 39. Available from: https://link.springer.com/article/https://doi.org/10.1186/s12905-016-0321-7.
24. Amentie M, Abera M, and Abdulahi M. Utilization of family planning services and influencing factors among women of child bearing age in Assosa district, Benishangul Gumuz regional state, West Ethiopia. Sci J Clin Med. 2015; 4(3): 52. Available from: http://www.sciencepublishinggroup.com/journal/paperinfo.aspx?journalid=159&doi=https://doi.org/10.11648/j.sjcm.20150403.11.
25. Kamal SM. Contraceptive use and method choice in urban slum of Bangladesh. Int Conf Fam Plann Res Best Pract. 2009;18:1–19. Available from: https://fpconference.org/2009/media/DIR_169701/15f1ae857ca97193ffff83a4ffffd524.pdf.
26. Ekpenyong MS, Nzute AI, Odejimi O, Abdullahi AD. Factors influencing utilisation of family planning services among female of reproductive age (15–45 years) in Bauchi local government area, Bauchi state. Nurs Palliat Care. 2018;3. https://doi.org/10.15761/NPC.1000180 Available from: https://www.oatext.com/pdf/NPC-3-180.pdf.
27. Bhandari R, Pokhrel KN, Gabrielle N, and Amatya A. Long acting reversible contraception use and associated factors among married women of reproductive age in Nepal. PLoS One. 2019; 14(3). Available from: https://doi.org/https://doi.org/10.1371/journal.pone.0214590.
28. Kasa AS, Tarekegn M, and Embiale N. Knowledge, attitude and practice towards family planning among reproductive age women in a resource limited settings of Northwest Ethiopia. BMC Res notes 2018; 11(1): 1–6. Available from: https://bmcresnotes.biomedcentral.com/articles/https://doi.org/10.1186/s13104-018-3689-7.

12

Patterns and determinants of modern contraceptive use and intention to use contraceptives among Malawian women of reproductive ages (15–49 years)

James Forty*, Serai Daniel Rakgoasi and Mpho Keetile

Abstract

Background: Malawi is one of the countries in SSA with the highest TFR. This study aimed to explore factors associated with modern contraceptive use and intention to use contraceptives among women of reproductive ages (15–49 years) in Malawi.

Methods: The study used secondary data from 2015 to 16 Malawi Demographic and Health Survey (MDHS) dataset. Logistic regression models were used to derive adjusted odd ratios as the measures of association between need, predisposing and enabling factors, and contraceptive use and the intention to use contraceptives among women. The sample constituted 24,562 women who were successfully interviewed during the MDHS. All comparisons are considered statistically significant at 5% level.

Results: Overall 54.8% of women were currently using contraceptives, while 69.1% had the intention to use contraceptives. The odds of contraceptive use were significantly low among, women aged 15–19 years, 20–24 years, 25–29 years, 30–34 years, 35–39 years and 40–44 years compared to women aged 45–49 years; women of Tonga ethnic group (OR = 0.60, CI = 0.43 0.84) compared to women of Nyanga ethnic group; women from poor households (OR = 0.78, CI = 0.68–0.90) and middle income households (OR = 0.84, CI = 0.74–0.95) compared to women from rich household. Nonetheless, women with no past experience of terminated pregnancy (OR = 1.50, CI = 1.34–1.68) were more likely to use contraceptives compared to women with past experience of terminated pregnancy. Similarly, Women with primary education (OR = 1.56, CI = 1.16–2.09) and secondary education (OR = 1.39, CI = 1.04–1.85) were more likely to use contraceptives compared to women with higher education. While the odds of intending to use contraceptives were significantly high with age only thus among women aged 15–19 years, (OR = 15.18, CI = 5.94–38.77); 20–24 years (OR = 16.77, CI = 7.46–37.71); 25–29 years (OR = 6.75, CI = 3.16–14.45); 30–34 years (OR = 7.75, CI = 3.61–16.65) and 35–39 years (OR = 5.05, CI = 2.29–11.12) compared to women aged 45–49 years.

Conclusion: As direct policy measure; information, education and communication programmes on family planning among poor and middle income women, and all women in reproductive ages should be strengthened.

Keywords: Determinants, Modern contraceptive use, Malawi, Women, Reproductive age

* Correspondence: fotejames@gmail.com
Department of Population Studies, University of Botswana, Private Bag UB, 00705 Gaborone, Botswana

Introduction

Family planning has improved the well-being of families and communities by preventing high risk pregnancy, abortion, and unplanned pregnancy and has the potential to reduce poverty and hunger as well as preventing maternal deaths and childhood deaths worldwide [1]. The main intervention in family planning is contraceptive use. The prevalence rates of contraceptive use tend to be higher in developed countries than in developing countries [2]. Among developing countries, the rates of contraceptive use vary widely and Sub-Saharan Africa (SSA) has the lowest prevalence rate of contraceptive use comparatively [3]. Lack of access to family planning services and concerns about the side effects associated with modern contraceptive methods are among the main reasons for the high unmet need of contraception in developing countries [4].

There are international commitments aiming at meeting the need to use contraceptives among women. Furthermore, there are important factors that help policy commitments to be realized. Studies done in developing nations, specifically in SSA found that contraceptive use and inte-ntion to use contraceptives were significantly associated with education, age, place of residence, religion, ethnicity, wealth index and husband's or partner's education [5–13]. Furthermore, women ever oriented on family planning by family planning workers and with past abortion experiences were also found to use contraceptive or with the intention to use contraceptives [8, 14, 15].

Malawi is committed to ensuring that contraceptive need and reproductive health needs in general are met. The country launched its first population policy in 1994. The current revised policy, now in its seventh year of implementation, was launched in 2013 and aims at addressing development challenges that emanate from unmanaged population growth and high levels of fertility and mortality [16]. According to Population policy and Family planning commitment (2020) there is an increase in contraceptive use. Thus, Malawi's contraceptive use prevalence rate increased from 7% in 1992 to 28% in 2004 and had reached 58% in 2015–16. Thus, by 2016, Malawi had nearly managed to attain 60% modern contraceptive prevalence rate as targeted by Family Planning Commitment (2020). Further, with estimated total fertility rate (TFR) of 4.2 in 2016 according to the Malawi Demographic Health Survey (MDHS,2015–16), Malawi was at the verge of attaining the target of National Sexual and Reproductive Health Strategy, 2011–2016 of 4.0 TFR by 2016.

Despite the progress, Malawi is one of the countries in SSA with the highest TFR but at the same time with higher contraceptive prevalence rate (CPR). For example, Malawi's TFR is 4.2 compared to South Africa's (2.6), Kenya's (3.9) and Gabon's (4.1) yet Malawi's CPR (58%) is similar to Kenya's and higher than those of the other nations [17]. This shows that Malawi has slow decline in TFR hence population continues to grow rapidly. It is against this background that this paper intends to establish factors that may inhibit realization of desired low fertility which can mainly be attained through contraceptive use. The realization of the factors that are distorting contraceptive use and its translation to desired fertility may help to come up with necessary interventions to deal with the same. Therefore, this study aims at finding determinants of modern contraceptives use and intention to use contraceptives.

Studies in Malawi found out contraceptive use is significantly associated with age, education, spouse approval by, number of living children, work status, visiting health facility and discussionbetween spouse and respondent, region, place of residence, parity, marital status and religion [18–21]. However, most studies, including Mandiwa et al. [19] focused on adolescents only. Meanwhile Palamuleni [20] focused on all women of reproductive ages, but the study used a 2010 MDHS dataset. On the other hand, Makupe et al. [18] focused on all women of reproductive age as well used the dataset that this study has used but there are differences in methods and in some explanatory variables used. For instance on finding the determinants, Makupe [19] used mixed effect model while this study used logistic regression. Furthermore, the two studies also differ in explanatory variables except on age, religion, region, place of residence and respondent education. Nonetheless, these common variables may be important for triangulating the results where two different method or models were used. Hence, this study is important in triangulating the findings of other studies and further finding other determinants that contribute to the prevailing high fertility irrespective of relatively high contraceptive prevalence rate in Malawi. Additionally, studies are scarce in Malawi pertaining intention to use contraceptives. Thus, the second aim of this study, as already alluded to, is to establish if the same explanatory variables under consideration are associated with intention to use contraceptives.

Conceptual framework

In order to assess the patterns and determinants of modern contraceptive use among women of reproductive ages in Malawi, this study adopted the theory of health-seeking behavior developed by Andersen and Newman [22]. The key focus was to examine the relationship between intra and inter-personal factors and contraceptive use. The main premise of the theory of health seeking behavior is that the use of health-care services is a function of three sets of individual characteristics; predisposing, enabling, and need factors. Predisposing factors are considered to be the individual and socio-cultural characteristics such as social structure, health beliefs and demographic factors [22]. Enabling factors for contraceptive use may include personal, family, place of residence and community resources which may increase accessibility to family planning resources. For instance; income, employment and the availability of family planning services could be categorized as enabling factors [22]. Need factors are self-perceptions and objective evaluations of general health conditions [23]. Several studies have suggested that abortion expe-rience and desire to have additional children are two crucial need factors related to contraceptive use [15, 24].

Figure 1 shows the pathways through which predisposing, enabling and need factors influence contraceptive use and intention to use contraceptives among women of reproductive age. For example the enabling factors like good knowledge of fertility awareness, household of higher wealth index, partners with higher education and living in urban [25, 26] can have some influence on the need of having few numbers of children which in turn affect contraceptive use. On the other hand, predisposing factors like education of women, age, religion and ethnicity tend to influence the decision on how many children a woman wants to have, which in turn affects contraceptive use [27–29]. Moreover, Malawi's 2013 population policy creates an enabling environment for increase in contraceptive use and intention to use contraceptives. For instance, the second specific objective of policy area 1 is the promotion of benefits of having few children [26]. The attainment of having few children is through the third and fourth specific objectives of policy area 1 which is ensuring reproductive health information and interventions are given and accessible to all irrespective of predisposing factors (age, ethnicity, religion and education) or enabling factors (wealth index, place of residence and partner education). Thus, such a policy has an overarching effect as it influences the need to have less number of children on both men and women irrespective of variations in predisposing and enabling factor.

Methods

The study area

Malawi is a landlocked, long stretched country in south-eastern Africa in the Great Rift Valley on the western shore of Lake Nyasa (Lake Malawi), the most southerly lake in the Great African Rift Valley system. Countries which borders with Malawi are Tanzania, Zambia and Mozambi-que. Malawi is one of the world's most densely populated nations with a population of about 17.6 million people according to 2018 Census report. Capital city is Lilongwe and English and Chichewa are the official languages. The nation is divided into three main regions: Northern, Central and Southern. Malawi's population is predominantly rural and is comprised of various ethnic groups that migrated from other parts of Africa. Based on its gross national income (GNI) the Republic of Malawi is one of the poorest country in Africa, its economy is agro-based. There is a small tourism sector which is being primed for growth. The former British protectorate of Nyasaland became the independent nation of Malawi in 1964. First democratic multiparty elections were held in 1994, after three decades of one-party rule.

Study design and data source

This study used secondary data cross sectional household data for women collected during the 2015–16

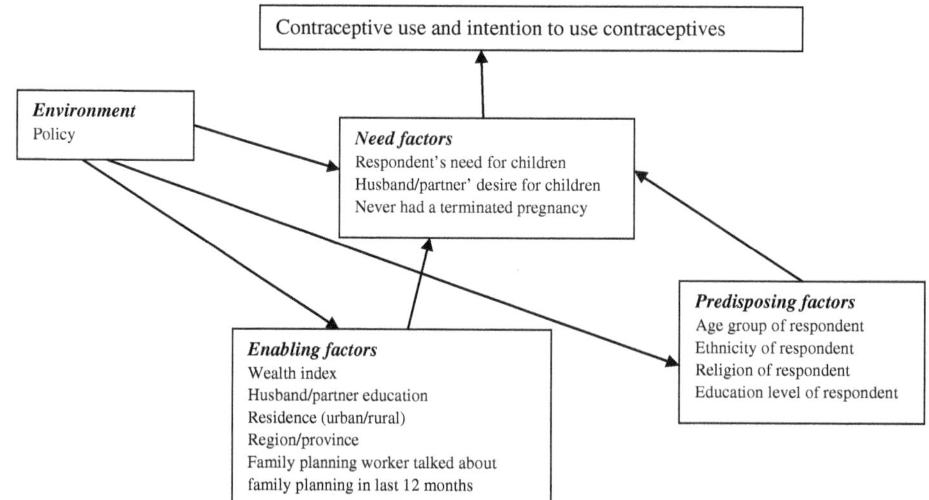

Fig. 1 Interaction of predisposing factors, enabling factors and needs factors and contraceptive use and intention to use

Malawi Demographic and Health Survey (MDHS). The data used in this analysis were collected using the women's individual questionnaire. The MDHS is designed to provide data for monitoring the population and health situation in Malawi [30].

The sampling frame used for the 2015–16 MDHS was derived from the Malawi Population and Housing Census frame (MPHC), conducted in Malawi in 2008, and provided by the Malawi National Statistical Office (NSO). The census frame is a complete list of all census standard enumeration areas (SEAs). SEA is a geographic area that covers an average of 235 households. The sampling frame contains information about the SEA location, type of residence (urban or rural), and the estimated number of residential households. The 2015–16 MDHS sample was stratified and selected in two stages. Each district was stratified into urban and rural areas; this yielded 56 sampling strata. Samples of SEAs were selected independently in each stratum in two stages. In the first stage, 850 SEAs, including 173 SEAs in urban areas and 677 in rural areas, were selected with probability proportional to the SEA size and with independent selection in each sampling stratum. A household listing operation was implemented in all the selected SEAs and the lists of households served as a sampling frame for the selection of households in the second stage.

In the second stage of selection, a fixed number of 30 households per urban enumeration area and 33 per rural enumeration area were selected with an equal probability systematic selection from the newly created household listing. All women aged 15–49 years who were either perma-nent residents of the selected households or visitorswho stayed in the household the night before the survey were eligible to be interviewed. Thus, in the 850 selected clusters, 26,564 households were occupied at the time of data collection of which 26,361 were successfully interviewed, yielding a household response rate of 99%. In total, 24,562 women were successfully interviewed andincluded in this analysis.

Study variables and measurements

Dependent variables

The outcome variables of this study are contraceptive use and intention to use contraceptives derived from questions which asked women "do you or your partner use contraceptives or intend to use contraceptives to delay or avoid getting pregnant". For contraceptive use, women who reported current use of either modern contraceptive method were given a code of **1** and **0** if otherwise. For the intention to use contraceptives, women who intended to use contraceptive were given a code of **1** and those who responded did not intend to use were coded **0**.

Independent variables

The independent variables were grouped into three categories; predisposing, enabling and need variables. Predisposing factors are individual and socio-cultural characteristics such as social structure, health beliefs and demographic factors [22]. Predisposing variables included age group (in categories of; 15–19 and 20–24, 25–29, 30–34, 35–39, 40–44 and 45–49), ethnicity (Mang'anjaChewa, Tubuka, Lomwe, Tonga, Yao, Sena, Nkhonde, Ngoni, and Nyanga), religion (Christians, Muslims, no religion) and education level (no education, primary, secondary and higher). This was done consistent with previous literature [9–12, 20, 31].

Enabling factors reflect the means or logistics required to obtain or increase accessibility to the services [22]. Enabling variables included wealth index (poor, rich and richest), husband/partner level of education (no education, primary, secondary and higher), residence (urban and rural), family planning worker visitation and having talked on family planning in last 12 months and region (northern, central and south). These variables were selected on the basis of reviewed literature [5–8, 10, 12, 31].

Need factors are self-perception of desired condition [23]. Need factors selected include desire for children (want the same, husband/partner wants more and husband or partner wants fewer) and experience of terminated pregnancy. Studies show past abortion experiences [24] and respondent or partner's desire for children are associated with contraceptive use [15].

Data analysis

Prior to data analysis, the data was cleaned and some variables; contraceptive use and intention to use, religion and wealth index were re-coded to suit the objectives of this study. Contraceptive use and the intention to use contraceptives were analyzed separately. Descriptive statistics was used to come up with summarized univariate data and the results were presented as proportions (%). Bivariate analysis was done where enabling, predisposing and need factors were crosstabu-lated with contraceptive use and the intension to use contraceptive. Pearson Chi-Square was usedto determine the significant explanatory factors for regression analysis. Binary logistic regression analysis was employed to identify predictors of contraceptive use and intention to use. Crude andadjusted odds ratios and their 95% confidence intervals (95% CI) were estimated. All statistical analyses were performed using Statistical Package for the Social Sciences (SPSS, IBM version 25) and statistical significance was set at P-value of less than 0.05.

Table 1 Distribution of sampled women by socioeconomic and demographic characteristics, Malawi DHS, 2015/16

Variable	N	%
Predisposing factors		
Age		
15–19	5273	21.5
20–24	5094	20.7
25–29	3976	16.2
30–34	3648	14.9
35–39	2988	12.2
40–44	2022	8.2
45–49	1561	6.4
Ethnicity		
Chewa	7317	30.8
Tumbuka	2612	11.0
Lomwe	4453	18.7
Tonga	942	4.0
Yao	2782	11.7
Sena	1153	4.8
Nkhonde	335	1.4
Ngoni	3085	13.0
Mang'anja	569	2.4
Nyanja	547	2.3
Religion		
Christian	21,685	88.4
Moslem	2726	11.1
Non-religious	123	0.5
Education level		
No education	2779	11.3
Primary	15,028	61.2
Secondary	6061	24.7
Tertiary	694	2.8
Enabling factors		
Wealth status		
Poor	8708	35.5
Middle income	9405	38.3
Rich	6449	26.3
Partner education level		
No education	1456	9.2
Primary	8377	53.2
Secondary	5008	31.8
Tertiary	915	5.8
Place of residence		
Urban	5247	21.4
Rural	19,315	78.6

Table 1 Distribution of sampled women by socioeconomic and demographic characteristics, Malawi DHS, 2015/16 *(Continued)*

Variable	N	%
Educated on family planning		
No	325	10.0
Yes	2926	90.0
Region		
Northern region	4803	19.6
Central region	8417	34.3
Southern region	11,342	46.2
Need factors		
Desire of children		
Both want same	8605	69.7
Partner wants more	2540	20.6
Partner wants fewer	1206	9.7
Ever terminated pregnancy		
No	22,102	90.0
Yes	2460	10.0
Outcome variables		
Contraceptive use		
No	9242	45.2
Yes	11,194	54.8
Intention to use contraceptive		
No	4126	30.1
Yes	9242	69.9
Total	24,562	100

Results

Sample description

Table 1 gives the summary statistics of the study population. The results indicate that 54.8% (11,194/24562) of women in the sample reported that they used contraceptives. Among those who indicated that they did not use any contraceptives, 69.1% (4126/9242) expressed the intention to use contraceptives. Age distribution of respondents shows that, the highest proportion of women in the sample was found in ages 15–19 and 20–24 years (21.5 and 20.7%, respectively). It was also noted that the Chewa ethnic group (30.8%), Christians (88.4%), primary education level (61.2%), middle income individuals (38.3%) and rural residents (78.6%) constituted the highest proportions in the sample. Moreover, the proportion of women whose partner had primary education (53.2%), were educated on family planning (90%), had the desire to have the same number of children as their partner (69.7%), and those who never terminated pregnancy (90%) were high in the sample.

Patterns of contraceptive use and intention to use

Contraceptive use

Contraceptive use was significantly associated with age group, ethnicity, religion, women education level, wealth index, husbands/partners' education level, type of place of residence (urban/rural), region and experience of terminated pregnancy (Table 2). For example, contraceptive use increased with age and was highest in the age group 45–49 years (81.1%). Furthermore, a high proportion (61.0%) of women who belonged to Mang'anja ethnic group, non-religious (58.0%), not educated (65.1%) and belonged to middle income households (55.9%) used contraceptive. Moreover, women whose partners had tertiary education (71.8%), resided in rural areas (55.4%), or resided in northern region (56.8%) and experienced terminated pregnancy (61.8%) used contraceptives.

Intention to use contraceptives

Intention to use contraceptives was significantly associated with age group, ethnicity, religion, women's education level, husbands/partners' education level, educated on family planning, region, desire for children and experience of terminated pregnancy (Table 2). For example, intention to use contraceptives decreased with age and was highest in age group 20–24 (84.1%) and lowest in age group 45–49 (17.1%%). Furthermore, a high proportion of women who belonged to Chewa ethnic group (73.6%), Christians (69.8%), poor households (69.7%) and secondary education (76.9%) intended to use contraceptive. Meanwhile, women whose partners had tertiary education (73.6%), resided in the Central region (75.7%), partner wanted fewer number of children (77.5%) and never experienced terminated pregnancy (69.7%) intended to use contraceptives.

Determinants of contraceptive use and intention to use

Table 3 shows the odds ratios for the likelihood of contraceptive use and intention to use contraceptives among women in Malawi.

Contraceptive use

After adjusting for covariates, women aged 15–19 years (OR = 0.13, CI = 0.10–0.16); 20–24 years (OR = 0.24, CI = 0.19–0.31); 25–29 years (OR = 0.37, CI = 0.29–0.46); 30–34 years (OR = 0.40, CI = 0.32–0.51), 35–39 years (OR = 0.55, CI = 0.43–0.70) and 40–44 years (OR = 0.73, P = 0.56–0.94) were less likely to use contraceptives compared to women aged 45–49 years. Furthermore, only women of Tonga ethnic group were less likely to use contraceptives (OR = O.60, CI = 0.43–0.84) compared to women of Nyanga ethnic group. Women with primary education (OR = 1.56, CI = 1.16–2.09) and secondary education (OR = 1.39, CI = 1.04–1.85) were more likely to use contraceptives compared to women with higher education. While women from poor households (OR = 0.78, CI = 0.68–0.90) and middle income households (OR = 0.84, CI = 0.74–0.95) were less likely to use contraceptives compared to women from rich households. On the other hand, women with no past experience of terminated pregnancy (OR = 1.50, CI = 1.34–1.68) were more likely to use contraceptives compared to women with past experience of terminated pregnancy.

Intention to use

Most variables were not significantly associated with intention to use contraceptives except age. Women aged 15–19 years (OR = 15.18, CI = 5.94–38.77); 20–24 years (OR = 16.77, CI = 7.46–37.71); 25–29 years (OR = 6.75, CI = 3.16–14.45); 30–34 years (OR = 7.75, CI = 3.61–16.65) and 35–39 years (OR = 5.05, CI = 2.29–11.12) were more likely to intend to use contraceptives compared to women aged 45–49 years.

Discussion

This study assessed the patterns and determinants of contraceptive use and intension to use contraceptives among women of reproductive ages in Malawi. The findings show that more than half of women reported that they were using contraceptives in 2015/16. This is an increase from the 2011 figure which was less than half (42%) [30]. The increase in contraceptive use observed in this study may have been contributed by, the USAID-funded Capacity-Plus Project implemented by IntraHealth International in collaboration with Christian Association of Malawi since January 2012 whose aim was to strengthen human resource management in affiliated health facilities in areas including contraceptives use [32]. Additionally, the inclusion of in-service training of health workers on long term family methods helped to reduce the shortage of health workers knowledgeable on contraceptives [32]. Thus, this may also have contributed to increase in CPR.

The results of the analyses show that contraceptive use increased with the age of women. For instance low contraceptive prevalence was observed among teenage women. The findings are consistent with previous findings which found that contraceptive use increased with age in Malawi [10, 20, 31, 33]. The low contraceptive prevalence among women in teen years may be due to the fact that most of these women especially aged below 18 may be shying away to seek contraceptives even if they are married as they fall below legal age (18 years) of marriage as well as not to be viewed as are indulging in premarital sex if they are not married.

On the other hand, intention to use contraceptives increased with age of women. This finding corroborates other findings in the region [20, 21]. The finding that women in teen years have higher intention to use contraceptives concurs with the already given explanation

Table 2 Prevalence of contraceptive use and intention to use contraceptives by predisposing, enabling and need factors, 2015–16 MDHS ($N = 24,562$)

Variable	*Contraceptive use*		*Intension to use contraceptives*	
	N	%	N	%
Predisposing factors				
Age				
15–19	810	19.2	3402	76.2
20–24	2377	51.0	2286	84.1
25–29	2295	63.7	1309	77.9
30–34	2136	66.7	1065	70.4
35–39	1807	71.1	698	59.1
40–44	1091	76.7	331	35.6
45–49	678	81.1	151	17.1
P-value	*< 0.001*		*< 0.001*	
Ethnicity				
Chewa	3499	55.5	2809	73.6
Tumbuka	1167	56.6	895	61.9
Lomwe	2176	56.8	1655	72.7
Tonga	345	47.1	387	64.8
Yao	1049	48.3	1125	64.9
Sena	495	52.3	452	68.7
Nkhonde	150	54.2	127	68.6
Ngoni	1411	54.8	1166	69.7
Mang'anja	288	61.0	184	65.5
Nyanja	226	52.8	202	62.9
P-value	*< 0.001*		*< 0.001*	
Religion				
Christian	10,107	55.6	8079	69.8
Moslem	1020	47.8	1112	65.2
Non-religious	51	58.0	37	59.7
P-value	*< 0.001*		*< 0.001*	
Highest education level				
No education	1319	65.1	708	48.5
Primary	7148	56.7	5468	69.4
Secondary	2456	47.0	2774	76.9
Tertiary	271	48.1	292	69.0
P-value	*< 0.001*		*< 0.001*	
Enabling factors				
Wealth group				
Poor	3884	54.9	3287	69.7
Middle income	4408	55.9	3471	69.5
Rich	2792	52.9	2484	67.9
P-value	*0.003*		*0.170*	
Partner education level				
No education	784	67.4	379	56.4
Primary	4999	68.4	2309	68.4

Table 2 Prevalence of contraceptive use and intention to use contraceptives by predisposing, enabling and need factors, 2015–16 MDHS ($N = 24{,}562$) *(Continued)*

Variable	*Contraceptive use*		*Intension to use contraceptives*	
	N	%	N	%
Secondary	2987	66.0	1542	76.3
Tertiary	574	71.8	225	66.0
P-value	*< 0.001*		*< 0.001*	
Type of place of residence				
Urban	2282	52.4	2077	70.1
Rural	8912	55.4	7165	68.9
P-value	*< 0.001*		*0.221*	
Educated on family planning				
No	144	56.7	110	60.8
Yes	1602	62.2	975	73.6
P-value	*0.087*		*< 0.001*	
Region				
Northern region	2168	56.8	1649	62.6
Central region	3969	54.1	3368	75.7
Southern region	5057	54.5	4225	62.7
P-value	*0.018*		*< 0.001*	
Need factors				
Desire of children				
Both want same	4839	64.3	2681	71.2
Partner wants more	1403	64.9	758	66.7
Partner wants fewer	727	66.2	371	77.5
P-value	*0.463*		*< 0.001*	
Ever terminated pregnancy				
No	9967	54.1	8456	69.7
Yes	1227	61.8	786	63.7
P-value	*< 0.001*		*< 0.001*	

Statistically significant at $P < 0.05$

that they had low contraceptive use while they intended to use contraceptives. The reduction in intention to use contraceptives among older women may be related to the fact that a good number of older women might be not sexually active or they have reduced their coital frequency. Additionally, most of them may rely on other traditional methods like string tie and they may not be willing or comfortable to talk about them in an interview hence reported to have lower intention to use contraceptives.

Women of Tonga ethnic group were found to be less likely to use contraceptives. Studies also show that there is variation in contraceptives use among ethnic groups [11, 34]. The possible explanation for low contraceptives use among the Tonga ethnic group could be because the grouping is more likely to spend more time schooling hence tend to marry at late age thus need of children after marriage become a priority. The explanation is supported by Palamuleni [21] who found that Tonga ethnic group, despite being one of the smallest ethnic groups, the grouping is among the top 3 most educated ethnic groups and spend most time schooling hence most of them secure jobs and live in urban areas and marry late.

Contrary to previous findings [9, 10, 12, 31, 35] which found that increase in education relates to increase in contraceptive use; we found that women with low level of education were more likely to use contraceptives. The most plausible explanation for this observation is that in Malawi there is good coverage of reproductivehealth interventions among all women regardless of their education level. Furthermore, most women with higher education are likely to be married by educated men of

Table 3 Adjusted odds ratios showing the likelihood of contraceptive use and intention to use among women (15–49 years) in Malawi

Variable	Contraceptive use				Intention to use contraceptives			
	Unadjusted Model		Adjusted Model		Unadjusted Model		Adjusted model	
	OR	95% C.I.	OR	95% C.I.	OR	95% C.I.	OR	95% C.I.
Age								
15–19	0.05***	0.04–0.06	0.13***	0.10–0.16	15.54***	12 .88–18.76	15.18***	5.94–38.77
20–24	0.23***	0.19–0.28	0.24***	0.19–0.31	25.71***	20.98–31.50	16.77***	7.46–37.71
25–29	0.39***	0.32–0.47	0.37***	0.29–0.46	17.06***	13.83–21.04	6.75***	3.16–14.45
30–34	0.45***	0.37–0.54	0.40***	0.32–0.51	11.55***	9.39–14.21	7.76***	3.61–16.65
35–39	0.58***	0.47–0.70	0.55***	0.43–0.70	7.01***	5.68–8.64	5.05***	2.29–11.12
40–44	0.73***	0.59–0.91	0.73***	0.56–0.94	2.67***	2.15–3.34	2.04	0.89–4.65
45–49	1.00		1.00		1.00		1.00	
Ethnicity								
Chewa	1.11	0.92–1.36	1.16	0.86–1.56	1.64***	1.29–2.08	0.97	0.20–4.15
Tumbuka	1.17	0.95–1.44	1.09	0.80–1.48	0.96	0.75–1.23	0.48	0.12–2.02
Lomwe	1.18	0.96–1.44	1.25	0.92–1.69	1.57***	1.23–2.00	0.83	0.18–3.87
Tonga	0.80	0.63–1.01	0.60***	0.43–0.84	1.09	0.82–1.44	0.46	0.10–2.10
Yao	0.83	0.68–1.03	1.01	0.73–1.40	1.09	0.85–1.40	0.43	0.08–2.18
Sena	0.98	0.78–1.23	0.87	0.63–1.21	1.29	0.98–1.71	0.65	0.11–3.84
Nkhonde	1.06	0.78–1.43	0.92	0.60–1.40	1.29	0.88–1.90	1.29	0.20–8.44
Ngoni	1.08	0.88–1.33	1.12	0.83–1.52	1.35***	1.05–1.74	0.80	0.17–3.67
Mang'anja	1.40***	1.07–1.83	1.43	0.97–2.10	1.12	0.88–1.56	0.52	0.06–4.61
Nyanja	1.00		1.00		1.00		1.00	
Religion								
Christian	0.91	0.59–1.39	1.07	0.62–1.86	1.56	0.94–2.60	1.02	0.61–1.82
Moslem	0.67	0.43–1.03	0.72	0.41–1.26	1.27	0.75–2.12	0.71	0.51–1.23
Non-religious	1.00		1.00		1.00		1.00	
Highest education level								
No education	2.01***	1.66–2.43	1.27	0.92–1.75	0.42***	0.34–0.53	0.75	0.16–3.65
Primary	1.41***	1.19–1.67	1.56***	1.14–2.09	1.02	0.82–1.26	0.72	0.16–3.18
Secondary	0.95	0.80–1.04	1.39***	1.04–1.85	1.50	1.20–1.87	0.77	0.18–3.34
Tertiary	1.00		1.00		1.00		1.00	
Enabling factors								
Wealth group								
Poor	1.08***	1.01–1.16	0.78***	0.68–0.90	0.98	0.81–1.16	0.74	0.68–1.35
Middle income	1.13***	1.05–1.21	0.84***	0.74–0.95	0.83	0.78–1.21	0.84	0.74–1.15
Rich	1.00		1.00		1.00		1.00	
Partner education level								
No education	0.81***	0.67–0.99	0.86	0.67–1.09	0.67***	0.51–0.87	1.08	0.34–3.38
Primary	0.85***	0.72–0.99	0.94	0.76–1.16	1.11	0.88–1.41	1.03	0.40–2.68
Secondary	0.76***	0.63–0.90	0.84	0.69–1.03	1.66***	1.30–2.12	1.14	0.18–2.92
Tertiary	1.000		1.000		1.00		1.000	
Type of place of residence								
Urban	0.88***	0.83–0.95	1.04	0.92–1.16	0.68	0.53–1.15	1.01	0.82–1.13
Rural	1.00		1.00		1.00		1.00	

Table 3 Adjusted odds ratios showing the likelihood of contraceptive use and intention to use among women (15–49 years) in Malawi *(Continued)*

Variable	Contraceptive use				Intention to use contraceptives			
	Unadjusted Model		Adjusted Model		Unadjusted Model		Adjusted model	
	OR	95% C.I.	OR	95% C.I.	OR	95% C.I.	OR	95% C.I.
Region								
Northern region	1.10***	1.02–1.19	1.09	0.91–1.30	0.82***	0.74–0.90	0.99	0.46–2.14
Central region	0.99	0.93–1.05	1.11	0.99–1.24	1.52***	1.40–1.66	0.66	0.36–1.23
Southern region	1.00		1.00		1.00		1.00	
Need factors								
Ever terminated pregnancy								
No	0.76***	0.69–0.83	1.50***	1.34–1.68	1.31	1.16–1.48	0.71	0.38–1.35
Yes	1.00		1.00		1.00		1.00	

***Statistically significant at $P < 0.05$

their levels who tend to understand the subject of contraceptives hence they also tend to be proactive in using contraceptives like condoms hence giving option for their women for less utilization of contraceptives.

Women of poor and middle income wealth quintiles were less likely to use contraceptives. This could be because women with less than tertiary education hardly get employment especially well paying jobs hence often times they depend on their husbands/partners who dominate in decision making including contraceptive use. This is exacerbated by patriarchal system which obstructs women in decision making thus most women, except in most cases tertiary educated, are at the mercy of their partners. However, the finding is consistent with other studies [6, 7, 10, 12, 31], and]. For instance, Rasooly et al. found that women from wealthiest households were more likely to use contraceptives than women from less wealth households.

Women with no experience of terminated pregnancy were found to be more likely to use contra-ceptives. The finding is consistent with the finding by Khanal et al. [24] who found that women with no experience of terminated pregnancy were found to be more likely to use contraceptives. Nevertheless, the use of experience of past terminated pregnancy as a factor needs further debate as is tricky since it could either be intended artificial terminated pregnancy or unintended natural terminated pregnancy (miscarriages).

Limitation of the study

Although our study provides vital insights on the association between predisposing, enabling and need factors and contraceptive use and on the intention to use contraceptives, it has some few limitations. For example, the outcome variables are explained based on women only yet most of them live with their husbands/ partners who most often are heads of households. As a result there is possibility of missing out on the male factor(s) that might have effect on contraceptive use and intention to use. Moreover, information was collected using self-reports, which can distort the accuracy of the results. Meanwhile, some variables on the influence of men on contraceptive use and intention to use contraceptives were included as need factors. For instance, partners desired number ofchildren. Despite these limitations, the study has shed some insights on the factors influencing contraceptive use and intention to use in Malawi among women aged 15–49 years.

Conclusions

The findings of this study indicate that more than half of women in reproductive ages use contra-ceptives, while more than two thirds among those who were not using contraceptives expressed intention to use contraceptives. The odds of contraceptive use were significantly high among women in higher age groups, with primary and secondary education, from rich households and who had experience of terminated pregnancy. On the other hand, the odds of intention to use contraceptive were significantly high among women in lower age groups. The findings of this study have far-reaching policy implications that can improve the use of contraceptives. Such policies must include strategies to address impediments associated with women in lower ages with use of contraceptive. The policies should also include economic empowering strategies to households and women in particular to reduce socio-economic disparities among households. Additionally, there should be strategies targeting women with no formal education with family planning messages that include the use of contraceptives.

Abbreviations

CI: Confidence Interval; CPR: Contraceptive Prevalence Rate; DHS: Demographic and Health Survey; GNI: Gross National Income; MDHS: Malawi Demographic and Health Survey; MPHC: Malawi Population and Housing Commission; NSO: National Statistical office; OR: Odds Ratio; SEA: Standard Enumeration Area; SSA: Sub-Sahara Africa; TFR: Total Fertility Rate

Acknowledgements

The authors thank the MEASURE DHS project for their support and for free access to the original data.

Authors' contributions

JF and MK did the analysis and wrote the initial draft of this paper. JF, MK and SDR gave feedbacks for revising the first draft. JF worked on the reviewed comments. All authors have reviewed and approved the final version of the manuscript.

References

1. Cleland J, Bernstein S, Ezeh A, Faundes A, Glasier A, Innis J. Family planning: unfinished agenda. Lancet. 2006;368(9549):1810–27. https://doi.org/10.1016/S0140-6736(06)69480-4.
2. Family Planning Worldwide. (2013). Data sheet. Population reference bureau 2013. http://www.prb.org/pdf13/family-planning-2013-datasheet.
3. United Nations. (2009). World contraceptive use 2009. http://www.un.org/esa/population/publications/ contraceptive2009/contracept2009wallchartfront.Pdf.
4. Cleland J, Harbison S, Shah IH. Unmet need for contraception: issues and challe-nges. Stud Fam Plan. 2014;45(2):105–22. https://doi.org/10.1111/j.1728-4465.2014.00380.x.
5. Adjiwanou V, Bougma M, LeGrand T. The effect of partners' education on wom-en' reproductive and maternal health in developing countries. J Soc Sci Med. 2017. https://doi.org/10.1016/j.socscimed.2017.11.054.
6. Finer LB, Henshaw SK. Disparities in rates of unintended pregnancy in the United States 1994 and 2001. Perspect Sex Reprod Health. 2006;38(2):90–6. https://doi.org/10.1363/3809006.
7. Grace K. Contraceptive use and intent in Guatemala. Demogr Res. 2010; 23(12):335–64. https://doi.org/10.4054/DemRes.2010.23.12.
8. Mboane R, Bhatta MP. Influence of a husband's healthcare decision making role on a woman's intention to use contraceptives among Mozambican women. Reprod Health. 2015;12(1):36. https://doi.org/10.1186/s12978-015-0010-2.
9. Mekonnen W, Worku A. Determinants of low family planning use and highunmetneed inButajira district, South Central Ethiopia. Reprod Health. 2011;8:37.
10. Nair PS, Navaneetham K. Patterns and determinants of modern contraceptive use in southern Africa. Demography India. 2015;44(1 & 2):40–9.
11. Obasohan PE. Religion, ethnicity and contraceptive use among reproductive age women in Nigeria. Int J Mater Child Health AIDS. 2015;3(1):63–73.
12. Rasooly MH, Ali MM, Brown NJ, Noormal B. Uptake and predictors of contraceptives use in afghan women. BioMedical Central Women's Health. 2015;15(1):9. https://doi.org/10.1186/s12905-015-0173-6.
13. Srikanthan A, Reid RL. Religious and cultural influences on contraception. J Obstet Gynaecol. 2008;30(2):129–37.
14. Ajong AB, Njotang PN, Kenfack B, Yakum MN, Mbu ER. Knowledge of women in family planning and future desire to use contraception: a cross sectional survey in urban Cameroon. BMC Res Notes. 2016;9(1):347. https://doi.org/10.1186/s13104-016-2155-7.
15. Okech T, Nelson W, Wawire NHW, Thom K, Mburu. Contraceptive use among women of reproductive age in Kenya's city slums. Int J Bus Soc Scientific Res. 2011;2(1):22–43.
16. Malawi Government. National Population Policy. Lilongwe: MOFEPD. Malawi Government; 2013. (2017)
17. DHS Program.(2019). Demographic and health survey. The DHS Program office, ICF, 530 Gaither road, suite 500 Rockville, MD 20850 USA.
18. Makupe DJ, Kumwenda S, Kazembe L. An application of mixed-effect models toanalyze contraceptive use in Malawian women. Contraceptive Reprod Med. 2019;4(1):12. https://doi.org/10.1186/s40834-019-0088-y.
19. Mandiwa C, Namondwe B, Makwinja A, Zamawe C. Factors associated with contraceptive use among young women in Malawi: analysis of the 2015–16 Malawi demographic and health survey data. ContraceptReprod Med. 2018; 3(1):12. https://doi.org/10.1186/s40834-018-0065-x.
20. Palamuleni ME. Socio-economic and demographic factors affecting contracepti-ve use in Malawi. Afr J Reprod Health. 2013;17(3):91–104.
21. Palamuleni ME. Trends and determinants of contraceptive use among female adolescents in Malawi. Transylvanian Rev. 2017; XXV(20):5239–50.
22. Anderson R, Newman JF. Societal and individual determinants of medical care utilization in the United States. Milbank Memorial Fund Quarterly. 1973; 51(1):95–124. https://doi.org/10.2307/3349613.
23. Gelberg L, Andersen RM, Leake BD. The behavioral model for VulnerablePopulations:application to medical care use and outcomes for homeless people. Health Serv Res. 2000;34(6):1273–302.
24. Khanal V, Joshi C, Neupane D, Karkee R. Practices and perceptions on co-ntraception acceptance among clients availing safe abortion services in Nepal. Kath-mandu Univ Med J. 2011;9(35):179–84.
25. Dibaba B, Mitike G. Factors influencing desired family size among residents ofAssela town. J Women Health Care. 2016;5:6.
26. Wei J, Xue J, Wang D. Socioeconomic determinants of rural women's desiredfertility: Asurvey in rural Shaanxi, China. PLoS One. 2018;13(9): e0202968. https://doi.org/10.1371/journal.pone.0202968.
27. Adsera A. Religion and changes in family-size norms in developed countries. Rev Relig Res. 2006;47(3):271–86.
28. Pearce LD, Brauner-Otto SR, Ji Y. Explaining religious differentials in family size preference: evidence from Nepal in 1996. Popul Stud. 2015;69(1):23–37. https://doi.org/10.1080/00324728.2014.995695.
29. Weinberger M. The relationship between Women's education and fertility: selected findings from the world fertility surveys. Int Fam Plan Perspect. 1987;13(2):35–46. https://doi.org/10.2307/2947826.
30. Malawi Government. (2017). Malawi Demographic and Health Survey2015/16. National Statistical Office and Macro International Inc., Zomba.
31. Rourke T. (2015). Association between socio demographic factors and knowledge of contraceptive methods with contraception use among women of reproductive age: a cross-section study using the 2013 Liberia DHS (Dissertation). Retrieved from http://urn.kb.se/resolve?urn=urn:nbn:se:uu:diva256717</div>.
32. African Institute for Development Policy. (2012). Assessment of Drivers of Progress in Increasing Contraceptive use in sub-Saharan Africa: Case Studies from Eastern and Southern Africa. www.afidep.org.
33. Asiimwe JB, Ndugga P, Mushomi J, Ntozi JPM. Factors associated with modern contraceptive use among young and older women in Uganda; a comparative analysis. BioMedical Central Public Health. 2014;14:926.
34. Addai I. Ethnicity and contraceptive use in sub-Sahara Africa: the case of Ghana. J Biosoc Sci. 1999;31(1):105–20. https://doi.org/10.1017/S0021932099001054.
35. Al-Riyami A, Afifi M, Mabry RM. Women's autonomy, education and employment in Oman and their influence on contraceptive use. Reprod Health Matter. 2004;12(23):144–54. https://doi.org/10.1016/S0968-8080(04)23113-5.

13

Utilization of long-acting and permanent contraceptive methods and associated factors among married women in Adama town, Central Ethiopia

Markos Desalegn[1*], Ayele Belachew[2], Muluken Gizaw[2], Gemechu Kejela[3] and Robsan Gudeta[3]

Abstract

Background: Long-acting and permanent contraceptive methods have clear advantages over short-acting methods of contraception that benefit both clients and health systems. Despite this importance, studies show that the proportion of women currently using long acting and permanent contraceptive methods are significantly lower than the proportion using short-acting methods.

Objective: The main aim of the study was to assess the level of utilization of long acting and permanent contraceptive methods and associated factors among married women in Adama town.

Methodology: Community Based Cross-Sectional Study was conducted in four kebeles of Adama town from April 15–30, 2015. Multistage sampling technique was used to select the study participants. The collected data was cleaned and entered using Epi info 3.5.3 and analyzed using statistical package for social science version 20.0. Factors associated with utilization of long acting and permanent contraceptive methods were identified using logistic regression model.

Result: In this study, the magnitude of long acting and permanent contraceptive methods was 20.9%. Implant, Intra-Uterine devices (IUDs) and tubal ligation accounted for 16.1, 4.6, and 0.2% respectively. Current use of long acting and permanent contraceptive methods was higher among women who had high knowledge (AOR = 5.26, 95% CI = 1.90–14.69), positive attitude (AOR = 3.25, 95% CI = 1.60–6.58) and women who had 3–4 children (AOR [95%CI] =2.3[1.14–4.63]) compared to those who had no child.

Conclusion: Current use of long acting and permanent contraceptive methods in Adama town was low. Level of knowledge, attitude about the methods, and number of children were factors affecting utilization of long acting and permanent contraceptive methods. Targeted Information Education Communication Intervention should be intensified to improve the utilization of these methods.

Keywords: Utilization, Long acting and permanent, Contraceptive methods

* Correspondence: markosdesalegn@gmail.com
[1]Department of Public health, College of medicine and health sciences, Jigjiga University, Jigjiga, Somali region, Ethiopia

Background

Family planning is a means by which individuals or couples space pregnancy and childbirth at intervals, mutually determined by both husband and wife in order to have the desired number of children [1].

Four contraceptive methods are categorized as Long-Acting and Permanent Contraceptive Methods (LAPCMs): Intra-Uterine Devices (IUDs), Implants, Tubal ligation, and Vasectomy. IUDs and Implants are long-acting methods; when removed, return to fertility is prompt. Copper-containing IUDs are effective for 10–12 years. Implants, depending on the type, last for 3–5 years. Tubal ligation and Vasectomy are permanent methods [2, 3].

LAPCMs have clear advantages over short-acting methods of contraception that benefit both clients and health systems. It increases the contraceptive method options that couples have, especially as their need evolve over time and is the best choice for couples both to space and limit childbirth and is the best way to protect women and couples against unwanted pregnancies [4].

Over time, the use of Long-acting and permanent contraceptive methods has not kept in pace with that of short-acting methods, such as oral contraceptives and injectables [5]. Surveys from four Sub-Saharan countries showed that, the proportion of women currently using LAPCMs is significantly lower than the proportion using short-acting methods, which accounts for less than 5 % [6]. Like other Sub-Saharan countries, Long-Acting and Permanent Contraceptive Methods use have lowest rates in Ethiopia (4.2%) for which IUD, Implant and Female sterilization contribute 0.3,3.4 and 0.5% respectively [7, 8].

The growing use of contraception around the world has given couples the ability to choose the number and spacing of their children and has had tremendous life-saving benefits [9]. Despite this, approximately 25% of Sub-Saharan African couples and 29% of Ethiopian couples, who need to space or limit births, are not using any form of modern contraception [7, 8].

Therefore, the aim of this study was to assess the utilization of LAPCMs and associated factors among married women.

Methods and materials

Study area

The study was conducted in Adama town, located to the east of Addis Ababa at the distance of 99 km. The town has 20 kebeles (the smallest administrative unit in Ethiopia with a geographical boundary of having a minimum of 1000 households). According to the 2007 Census conducted by the Central Statistical Agency of Ethiopia (CSA), the city has a total population of 220, 212. About 60,174 households were counted in the city, which results in an average of 3.66 persons to a household, and 59,431 housing units [10]. Adama town has one government hospital, three private hospitals; six government health centers, one private clinic, one maternal health clinic (Marie Stopes), one Family Guidance Association of Ethiopia (FGAE) and 72 drug shops. From these health institutions, family planning service is being delivered in all hospitals, health centers, FGAE, and Marie Stopes clinics.

Study period

The study was conducted from April 15–30, 2015.

Study design

Community-based cross-sectional survey was conducted to assess the utilization of LAPCMs and associated factors among married women aged 15–49 in Adama town.

Source population

The source populations of the study were all married women aged 15–49 years who live in Adama town during the study period.

Study subject

The study subject in this study was a sampled married women of age 15–49 years who live in Adama town during the study period.

Sample size determination

To estimate the sample size, a single population proportion formula with the following assumptions was used.

$$n = \frac{(Z\alpha/2)^2 P\,(1-(P)}{d^2}$$

Assumptions

Desired precision (d) = 5%.

Proportion of long acting and permanent contraceptive methods clients from the previous study done in Adigrat and Debre Markos town was 19.5% each [11, 12].

Confidence level = 95%, which means α set at 0.05 and Zα/2 = 1.96 (value of Z at α 0.05 or critical value for normal distribution at 95% CI [13].

$$n = \frac{(Z\alpha/2)^2 P\,(1-(P)}{d^2}$$

$$n = \frac{(1.96)^2 0.195(1-(0.195)}{(0.05)^2} = 241$$

Using a design effect of 2(since it is a multistage sampling) and a 10% non-response rate, the calculated minimum sample size was 530.

Sampling procedures

A multi-stage sampling technique was used to select the study participants. The town has 20 kebeles. Out of this, four kebeles were selected using simple random sampling. Then, the number of households with reproductive-age women in each selected kebele were identified and proportionally allocated for the sample size. Sampling fraction was calculated for each kebele and initial household with eligible married women was picked randomly. Finally, study samples were selected using a systematic sampling method. Only one woman was interviewed for households having two or more married women on random to avoid intra-class correlation [13]. In the absence of married women in the sampled household, interviewer jumped to the next house.

Inclusion and exclusion criteria

Married women of reproductive age group (15–49), women who have lived in the town for more than six months were included. Women having a serious illness and mental disorder were excluded.

Data collection and questionnaire

A structured interviewer-administered questionnaire was used. The questionnaire was adopted from similar studies done in Mekelle and Adigrat town [11, 13]. It was modified based on the situation of the study to collect information on the utilization of long acting and permanent contraceptive methods and associated factors from married women in Adama town. The questionnaire was prepared in English, translated to Amharic language and translated back to English by another person in order to check its consistency.

The questionnaire has five sections: socio- demography (9 items), reproductive history (6 items), knowledge (18 items), attitude (10 items) and practice of modern contraception (12 items).

The questionnaire was pretested before actual data collection among 28 respondents (5% of the calculated sample size) in Modjo town. Because population residing in Modjo town share almost similar characteristics with the population in the study area.

Five health extension workers were trained for data collection on the content of the questionnaire and approach to participants during data collection. They were selected based on their ability to speak and write Afan Oromo and Amharic languages.

During data collection, one supervisor was selected to supervise the data collector's activity, checking the completeness of the questionnaire and receive the collected and completed questionnaire. Participants were interviewed, where they were free to express their idea freely. Moreover, on occasions when the sampled women were not be accessed for absence, up to two attempts was endeavored for interviewing to lessen the non-response rate.

Data processing and analysis

Data were coded, entered into Epi info version 3.5.3 and exported to SPSS version 20.0 for analysis. Descriptive statistics were computed to determine the frequency and percentages. Binary logistic regression was conducted and COR, with 95% CI was estimated to select the candidate variables for the final model. Then, variables with a p-value of < 0.2 at binary logistic regression were taken into a multivariable logistic regression to control confounding. Hosmer-Lemeshow goodness-of-fit with stepwise (backward elimination) logistic regression was used to test for model fitness. AOR with 95% CI was estimated to assess the presence of association at multivariable logistic regression. Finally, variables with a p-value of < 0.05 were considered as statistically significant predictors of the outcome variable.

Operational definition

Utilization of LAPCMs

Is the current use of contraceptive implants or IUDs or Tubal Ligation by the women (study participant) or Vasectomy (male sterilization) by her husband.

User of LAPCMs

Women who were using either contraceptive implants or IUDs or Tubal Ligation by herself or Vasectomy (male sterilization) by her husband during the data collection period.

Non-user of LACMs

Were women who were not using contraceptive implants, either IUDs or Tubal Ligation by herself or Vasectomy (male sterilization) by her husband during the data collection period.

Attitude of LAPCMs

Refers to one's own opinion, belief and perception about LAPCMs. In this study, the attitude of the respondent was measured by attitude statements like using Implant do not lead to abnormal bleeding, Implant and IUD do not move/escape in the body after insertion and using LAPCMs do not lead to abnormal bleeding. It was labeled as a positive and negative attitude where those who have scored above mean of attitude questions was grouped as a positive attitude and mean or below mean was grouped as negative attitude [13].

Knowledge of LAPCMs

Refers to one's own awareness and familiarity with LAPCMs. Ten knowledge questions were used to grade the knowledge of LAPCMs. It was graded as low knowledge; those who have answered less than 60% of knowledge question; Moderate knowledge; those who have answered 60–79% of knowledge question; High knowledge: those who have answered above or 80% of knowledge question [13].

Kebele
is the smallest administrative unit in Ethiopia with a geographical boundary of having a minimum of 1000 households.

Zone
Is small administrative subdivision within the kebele.

Data quality management
To assure the quality of the data, structured interviewer-administered questionnaire was used to collect information. Before the actual data collection, pre-test had been conducted. Data collectors were trained for one day and they have been informed about how to approach the respondents, how to apply the designed data collection method, how to ask each of the questions, follow the instructions of the questionnaire and to keep the confidentiality of the respondents. One supervisor was assigned to check the completeness of the questionnaire every night with the principal investigators.

Table 1 Socio-demographic characteristics of the study participants, Adama town, April 2015

S/No	Socio demography	frequency	Percentage
1	Age		
	15–24	128	24.3
	25–34	297	56.5
	35–44	87	16.5
	> 45	14	2.7
2	Religion		
	Orthodox	297	56.5
	Muslim	130	24.7
	Protestant	99	16.9
	Others*	10	1.9
3	Educational status		
	No education	49	9.3
	Only read and write	30	5.7
	Elementary [1–8]	161	30.6
	Secondary [9, 10]	107	20.3
	Senior secondary [11, 12]	66	12.5
	Diploma and above	113	21.5
4	Family size		
	2–3	246	46.8
	4–5	213	40.5
	> 5	67	12.7

Others*: catholic and Adventist

Table 2 Reproductive history of the study participants, Adama town, April 2015

S/No	Reproductive history	Frequency	Percentage
1	Ever gave birth (n = 526)		
	yes	435	82.7
	No	91	17.3
2	Number of birth (n = 435)		
	1–2	283	65.1
	3–4	117	26.9
	> 4	35	8
3	Number of living children (n = 435)		
	0	2	0.5
	1–2	293	67.4
	3–4	110	25.3
	> 4	30	6.9
4	An additional number of the child they need (n = 435)		
	0	151	34.7
	1–2	236	54.3
	> 2	48	11
5	Discussion about modern contraception (n = 526)		
	Yes	474	90.1
	No	52	9.9

Table 3 knowledge of modern contraceptive methods among study participants

S/No	Variables	Frequency	Percentage
1	Ever heard of modern contraceptive method (n = 526)		
	Yes	512	97.3
	No	14	2.7
2	Type of contraceptive method known (n = 512)		
	Pill	479	93.6
	Injectable	508	99.2
	Implant	433	84.6
	IUD	130	25.4
	Tubal ligation	76	14.8
	Vasectomy	368	71.9
	Condom	388	71.9
3	Source of information(n = 512)		
	Friend, neighbor, and relatives	137	26.8
	Husband	54	10.5
	Health professionals	453	88.5
	Mass media	423	82.6

Each of the percentages does not add up to 100.00 because respondents could choose several responses, which could be spontaneous or prompted

Table 4 knowledge level of the study participants, Adama town, April 2015

	Knowledge variables (n = 512)	knowledge level			
		True		False	
		Frequency	percent	frequency	Percent
1	IUD prevent pregnancy for > 10 years	404	78.9	108	21.1
2	IUD is not good for women at risk of STI	246	48	266	52
3	IUD has no effect on sexual desire	349	68.2	163	31.8
4	Pregnancy is possible after the removal of IUD	362	70.7	150	29.3
5	Implant prevent pregnancy for > 5 years	423	82.6	89	17.4
6	Implant has no effect on sexual desire	409	79.9	103	20.1
7	Pregnancy is immediate after removal of the implant	379	74	133	26
8	Vasectomy has no effect on sexual desire	205	40	307	60
9	Pregnancy is not possible after tubal ligation	312	60.9	200	39.1

Results

Socio-demographic characteristics of the respondents

Five hundred twenty-six married women were interviewed, making response rate of 99.25%. The mean age of the respondents was 29 years (+SD 6.31), majority 297(56.5%) of which belong to the age group of 25–34. Many of the participants were Oromo 220 (41.8%) in ethnicity (data not shown in the table). More than half of the respondents were Orthodox 297 (56.5%) in religion. Most of the married women interviewed were educated 477(92.2%), whereas by occupation, 127 (51.5%) of the participants were home-maker. The mean family size of the respondents was 4 (3.9 + SD). The majority, 246 (46.8%) of the study respondents have family sizes of 2–3 (Table 1).

Reproductive characteristics of the participants

About 151 (34.7%) of the respondents did not need to have more children and 236 (54.3%) of the participants need to have 1–2 more children. From all participant, 234(44.6%) want to have a child in the next two years and 292 (55.4%) did not want to have a child in the next two years (Table 2).

Knowledge of the participants about long acting and permanent contraceptive methods

From the total respondents, 512(97.3%) have heard at least one modern contraceptive methods. About 479 (93.6%), 508 (99.2%), 433 (84.6%), 130 (25.4%) and 76 (14.8%) of respondents have heard Pill, Injectable, Implant, Tubal ligation and Vasectomy as contraceptive methods respectively. The major source of information was the health profession 453(88.5%) followed by mass media 423(82.6%).

Four hundred thirty-five (87%) of the respondents knew about long acting and permanent contraceptive methods. Majority of them (66.3%) knew that IUD prevents pregnancy for more than 10 years. About 69 and 72.1% knew that pregnancy is possible immediately after removal of IUD and implant respectively. Eighty-seven percent of them had awareness of LAPCMs; 63.7% as it prevents

Table 5 Attitude of study participants about LAPCMs, Adama town, April 2015

S/No	Perception statement($n = 525$)	Level of agreement					
		Agree		Not sure		Disagree	
		frequency	Percent	frequency	percent	frequency	percent
1	Implant do not lead to bleeding	137	26.1	162	30.9	226	43
2	Insertion of IUD does not lead to loss of privacy	212	40.4	172	32.8	141	26.8
3	IUD does not move through the body	85	16.2	163	31	277	52.8
4	IUD do not prevent ordinary activity	93	17.7	134	25.5	298	56.8
5	IUD do not lead to excessive bleeding ($n = 524$)	93	17.7	183	35	248	47.3
6	Operation of Tubal ligation is not dangerous	50	9.5	307	58.5	168	32
7	Insertion and removal of implant is painful	52	9.9	165	31.4	308	58.7
8	Implant do not move through the body	67	12.8	127	24.2	331	63
9	spouse cannot decide on wife's FPM choice	253	48.2	36	6.8	236	45
10	HP cannot decide on method choice of FP.	142	27	19	3.7	364	69.3

Table 6 Utilization, the reason for not using and service center of modern contraceptive methods of the study participants, Adama town, April 2015

S/No	Variables	Frequency	Percentage
1	Current use of methods ($n = 315$)		
	pill	41	7.8
	Injectables	159	30.1
	Implant	85	16.1
	IUD	24	4.6
	Tubal ligation	1	0.2
	Condom	5	1
3	Service center (n = 315)		
	Health center	165	52.4
	Hospitals	51	16.2
	Private clinic	60	19.0
	Pharmacy	4	1.3
	HEW	3	1.0
	Relatives	1	0.3
	Others****	31	9.8

Others****: Mariestops and FGAE

possible child and maternal death; 69.5% as it spaces childbirth and 91% as it limits the family size. Concerning the level of knowledge, 46.8% of the participant had high knowledge, 24.5% had moderate knowledge and 28.7% had low knowledge (Tables 3 and 4).

The attitude of participants about long acting and permanent contraceptive methods

Only 137 (26%) of the participant agreed that Implant does not bring about excessive bleeding. Three hundred thirteen (59.6%) of them perceived that insertion of IUD exposes once own privacy and 432 (82.3%) perceived that IUD block ordinary activities. Four hundred fifty-eight (87%) of the participants perceived that Implant moves and escapes in the body while most of them perceive that insertion and removal of the Implant is pain full. Concerning the respondent's general attitude status, 55.1% of the participant had a positive attitude towards LAPCMs while the rest 44.9% had a negative attitude (Table 5).

Utilization of long-acting and permanent contraceptive methods among respondents

Ever use of modern contraceptive methods

The ever use of the modern contraceptive methods in this study area was 87.1%. The most ever used method was Injectable (66.3%).

Current use of modern contraceptive methods

Current modern contraceptive use was 59.8%. The most preferred method was Injectable 159(30.1%) and Implants 85(16.1%). The rest were using Pill 41(7.8%), IUD 24(4.6%), Condom 5(1%) and Tubal ligation 1(0.2%).

None use of modern contraceptive methods and the reasons for nonuse

About 40.2% of the respondents were not using any modern contraceptive methods (Table 6). Sixty-three point 5 % (63.5%) of them reported that they were not using modern contraceptive methods because of fear side effects (Fig. 1).

The overall prevalence of the LAPCMs was 20.9%. Majority of them use Implant (16.1%) and IUD (4.6%). The rest 0.2% use tubal ligation. Health center was where majority of the users get the service (52.4%) while others get service from other government organization (16.2%) and private clinic (19%).

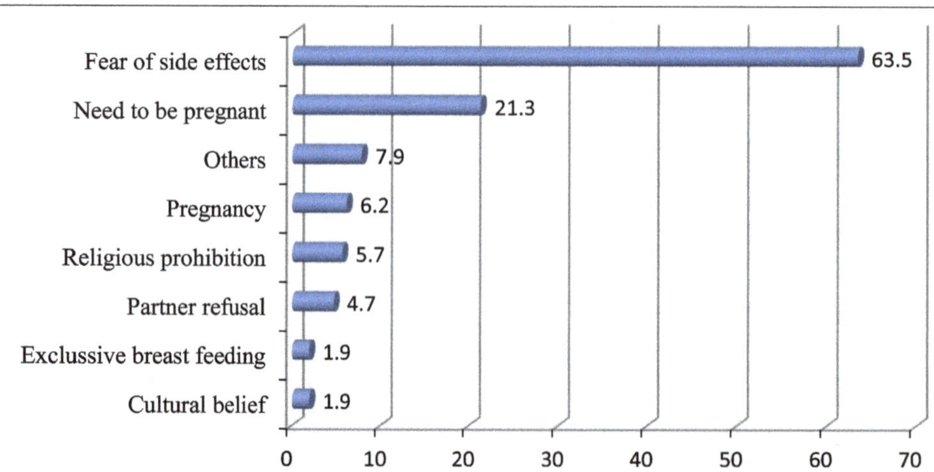

Fig. 1 Reason for not using modern contraceptive method among study participants, Adama tow, April 2015

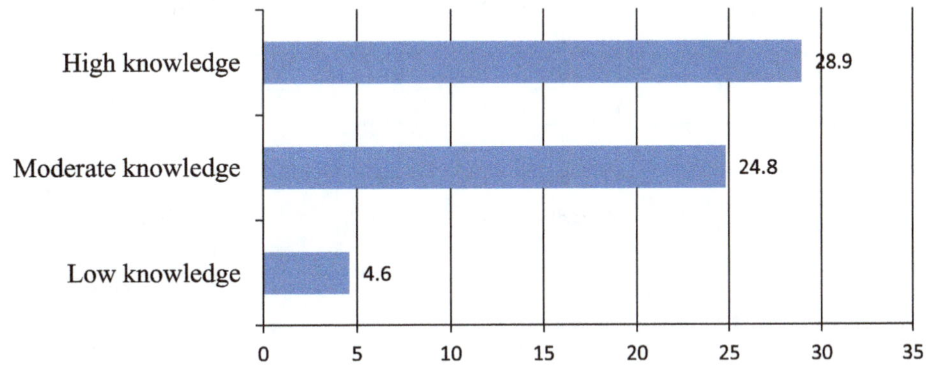

Fig. 2 Current use of LAPCMs by knowledge level of the study participants, Adama town, April 2015

Utilization of LAPCMs among married women who had no formal education was 2 and 28.3% among diploma and above. Current use of LAPCMs was 4.4% among married women who did not give birth. However, 37.6 and 25.7% of married women who gave birth to 3–4 and > 4 children were using LAPCMs respectively.

Current use of LAPCMs among those with low knowledge and negative attitude was, 4.6 and 6.8% respectively. However, current use among those with high knowledge and positive attitude was 28.9 and 32.4% respectively (Figs. 2 and 3).

Factors associated with utilization of long-acting and permanent contraceptive methods

The result of multivariate analysis revealed that knowledge level was one of the predictors of the current use of LAPCMs. Married women with high knowledge use LAPCMs 5 times more likely than those with low knowledge (AOR [95% CI] = 5.26[1.90–14.69]), and those with moderate knowledge use 3 times more likely compared to those with low knowledge (AOR [95%CI] = 3.27[1.12–9.52]). The attitude of the respondent was also known to predict the current use of LAPCMs in which those who had a positive attitude about LAPCMs use the methods 3 times more likely compared to those who had a negative attitude (AOR [95%CI] =3.25[1.60–6.58]). In this model, married women who gave birth to 3–4 children use LAPCMs 2 times more likely compared to those who had given birth to 1–2 children (AOR [95%CI] = 2.3[1.14–4.63]). Participants who need to have 1–2 more children had 67% lesser odds of using LAPCMs compared to a participant who didn't need any more children (AOR [95%CI] = 0.33[0.16–0.66]) (Table 7).

Discussions

The magnitude of the current use of LAPCMs in this study was 20.9%. This result was in line with studies conducted in Adigrat and Debra Markos (19.5%) each [11, 12]. The most preferred method was Implant (16.1%) followed by IUD (4.6%) and Tubal ligation (0.2%). This finding was greater than the study conducted in Nigeria (24.7%) [14].

In multivariate analysis, knowledge level, attitude status, and a number of children were found to affect the current use of LAPCMs among respondents.

Participants who had high knowledge and moderate knowledge used LAPCMs five and three times more likely compared to the participant of low knowledge. Similarly, a study done in Mekelle revealed, participant of high knowledge had used LAPCMs 8 times more likely compared to low knowledge level. Those who had moderate knowledge used LAPCMs 3 times more likely

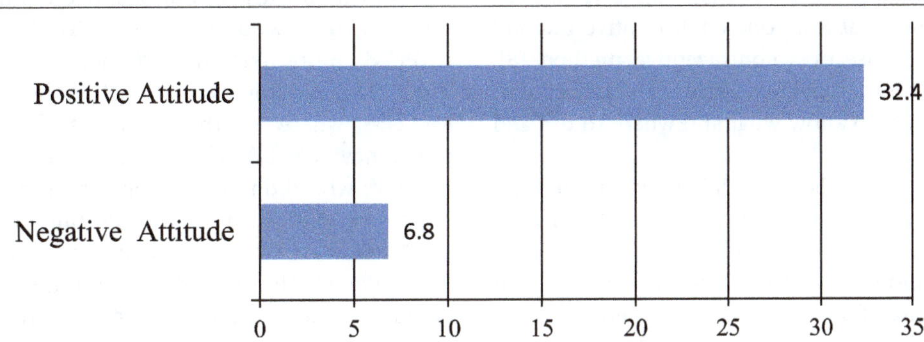

Fig. 3 Current Use of LAPCMs by Attitude status of the study participants, Adama town, April 2015

Table 7 Multivariate and Bivariate analysis of selected variables affecting utilization of LAPCMs among married women aged 15–49 years, Adama town, April 2015

Variables	Total	Utilization of LAPCMs			
		Yes	No	COR,(95% CI)	AOR,(95 CI)
Age of married women					
15–24	66	9 (13.6)	57 (86.4)	1.0(ref)	
25–34	269	64 (23.8)	205 (76.2)	2,(0.93–4.22)	1.43,(0.57–3.60)
35–44	87	33 (37.9)	54 (62.1)	3.87,(1.70–8.84)	1.60,(0.51–5.00)
> 45	13	2 (15.4)	11 (84.6)	1.15,(0.22–6.07)	1.13,(0.14–9.13)
Occupation of women					
Housewife	235	53 (22.6)	182 (77.4)	1.0(ref)	
Gov't employee	76	26 (34.2)	120 (78.9)	1.79 (1.02–3.14)	0.90,(0.42–1.94)
Daily labourer	39	4 (10.3)	35 (89.7)	0.4 (0.13–1.15)	0.34,(0.10–1.16)
Merchant	53	14 (26.4)	39 (73.6)	1.24 (0.62–2.44)	0.84 (0.36–1.94)
Student	18	4 (22.2)	14 (77.8)	0.98 (0.3–3.10)	0.76 (0.18–3.18)
NG0s	14	7 (50)	7 (50)	3.4 (1.15–10.2)	4,(1.04–16.20)*
No of birth					
1–2	283	53 (19.4)	230 (80.6)	1.0(ref)	
3–4	117	44 (37.6)	73 (62.4)	2.5,(1.55–4.02)	2.30,(1.14–4.63)*
>4	35	9 (25.7)	26 (74.3)	1.44,(0.64–3.24)	1.43,(0.35–5.92)
Knowledge level					
Low knowledge	123	7 (5.7)	144 (94.3)	1.0(ref)	
High knowledge	202	69 (34.2)	133 (65.8)	8.6 (3.8–19.45)	5.26 (1.9–14.6)*
Moderate knowledge	110	32 (29.1)	78 (70.9)	6.8 (2.86–16.17)	3.27 (1.12–9.52*
Attitude status					
Negative attitude	187	16 (8.6)	171 (91.4)	1.0(ref)	1
Positive attitude	248	92 (37.1)	156 (62.9)	6.3 (3.55–11.18)	3.25 (1.60–6.58)*
Number of the child they wanted					
0	151	59 (39.1)	92 (60.9)	1.0(ref)	1
1–2	236	40 (16.9)	196 (83.1)	0.32 (0.20–0.50)	0.33 (0.16–0.66)*
>2	48	9 (18.8)	39 (81.2)	0.36 (0.16–0.80)	0.5 (0.17–1.48)

*Respective variables are statistically significant

compared to the participant of low knowledge [13]. In addition, finding in Uganda revealed, knowing the duration of protection of IUD and Implant was positively associated with the use of LAPCMs [15]. EDHS 2011 showed, even knowing at least one contraceptive method was prerequisite for use of a contraceptive method [8]. This might be due to the knowledge of contraceptive method helps women to know what and where to use and get the method.

Current use of LAPCMs was higher among participants who had a positive attitude about LAPCMs than those who had a negative attitude. This finding was similar to other findings in Ethiopia where women with positive perceptions about contraceptive methods used contraceptive methods more likely [16, 17]. In Malaysia practice of LAPMs was surrounded by fear and misperception about a modern contraceptive method like IUD that it had to harmful effects on the health [18]. This might be due to, having a positive attitude was prerequisite for using contraceptive method [8, 17].

Participants who gave birth to 3–4 children used LAPCMs more likely than participants who did not give birth. This finding was almost in line with finding in Mekelle where mothers who had more than two pregnancy use LAPCMs three times more likely than mothers who didn't experience any pregnancy [13]. This might be due to fear of infertility after removal of LAPCMs. Participants who need to have more children [1, 2] had 67% lesser odds of using LAPCMs. This might be due to a significant amount of the respondents in this study did not know that pregnancy is immediate after removal of IUD (31.2%) and Implants (27.9%).

Conclusion and recommendation

The study showed that the utilization of LAPCMs is low despite several efforts made by the federal ministry of health and other stakeholders to escalate it. The main reason for not using the method was the fear of side effects. Knowledge level, attitude status, and parity were found to be associated with utilization of LAPCMs. Information education communication should be intensified and further research should be conducted to explore for other factors associated with utilization of LAPCMs.

Abbreviations

ACIPH: Addis Continental Institute of Public Health; BRDC: Birhan Research and Development Consultancy; CPR: Contraceptive Prevalence Rate; CSA: Central Statistical Agency; EDHS: Ethiopian Demographic Health Survey; FGAE: Family Guidance Association of Ethiopia; FGD: Focus Group Discussion; FMOH: Federal Ministry of Health; FP: Family Planning; HEW: Health Extension Workers; IDHS: Indonesia Demographic Health Survey; IUD: Intra-Uterine Device; KAP: Knowledge, Attitude and Practice; LACMs: Long-Acting Contraceptive Method; LAPCMs: Long-Acting and Permanent Contraceptive Methods; MSI: Marie Stopes International; NPC: National Population Commission; OCs: Oral Contraceptives; PMs: Permanent Methods; SNNP: Southern Nation Nationality and Peoples; TFR: Total Fertility Rate; USAID: United State Agency for International Development; WHO: World Health Organization

Acknowledgments

The authors acknowledged Addis Ababa University, school of public health and their library for their support. In addition, the authors would like to thank the study participants, data collectors, and supervisors.

Authors' contribution

MD involved in the proposal development, analysis and interpretation of the data and prepared the manuscript. AB and MG involved in conceptualization of the study and analysis of the data. RG and GK involved in the preparation of the manuscript and reviewing the paper. All authors read and approved the final manuscript.

Author details

[1]Department of Public health, College of medicine and health sciences, Jigjiga University, Jigjiga, Somali region, Ethiopia. [2]School of public health, college of health sciences, Addis Ababa University, Addis Abeba, Ethiopia. [3]Department of public health, Institute of health sciences, Wollega University, Oromia region, Nekemte, Ethiopia.

References

1. Mayhew S, Osei I, Bajos N. Provider Attitudes to Emergency Contraception in Ghana and Burkina Faso. Population (English Edition). 2013;68(1):115–39.
2. Bureau. PR. By contrast, more than seven of every 10 women in Northern and Western Europe use modern contraception Washington, DC: *World Population Data Sheet*. 2006.
3. USAID. Long-Acting and Permanent Methods of Contraception: Meeting Clients' Needs: United State International Agency for Development At http://WWW.poptechproject.com/pathfainder, 2006.
4. World Health Organization. Reproductive H. Medical eligibility criteria for contraceptive use: World Health Organization, 2015.
5. Pile JM, Ndede F, Ndong I, Jacobstein R, Johri N. Investing in the future-the case for long-acting and permanent contraception in sub-Saharan Africa. Arusha, Tanzania: *Paper submitted to the* Union for African Population ConferenceDecember 2007.
6. Trussell J, Guthrie K. Choosing a contraceptive: efficacy, safety, and personal considerations. Hatcher RA, Trussell J, Nelson AL, Cates W, Stewart FH, Kowal D Contraceptive technology 19th revised ed New York (NY): Ardent Media, Inc2007:19–47.
7. Dr. Zaheen B DJH, Dr. Sarah S. Factors affecting hormonal and nonhormonal contraceptive method use in women presenting to Reproductive Health.*IOSR Journal of Dental and Medical Sciences (JDMS)Sep-Oct. 2012*;volume 2(*Issue1*).
8. CSA [Ethiopia], ICF [International]. Ethiopia Demographic and Health Survey 2011. Addis Ababa, Ethiopia, and Calverton, Maryland, USA: Central Statistical Agency and ICF International, 2012.
9. Darroch JE, Singh S. Trends in contraceptive need and use in developing countries in 2003, 2008, and 2012: an analysis of national surveys. Lancet; 381(9879):1756–62.
10. Ethiopia CSA. National population and housing census. Addis Addis Ababa2007.
11. Gebremariam A, Addissie A. Intention to use long acting and permanent contraceptive methods and factors affecting it among married women in Adigrat town, Tigray, northern Ethiopia. Reprod Health. 2014;11(1):24.
12. Bulto GA, Zewdie TA, Beyen TK. Demand for long acting and permanent contraceptive methods and associated factors among married women of the reproductive age group in Debre Markos town, north West Ethiopia. BMC Womens Health. 2014;14(1):46.
13. Alemayehu M, Belachew T, Tilahun T. Factors associated with the utilization of long acting and permanent contraceptive methods among married women of reproductive age in Mekelle town, Tigray region, North Ethiopia. BMC pregnancy and childbirth. 2012;12(1):6.
14. Eko Jimmy E, Osonwa Kalu O, Osuchukwu Nelson C, Offiong Dominic A. Prevalence of Contraceptive use among women of reproductive age in Calabar Metropolis, Southern Nigeria. *International Journal of Humanities and Social Science Invention* ISSN (Online): 2319–7722, ISSN (Print): 2319–7714 www.ijhssi.org Volume 2 Issue 6 ll June. 2013ll PP.27–34.
15. Anguzu, al.: e. Knowledge and attitudes towards the use of long acting reversible contraceptives among women of reproductive age in Lubaga division, Kampala district, Uganda. BMC Research Notes2014;7:153.
16. Lee T, Lee H, Ahn HM, Jang Y, Shin H, Kim MS. Perceptions about family planning and contraceptive practice in a marital dyad. J Clinical Nursing. 2014;23(7–8):1086–94. https://doi.org/10.1111/jocn.12348 Epub 2013 Sep 6.
17. Lee H, Lee T, Shin H, Ahn H, Kim M, Lee M. Patterns and predictors of none use of family planning methods in Ethiopian women: a panel survey. Int Nurs Rev. 2013;60(3):335–43.
18. FSA N, Rahman HA, Juni MH. Barriers to Modern Contraceptive Practices among Selected Married Women in a Public University in Malaysia. Global J Health Sci. 2013;3(2).

14

Prevalence and determinants of unmet need for family planning among married women in Ghana-A multinomial logistic regression analysis of the GDHS, 2014

Joseph K. Wulifan[1], Jacob Mazalale[2], Christabel Kambala[3], William Angko[4], Job Asante[5], Stephen Kpinpuo[1†] and Albino Kalolo[6*†]

Abstract

Background: Documentary evidence points to high unmet need for family planning across sub-Saharan Africa. Modern contraceptive use has been staggering over decades with unacceptable marginal increases given that one in three women still report unmet need in Ghana. This study sought to re-examine through a further analysis on the prevalence and determinants of unmet need for family planning in Ghana using married women extracted from the recent 2014 Ghana Demographic and Health Survey.

Method: Data was analyzed using univariate, bivariate, logistic and multinomial logistic regression models.

Results: Of the 4527 women, more than a third (35.17%) experienced unmet need of which 20.19% had unmet need for spacing while 14.98% reported unmet need for limiting. The logistic results showed that older aged women, being employed and women with higher ideal number of children were less likely to experience unmet need. However, women who did not know the couples' preferred number of children, women who had more than one union and those with higher number of living biological children were more likely to report unmet need. From the multinomial model, an increase in age, residing in a rural area, and being employed were associated with lower risk of unmet need for spacing. Additionally, Women who did not know the couples' ideal number of children, women who had higher age when they got married, and women with higher number of biological children were more likely to report unmet need for spacing. Women who had a higher number of ideal children, women who had secondary or higher education, women from higher socio-economic households, were less likely to report unmet need for limiting. .

Conclusions: We recommend the strengthening of contraception services in order to address the various age specific needs and women within the different socio-demographic sects so as to reduce unmet need. Addressing the needs of women with increasing number of living biological children is equally paramount.

Keywords: Unmet need, Spacing, Limiting, Demographic and health survey, Multinomial regression, Ghana

* Correspondence: kaloloa@gmail.com
[†]Stephen Kpinpuo and Albino Kalolo contributed equally to this work.
[6]Department of Public Health, St. Francis University College of Health and Allied Sciences, P.O.Box, 175, Ifakara, Tanzania

Background

Globally, in 2014 alone nearly 290,000 women within the reproductive age (15–49 years) died from preventable pregnancy related complications of which sub-Saharan Africa accounted for 65% (179,000) of the deaths [1–3]. Women from low and middle income countries-LMICs are consistently more likely (1 in 30) to die of pregnancy and unsafe abortion related complications compared to (1 in 9500) women from the developed world [3]. Adherence to contraceptive use has witnessed a significant reduction in maternal mortality rate by 40% in LMICs over the last two decades [4]. Contraception adoption invariably lengthens inter-pregnancy intervals and ultimately improves child survival and maternal health outcomes [3]. A conscious management of one's desired fertility can improve household scarce resources and family welfare [5].

Most family planning interventions aim at reducing unmet need for modern contraception which has been the fundamental cause of unintended pregnancies. Following the Ghana demographic and health survey (GDHS, 1993), nearly 40% of married women reported unmet need for family planning and by 2014, the GDHS reported an unmet need of 30%. This means the change over the two decades has been very slow than previously anticipated [6]. Conceptually, scholars define unmet need for family planning to encompass the discrepancy between a woman's reproductive intensions and contraception behaviour [7–10]. Unmet need arises from two categories of women-thus pregnant women whose pregnancies were mistimed or unwanted because they were not using any contraception method before the pregnancy and fertile non-pregnant women who currently are not using any method of contraception who do not intend to give birth in the next 2 years or are undecided whether they wanted another pregancy [7, 11]. A woman is said to have unmet need for family planning if desired to delay the next child birth by at least 2 years but no using any method of family planning [12]. A pregnant woman has unmet need if she desired to have had her current pregnancy later (unmet need for spacing/mistimed pregnancy) or did not want the pregnancy at the time she got pregnant (Unmet need for limiting/unwanted pregnancy) but retrospectively did not use any contraception before the pregnancy [13]. The non-pregnant fertile woman has unmet need if she equally prefers to have the next child in at least 2 year's time (unmet need for spacing), isn't sure when to have the next child (unmet need for spacing) or reports not wanting any more children (unmet need for limiting) but using any contraception [7]. Given the high failure rate associated with traditional methods, women who use traditional method of contraception are regarded as having unmet need for family planning [14].

In Ghana, contraceptive prevalence rate (CPR) among currently married women of reproductive age rose from 10% each for traditional and modern methods of contraception to 7 and 22% respectively in 2014 [15]. Unmet need for family planning has important public health concerns as it often associated with unintended pregnancies [16]. Unintended pregnancies carry serious consequences for the woman and their families including the likelihood of unsafe abortion, delayed prenatal care, poor maternal and child health outcomes [16, 17]. Till date, it is still not very clear which single factor(s) operate to influence the persistent low contraceptive use and the corresponding high unmet need given that one in three women still report unmet need for contraception in Ghana [6, 18]. In recent years, unmet need for family planning has gained prominence in policy and academia hence its inclusion in the just ended millennium development goals (MDGs 2015) and by extension the space it occupies in the proposed sustainable development goals (SDGs 2030) [19, 20]. Currently there is no study that examined unmet need for modern contraception among currently married women in Ghana at the three analytical levels using the recent 2014 DHS data. Given this background, an assessment of the individual, household and facility factors that are associated with unmet need for family planning is not only timely but also appropriate. Our study therefore sought to examine which factors are associated with unmet need among married women in Ghana looking specifically at the levels of unmet need for spacing, limiting as well as the characteristics of women with unmet need for contraception.

Methods

Data extraction

We used the 2014 Ghana Demographic and Health Survey (GDHS) data for this manuscript. The data was extracted from the Measure DHS web platform after explicit permission sought to use the data was granted by the data originators (https://dhsprogram.com/). The entire survey covered a sample of 9396 women of reproductive age (15–49 years). The survey employed multi-stage sampling technique. Details of the data sampling techniques, data collection procedures, research assistant's training and pre-test details are outlined in the report [15]. The primary purpose of the GDHS was to generate recent and reliable data on fertility, family planning, maternal and child health, infant and child mortality and nutrition [21].

Study design

The 2014 GDHS was cross-sectional in design in which men and women who met the survey criteria were interviewed using a structured questionnaire. The analyses in this manuscript was restricted to currently married women of reproductive ages (15–49 years), fecund but reported their desire to space childbirth for at least 2 years or limit childbirth to their desired number but were not using any contraceptive method. In our analysis, we excluded women who had never had sexual intercourse, infecund and menopausal women. Given this criteria, we reduced the number of women to 4527 of which 1592 reported unmet need for family planning.

Study variables

The outcome variables for this study, which was unmet need for family planning, was derived from a series of specific questions in the section under contraception in the individual woman's questionnaire. Unmet need was defined as a dichotomous variable, differentiating between women with unmet need for family planning (coded as 1) and women without unmet need (coded as 0). Women in the non-contraceptive users' category were separated into pregnant women and non-pregnant women. A pregnant woman was defined as having unmet need if she indicated that her pregnancy was either wanted later (mistimed pregnancy) or she did not want to be pregnant (unwanted pregnancy) but was not using any method of contraception before the pregnancy. Women with mistimed pregnancies were classified as having unmet need for spacing while those with unwanted pregnancies were classified as having unmet need for limiting. At the non-pregnant fertile women category, women were further separated into women who desired to have a child in at least after 2 years (unmet need for spacing), women who were not sure when to have their next child (unmet need for spacing) and women who indicated they didn't want additional children (unmet need for limiting). The two categories of women from pregnant and fertile non-pregnant women together (unmet need for spacing and unmet need for limiting) are referred to total women with unmet need for family planning consistent with prior scholarly studies [7, 8, 10–12].

The independent variables were selected for inclusion in the analysis based on their significance in prior studies on factors which influence unmet need for family planning. These variables were identified under four categories comprising demographic, socio-eco-cultural, proximate, programme and health facility related. All variables included in the analysis were carefully selected from the women's questionnaire. For meaningful analysis and interpretation, a few of the variables were regrouped from their original categories in the main dataset which are explained in the subsequent paragraphs consistent with prior studies [22].

The demographic variables included were age of woman, age at first marriage and number of living children. Age was regrouped into the conventional five standard age groupings as 15–19, 20–24, 24–29, 30–34, 35–39, 40–44 and 45–49. Age at first marriage and number of living children maintained their original continuous variables structure. The socio-eco-cultural variables included in the analysis were religion, number of unions, residence, woman's level of education, household wealth, occupation and status of been registered under the national health insurance scheme. Religion was regrouped into Christianity, Islam and others/no religion [23]. Variables related to programme and health facility included sources from which individual heard information on family planning (radio, T.V and newspapers), whether the individual visited a health facility in the prior 12 months, whether the individual was visited by a health worker and if the individual knows a modern family planning method.The last category of variables which most prior studies classify as proximate/attitudinal variables [11, 22] included couple desire for children and ideal number of children. Table one presents the variables, their measurements and our hypothesis on association with unmet need.

Analytical approach

We analyzed the data at three (3) levels. At the first level we employed univariate analysis which included an assessment of the level of unmet need, and a sample description using the demographic, socioeconomic proximate and programme/facility variables. Frequencies and percentages were used to guide the sample description. The second level applied bivariate analysis which focused on establishing the unadjusted relationship between the explanatory variables and the outcome variable - unmet need. This approach provided a preliminary assessment of unmet need levels across the individual explanatory variables and a further overview of the characteristics of women with unmet need for contraception. The third level of analysis focused on multivariate analysis to assess adjusted association of the explanatory variables with unmet need. We used a logistic regression model and the multinomial logistic regression model at the multivariate level to assess how the factors are associated with unmet need. The binary logistic regression was used because the outcome variables for total unmet need was dichotomous (no unmet need coded as 0, and unmet need coded as 1). The multinomial logistic regression was applied because the second categorical dependent variable of unmet need had three categories (no unmet need coded as 1, unmet need for spacing coded as 2, and unmet need for limiting coded as 3).

The multivariate analysis was based on an accurate representative of the population from which the sample was taken. The dichotomous relationship between unmet need for family planning and the various explanatory variables were analyzed using the logistic regression. The multinomial regression model was used to examine the association between selected explanatory variables on unmet need for spacing and unmet need for limiting. This was possible because the outcome variables had three categories (spacing, limiting and met need). This means that two dichotomies were compared (unmet need for limiting to no unmet need and unmet need for spacing to no unmet need) rather than one.

Results

Univariate analysis

Table 1 reports the distribution of selected background characteristics of respondents. A total of 4527 women were interviewed with 35.17% women reporting unmet need which was further split into unmet need for spacing (20.19%) and unmet need for limiting (14.98%). Majority of the women (23.0%) were found between 25 and 29 years while the least proportions of women were in age categories 15–19 and 45–49 years (3.0 and 6.0%) respectively. Pentecostal Protestants formed the majority (36.0%) of the religious sect and the minority (7.0%) being respondents without a religion or practised traditional religion. Majority of women (79.0%) belonged to the category of women who reported ever been engaged in a single union compared to their counterparts (21.0%) who had more than one marriage unions. Majority of the respondents were from rural areas. On educational status, majority (47.0%) had at least secondary education. Women from the poorest households formed a third (30.0%) while women from the richest category were (16.0%). The proportion of women with employment status was the highest (83.0%) as against 17.0% who reported not having an employment. Pertaining to information on family planning, 57.0% women reported they heard of family planning from the radio, 56.0% mentioned T.V while 5.0% identified the newspaper. 64.0% of the women reported having visited a health facility in the past 12 months while 14.0% confirmed also been visited by a health worker. The number of women who knew a family planning method was almost universal (99.0%). Majority of women (70.0%) reported being subscribed members under the Ghana national health insurance scheme (NHIS). The bivariate are presented in Table 2 in the appendix.

Bivariate analysis

The bivariate distribution of currently married women who reported unmet need for contraception according to selected background characteristics are presented in Table 2. The Pearson's Chi-square test reported statistically significant variation in age of woman and total unmet need (X^2 = 77; $P < 0.001$), unmet need for spacing (X^2 = 96; $P < 0.001$) and unmet need for limiting (X^2 = 451; $P < 0.001$). There was a significant difference between woman's religion and unmet need for limiting (X^2 = 31; $P < 0.001$) but no significant variation was observed between woman's religion and total unmet need as well as unmet need for spacing. Significant difference was observed in number of unions and total unmet need (X^2 = 21; $P < 0.001$) as well as unmet need for limiting (X^2 = 68; $P < 0.001$) but not unmet need for spacing. On socioeconomic status, the results showed a significant difference between household wealth and all the three levels of unmet need (total unmet need, unmet need for spacing and unmet need for limiting). The results equally showed a significant difference in woman's occupation and the three levels of unmet need. Statistically significant variation was observed between women who heard of family planning message on the T.V and total unmet need (X^2 = 5; $P < 0.002$) as well as unmet need for spacing (X^2 = 4; $P < 0.005$). Statistically significant variation was equally observed between women who visited a health facility in the past 12 months and both total unmet need (X^2 = 6; $P < 0.002$) as well as unmet need for limiting (X^2 = 11; $P < 0.001$). We observed a statistical significant change in the proportion of women with both total unmet need (X^2 = 20; $P < 0.001$) and unmet need for spacing (X^2 = 21; $P < 0.001$) by couple's desire for children but not unmet need for limiting. Significant variation was observed between women who subscribed to the Ghana National health insurance scheme (NHIS) and both total unmet need and unmet need for limiting. The t-test results detected a significant difference between mean age of woman at first marriage and total unmet need (t = 4; $P < 0.001$), unmet need for spacing (t = 3; $P < 0.001$) and unmet need for limiting (t = 4; $P < 0.001$). Lastly, we also observed a significant difference between number of living biological children and the three levels of unmet need for family planning.

Multinomial regression results

Table 3 presents the logistic regression (Model I) estimates of odds ratio and the multinomial regression (Model II) estimates of relative risk ratios (RRR) for selected variables of currently married women on the three levels of unmet need (total unmet need, unmet need for spacing and unmet need for limiting). Model I reveals that for total unmet need, women with higher age were less likely to report unmet need for family planning compared to women aged 15–19 years. No significant difference was detected across the various religious faiths. Women who had more than one marriage union were more likely (OR = 1.21; CI 1.03–1.42) to report unmet need for family planning compared with their colleagues who had one marriage union. No significant difference was observed across socioeconomic status. Only women from second quintile were more likely to report unmet need (OR = 1.28; CI 1.05–1.56) compared with women from poorest households. Women who reported having employment were less likely (OR = 0.79; CI 0.66–0.93) to report unmet need compared to their colleagues who had no employment. Couple who did not know the preferred number of children were more likely (OR = 1.37; CI 1.14–1.66) to experience unmet need compared to women who reported the couple desired the same number. Women who had an additional living biological child were more likely (OR = 1.36; CI 1.28–1.43) to report unmet need. Also, women who had

Table 1 Variable measurements and their respective expected sign on unmet need

Variable	Measurement	$n = 4527$	%	Hypothesized/expected coefficient
Age				
	1 = 15–19	118	3	+
	2 = 20–24	632	14	
	3 = 25–29	1038	23	
	4 = 30–34	967	21	
	5 = 35–39	891	20	
	6 = 40–44	592	13	
	7 = 45–49	289	6	
Religion				
	0 = no or traditional. religion	314	7	+
	1 = catholic	651	14	
	2 = non-Pentecostal protestant	987	22	
	3 = Pentecostal protestant	1614	36	
	4 = Islam	961	21	
Number of unions ever engaged in				
	1 = once	3557	79	–
	2 = more than once	970	21	
Residence				
	1 = urban	1995	44	–
	2 = rural	2532	56	
Education				
	0 = no education	1528	34	+
	1 = primary	868	19	
	2 = secondary +	2131	47	
SES				
	1 = poorest	1339	30	+
	2 = poorer	878	19	
	3 = middle	823	18	
	4 = richer	768	17	
	5 = richest	719	16	
Occupation				
	0 = no	779	17	+
	1 = yes	3748	83	
Heard FP methods on the radio				
	0 = no	1951	43	+
	1 = yes	2576	57	
Watched FP messages on the TV				
	0 = no	2550	56	+
	1 = yes	1977	44	
Read FP messages in newspapers				
	0 = no	4314	95	+
	1 = yes	213	5	
Woman visited a health facility in the past 12 months				
	0 = no	1617	36	+

Table 1 Variable measurements and their respective expected sign on unmet need *(Continued)*

Variable	Measurement	*n* = 4527	%	Hypothesized/expected coefficient
	1 = yes	2910	64	
FP worker visited woman				
	0 = no	3879	86	+
	1 = yes	648	14	
Woman knows modern FP methods				
	0 = doesn't know modern FP methods	50	1	+
	1 = knows modern FP methods	4477	99	
Couple's congruence of desire for children				
	1 = both want same	2101	46	-
	2 = husband wants more	1178	26	
	3 = husband wants fewer	402	9	
	8 = don't know	846	19	
Woman is member of any health insurance				
	0 = no	1350	30	+
	1 = yes	3177	70	

an additional ideal child were less likely (OR = 1.86; CI 1.81–1.92) to experience unmet need.

In Model II, women with higher age were relatively less likely to report unmet need for spacing compared to women within age group 15–19 years. No significant difference was observed across the age categories and unmet need for limiting. Women from rural areas were relatively less likely (RRR = 0.78; CI 0.63–0.97) to report unmet need for spacing compared to their colleagues from urban areas. Women who had at least secondary education were relatively more likely (RRR = 1.53; CI 1.13–2.06) to report unmet need for limiting compared to women who had no education. Women from higher socioeconomic status households were relatively more likely to report unmet need for limiting compared with women from poorest households. Women who were employed were relatively less likely (RRR = 0.70; CI 0.59–0.84) to report unmet need for spacing compared to unemployed women. Couple who reported they did not know the desired number of children were more likely (RRR = 1.50; CI 1.22–1.83) to report unmet need for spacing relative to couple who both want the same number of children. From the continuous variables, women who had an additional age at first marriage were relatively more likely (RRR = 1.02; CI 1.00–1.04) to report unmet need for spacing. Women who had an additional number of living biological child were relatively more likely to report both unmet need for spacing (RRR = 1.11; CI 1.03–1.19) and unmet need for limiting (RRR = 1.77; CI 1.63–1.92). Finally women who had an additional ideal child were relatively less likely (RRR = 0.72; CI 0.66–0.80) to report unmet need for limiting.

Discussion

This study assessed the associations between selected explanatory variables and unmet need in Ghana. The patterns of high unmet need as reported in unmet need prevalent country like ours (35.17%) reveals that, unmet need increased among Pentecostal Protestants, women who had more than one marriage unions, women who did not know couple's desired number of children and women who had an additional number of living biological child. Unmet need decreased among women as they grew older, among those employed and women with an additional number of ideal child. Unmet need for spacing was positive among women who did not know couple's desired number of children, as the age of women getting married increases and women who had additional living biological child. Unmet need for spacing decreased as women grew older, among rural women and women employed. Unmet need for limiting was positive among women who had at least secondary education, women from wealthier households and among women with an additional living biological child. Unmet need for limiting decreased as women had an additional ideal child.

The results suggest that unmet need for spacing and total unmet need were negatively associated with age. As women grew older, both unmet need for spacing and total unmet need decreased but no significant association was observed across ages under unmet need for limiting. This is expected in that, younger mothers might have not reached the desired fertility and hence preferred to space childbirths than limit [11, 24]. These findings are consistent with three other studies from SSA focusing on women's fertility choices.

Table 2 Descriptive statistics

	Univariate			Bivariate											
	Overall sample ($n = 4527$)			Women with unmet need - total ($n = 1592$) = 35.17%				Women with unmet need for spacing ($n = 914$) = 20.19%				Women with unmet need for limiting ($n = 678$) = 14.98%			
Variable	Measurement	n	%	n	%	Chi2	*p*-value	n	%	Chi2	*p*-value	n	%	Chi2	*p*-value
Age															
	15–19	118	3	56	47	77	0.00	54	47	96	0.00	2	3	451	0.00
	20–24	632	14	201	32			189	30			12	3		
	25–29	1038	23	306	29			265	27			41	5		
	30–34	967	21	295	31			180	21			115	15		
	35–39	891	20	337	38			153	22			184	25		
	40–44	592	13	260	44			59	15			201	38		
	45–49	289	6	137	47			14	8			123	45		
Religion															
	None or traditional religion	314	7	118	38	7	0.14	66	25	5	0.25	52	21	31	0.00
	Catholic	651	14	212	33			131	23			81	16		
	Non-Pentecostal protestant	987	22	352	36			169	21			183	22		
	Pentecostal protestant	1614	36	594	37			328	24			266	21		
	Islam	961	21	316	33			220	25			96	13		
Number of unions															
	One	3557	79	1191	33	21	0.00	743	24	0	0.65	448	16	68	0.00
	More than one	970	21	401	41			171	23			230	29		
Residence															
	Urban	1995	44	686	34	1	0.33	398	23	0	0.58	288	18	1	0.32
	Rural	2532	56	906	36			516	24			390	19		
Education															
	no education	1528	34	544	36	4	0.15	318	24	3	0.19	226	19	2	0.45
	primary	868	19	326	38			187	26			139	20		
	secondary +	2131	47	722	34			409	22			313	18		
SES															
	Poorest	1339	30	450	34	23	0.00	284	24	12	0.02	166	16	23	0.00
	2	878	19	355	40			195	27			160	23		
	3	823	18	314	38			170	25			144	22		
	4	768	17	250	33			139	21			111	18		
	Least poor	719	16	223	31			126	20			97	16		

Table 2 Descriptive statistics *(Continued)*

	Univariate			Bivariate											
	Overall sample ($n = 4527$)			Women with unmet need - total ($n = 1592$) = 35.17%				Women with unmet need for spacing ($n = 914$) = 20.19%				Women with unmet need for limiting ($n = 678$) = 14.98%			
Variable	Measurement	n	%	n	%	Chi2	*p*-value	n	%	Chi2	*p*-value	n	%	Chi2	*p*-value
Occupation															
	Unemployed	779	17	301	39	5	0.03	225	32	32	0.00	76	14	11	0.00
	Employed	3748	83	1291	34			689	22			602	20		
Heard FP messages on radio															
	No	1951	43	706	36	2	0.21	418	25	3	0.08	288	19	0	0.98
	Yes	2576	57	886	34			496	23			390	19		
Heard FP messages on TV															
	No	2550	56	933	37	5	0.02	538	25	4	0.05	395	20	2	0.13
	Yes	1977	44	659	33			376	22			283	18		
Read FP messages in newspaper															
	No	4314	95	1529	35	3	0.08	880	24	3	0.09	649	19	1	0.37
	Yes	213	5	63	30			34	18			29	16		
You visited health facility in the past 12 months															
	No	1617	36	605	37	6	0.02	326	24	0	0.51	279	22	11	0.00
	Yes	2910	64	987	34			588	23			399	17		
FP worker visited you in the past 12 months															
	No	3879	86	1354	35	1	0.37	766	23	3	0.10	588	19	0	0.64
	Yes	648	14	238	37			148	27			90	18		
Knows modern FP methods															
	No	50	1	14	28	1	0.29	10	22	0	0.75	4	10	2	0.15
	Yes	4477	99	1578	35			904	24			674	19		
Couple's desire for children															
	Both want the same	2101	46	678	32	20	0.00	385	21	21	0.00	293	17	6	0.09
	Husband wants more children	1178	26	419	36			231	23			188	20		
	Husband wants fewer children	402	9	150	37			84	25			66	21		
	Does not know	846	19	345	41			214	30			131	21		
Membership to any health insurance scheme															
	Not member	1350	30	505	37	4	0.04	266	24	0	0.86	239	22	11	0.00
	Member	3177	70	1087	34			648	24			439	17		
Continuous variables															

Table 2 Descriptive statistics *(Continued)*

	Univariate			Bivariate											
	Overall sample ($n = 4527$)			Women with unmet need - total ($n = 1592$) = 35.17%				Women with unmet need for spacing ($n = 914$) = 20.19%				Women with unmet need for limiting ($n = 678$) = 14.98%			
Variable	Measurement	n	%	n	%	Chi2	*p*-value	n	%	Chi2	*p*-value	n	%	Chi2	*p*-value
Overall sample ($n = 4527$)				Total unmet need ($n = 1592$)				Unmet need for spacing ($n =$ 1154)				Unmet need for limiting ($n = 696$)			
		mean	Sd	mean	sd	t-statistic	p-value	mean	sd	t-statistic	*p*-value	mean	sd	t-statistic	*p*-value
Age at first marriage	Yes	19.72	5	19.34	4.34	4.07	0.00	19.46	4	3	0.01	19.17	4	4	0.00
	No			19.2	4.7			19.92	5			19.92	5		
Number of living biological children	Yes	3.13	2	3.63	2.04	−12.78	0.00	2.66	2	3	0.00	4.94	2	−26.08	0.00
	No			2.86	1.90			2.86	2			2.86	2		
Ideal number of children	Yes	4.44	1	4.43	1.25	0.62	0.54	4.41	1	1	0.37	4.45	1.31	−0.01	0.99
	No			4.45	1.26			4.45	1			4.45	1.26		

Table 3 Determinants of unmet need for family planning

Regression results (*n* = 4527)									
Variable and measurement	Model I [Logistic]			Model II [Multinomial]					
	Women with unmet need-total (*n* = 1592)			Women with unmet need for spacing (n = 914)			Women with unmet need for limiting (n = 678)		
	OR	95% CI		RRR	95% CI		RRR	95% CI	
Age									
15–19	1			1			1		
20–24	0.448***	0.296	0.680	0.481***	0.314	0.736	0.634	0.140	2.875
25–29	0.332***	0.218	0.506	0.376***	0.242	0.586	0.882	0.207	3.757
30–34	0.255***	0.163	0.399	0.251***	0.155	0.406	1.557	0.373	6.491
35–39	0.284***	0.177	0.456	0.231***	0.137	0.390	2.23	0.527	9.430
40–44	0.279***	0.171	0.456	0.132***	0.075	0.233	2.88	0.683	12.150
45–49	0.308***	0.180	0.530	0.065***	0.031	0.140	3.98	0.930	17.030
Religion									
none or trad. Religion	1			1			1		
Catholic	0.924	0.692	1.234	0.891	0.652	1.219	0.89	0.545	1.453
Non-Pentecostal protestant	0.952	0.716	1.266	0.787	0.569	1.088	1.159	0.726	1.849
Pentecostal protestant	1.076	0.829	1.396	0.974	0.732	1.294	1.172	0.748	1.838
Islam	0.968	0.729	1.283	0.967	0.720	1.299	0.768	0.457	1.290
Number of unions									
One	1			1			1		
More than one	1.212*	1.033	1.423	1.214	0.992	1.486	1.204	0.960	1.510
Residence									
Urban	1			1			1		
Rural	0.831	0.687	1.007	0.784*	0.630	0.977	0.892	0.661	1.203
Education									
no education	1			1			1		
primary	1.034	0.856	1.249	0.942	0.758	1.172	1.143	0.845	1.546
secondary +	1.099	0.910	1.327	0.888	0.710	1.112	1.531**	1.138	2.060
SES									
Poorest	1			1			1		
2	1.284*	1.057	1.561	1.191	0.955	1.485	1.627**	1.195	2.216
3	1.242	0.974	1.583	0.991	0.756	1.300	2.012***	1.367	2.961
4	1.042	0.786	1.383	0.804	0.574	1.126	1.856**	1.186	2.904
Least poor	1.077	0.777	1.493	0.848	0.572	1.258	1.809*	1.096	2.986
Occupation									
Unemployed	1			1			1		
Employed	0.789**	0.666	0.934	0.707***	0.592	0.845	0.964	0.703	1.320
Heard FP messages on radio									
No	1			1			1		
Yes	0.933	0.797	1.093	0.949	0.793	1.136	0.918	0.717	1.176
Heard FP messages on TV									
No	1			1			1		
Yes	0.974	0.814	1.164	1.00	0.812	1.232	0.912	0.702	1.185
Read FP messages in newspaper									
No	1			1			1		

Table 3 Determinants of unmet need for family planning *(Continued)*

Regression results ($n = 4527$)									
Variable and measurement	Model I [Logistic]			Model II [Multinomial]					
	Women with unmet need-total ($n = 1592$)			Women with unmet need for spacing (n = 914)			Women with unmet need for limiting (n = 678)		
	OR	95% CI		RRR	95% CI		RRR	95% CI	
Yes	0.974	0.722	1.313	0.788	0.528	1.177	1.393	0.920	2.107
You visited health facility in the past 12 months									
No	1			1			1		
Yes	0.883	0.767	1.017	0.872	0.737	1.032	0.93	0.752	1.150
FP worker visited you in the past 12 months									
No	1			1			1		
Yes	1.101	0.915	1.326	1.205	0.971	1.494	1.017	0.769	1.343
Knows modern FP methods									
No	1			1			1		
Yes	1.158	0.556	2.415	1.428	0.664	3.070	0.861	0.259	2.865
Couple's desire for children									
Both want the same	1			1			1		
Husband wants more children	1.081	0.923	1.267	1.093	0.905	1.320	1.094	0.850	1.408
Husband wants fewer children	1.214	0.948	1.555	1.289	0.975	1.704	1.176	0.813	1.702
Does not know	1.376***	1.141	1.660	1.5***	1.225	1.837	1.134	0.823	1.561
Membership to any health insurance scheme									
Not member	1			1			1		
Member	1.006	0.871	1.161	1.002	0.845	1.188	1.005	0.802	1.258
Age at first marriage	1.008	0.990	1.025	1.023*	1.001	1.045	0.98	0.956	1.004
Number of living biological children	1.36***	1.286	1.438	1.111**	1.038	1.189	1.775***	1.636	1.927
Ideal number of children	0.863***	0.810	0.920	0.957	0.888	1.032	0.722***	0.656	0.795

*** $p < 0.001$, ** $p < 0.01$, * $p < 0.05$

These studies posit that, whereas the need for spacing childbirth was more likely not to be met among younger women who had not yet achieved their desired fertility goals and for that matter would be more interested in spacing future pregnancies, the unmet need for limiting was negative during later reproductive years once their desired family size was achieved and no further pregnancies are desired [25–27]. It will therefore be beneficial for policies targeting unmet need to address women according to their age specific needs.

We anticipated that given the underlying Catholic doctrines, Catholics compared to traditional religion were expected to be more likely to report unmet need but the results pointed no significant difference across the various religious faiths. In the current study, Pentecostal Protestants women had higher odds of unmet need compared to traditional religion but was equally not statistically significant. In a prior study, Muslim women had lower odds of unmet need compared to orthodox Christians and this might be attributable to the tendency of Muslim women to have higher total fertility compared to Christians [28]. In a reviewed study on determinants of unmet need from selected studies in LMICs the influence of religious beliefs on family planning decisions appeared a little complex [11]. Data from six quantitative studies examining the role of a woman's religious belief detected significant associations with unmet need for contraception [11]. In a Nepal study, Muslim belief was positively associated with an increase in unmet need when compared to Hinduism [29]. In another study on unmet need in Ghana, Catholicism was identified to be negatively associated with unmet need when compared to other religious sects [30]. A qualitative study from Uganda on determinants of unmet need findings were consistent as they identified Anglicans to be more positive towards contraceptive use compared to Muslims and Catholics [11, 31]. In an Indian study for instance, Hindu traditions identified selected menstrual taboos amongst which required relatives close observation of a woman's fertility and thus made contraceptive use limited [32].

Our study detected that unmet need was dominant among women who had more than one marriage unions. A study reported that, marital instability can potentially propel women to re-marry and have additional children from the new matrimonial home hence increasing the woman's total fertility beyond her initial fertility intensions given that the initial marriage was note terminated [33]. The desire to have additional children in the new matrimonial home can trigger unmet need for contraception. Consistent with this finding, a review of selected studies on Male attitude and behavior on family planning in Africa reported that new unions propel higher parity progression since in the African context, it is believed that any marriage should be graced with at least a child to symbolize effective marriage union even if the woman had given birth to her desired number of children in the previous marriage [34, 35].

Place of residence did not exhibit any significance for total unmet need and unmet need for limiting except for only unmet need for spacing where rural dwellers were less likely to report unmet need in the multinomial analysis. The outcome is inconsistent with prior studies in Uganda and Ethiopia which reported higher odds on unmet need among rural women [22, 36]. The lower levels of unmet need relative to their urban counterparts is again inconsistent with another Ethiopian study in the fact that rural women relatively have lower decision making power on contraceptive use and could not report substantial contraceptive use level to reflect the reduction in unmet need reported [28].

Our multinomial results detected that women with at least secondary education were more likely to report unmet need for limiting. Unmet need is often higher among women with a primary school education. This is because women with higher education are relatively more likely to report contraceptive use and women with no education generally want more children [33, 37]. This results are inconsistent with results from Burkina Faso and Malawi which reported higher likelihood of unmet need among rural women with lower educational levels [16, 33].

Our model I did not detect any significant levels across the socioeconomic status except for our Model II which reported positive association with unmet need for limiting as household wealth increases. Higher unmet need for limiting was reported among the less poor households. Unlike in most prior studies where lower wealth quintiles associated positively with unmet need for contraception [22, 28], our findings reported a contradiction in that women from higher wealth quintiles were more likely to report unmet need against the view that women with wealthier background ought to have better decision making power on contraceptive use and should therefore report lower levels of unmet need [11, 28, 33].

Woman's occupational status was identified to be negatively associated with unmet need and unmet need for spacing. Previous studies suggests that female occupation and an independent income positively enhances a woman's autonomy by improving financial decision-making within a household which can lead to better contraceptive use decision [38, 39]. Also professionals/ clerical occupations workers were observed in a Zambian study to be significantly less likely to report unmet need for spacing compared to their non-working colleagues, where as all other occupations except those in Agriculture were equally significantly less likely to report unmet need for limiting compared to their unemployed companions [24]. This means that there were differences in contraceptive use among the different occupational groupings. Given that woman's autonomy in employment can contribute to an increase in the contraceptive use and thus a reduction in unmet need, policies should focus on assisting women acquire gainful employment.

Total unmet need and unmet need for limiting were negative among married women who desired an additional child. This trend was expected as some of the currently married women who mentioned and additional child as their ideal number might have not had this desired number either presently or in the past and are less willing to limit child bearing but have no access to consistent modern contraceptive use. Alternatively previous studies attest that, their colleagues who desired additional children were probably in active child bearing and for that matter might prefer contraception to space future childbirths [33]. In rural settings in Ghana like many parts in SSA, contraception to limit childbearing is scarce compared to other modern methods which are more available. Long acting contraceptive method use decisions are difficult to reach than other methods [14]. Our findings are consistent with previous studies which equally suggest lower unmet need detected among married women who reported higher number of children as their ideal preference [40].

Methodological considerations

The study population consisted of currently married fertile women at the time of the study. This means that the prevalence of unmet need should not be misconstrued and generalized to cover the entire population of women in Ghana as the method for calculation did not cover all women. Following the objective of our study, we carefully selected the category of currently married women who are consistently referred to in literature as being at extremely higher risk of unmet need [7]. Also given the cross-sectional design nature of the study, all variables included in the regression analysis were information obtained at the time of the survey which only provides evidence of statistical associations between the predictor and dependent variables and cannot show cause-effect relationship.

Conclusion

The results showed that an increase in age, residing in a rural area, and being employed were associated with lower risk of unmet need for spacing. Additionally, Women who did not know the couples' ideal number of children, women who had higher age when they got married, and women with higher number of biological children were more likely to report unmet need for spacing. Women who had a higher number of ideal children, women who had secondary or higher education, women from higher socio-economic households, were less likely to report unmet need for limiting.

The unmet need for contraception reported in this study is high compared to other LMICs with similar socio-demographic characteristics given the more than one in three married women reporting unmet need is a major concern. The study recommend that continuous health education on the significance of family planning both at the individual and household level is an important strategic measure to adopt if contraceptive use decisions are to be enhanced so as to reduce the lagging persistent unmet need for family planning in Ghana. Community based family planning programmes should be strengthened and expanded to serve all rural communities. A recent study in Ethiopia reported majority of contraceptive users preferred child spacing to limiting which supports many studies in SSA and by extension Ghana [41, 42]. The findings are crucial and points the need for programmes to incorporate access to contraceptive services and raise educational levels to bring about behavioral and attitudinal change among the affected women so as to lower the nagging desire for additional children. Specific emphasis should be accorded to educated women and women within the various socioeconomic levels. Qualitative research is needed to understand the reasons for the underlying trend.

Abbreviations

CI: Confidence interval; FP: Family planning; GDHS: Ghana demographic health survey; LMICs: Low and middle income countries; NHIS: Nation health Insurance scheme; OR: Odds ratio; RRR: Relative risk ratio; SES: Socioeconomic status; SSA: Sub-Saharan Africa; T.V: Television

Acknowledgements

The authors wish to express their great debt of gratitude to the ICF Macro Calverton, Maryland, USA, for releasing the data for 2014 and also granting the author access to their DHS web platform for this study. We also appreciate the efforts of the Ghana statistical service and the Government of Ghana for coordinating and conducting these surveys.

Authors' contributions

JKW conceived the study, carried out the GDHS data extraction from the Measure DHS web platform. JM run the initial analysis. JKW, JM critically appraised the data and tables. JKW carried out the initial draft and was complimented by JM, AK, CK, WA JA and SK. JM, AK, CK, WA, JA and SK proof read the draft manuscript to ensure consistency. JA and AK contributed equally. All authors read through subsequent versions of the manuscript and approved the final version.

Author details

[1]School of Business and Law, Department of Administration and Management Studies, University for Development Studies, Box UPW 36, Wa-campus, Wa, Ghana. [2]Department of Economics, University of Malawi, Chancellor College, P.O Box 280, Zomba, Malawi. [3]Environmental Health Department, The Malawi Polytechnic, University of Malawi, P/B 303, Chichiri, Blantyre 3, Blantyre, Malawi. [4]School of Business and Law, Department of Banking and Finance, University for Development Studies, Wa-campus, Wa, Ghana. [5]Faculty of Integrated Development Studies, Campus Officer, University for Development Studies, Wa-campus, Wa, Ghana. [6]Department of Public Health, St. Francis University College of Health and Allied Sciences, P.O.Box, 175, Ifakara, Tanzania.

References

1. Say L, Chou D, Gemmill A, Tunçalp Ö, Moller A-B, Daniels J, et al. Global causes of maternal death: a WHO systematic analysis. Lancet Glob Health. 2014;2:e323–33.
2. WHO Trends in Maternal Mortality. 1990 To 2013 - estimates by WHO, UNICEF, UNFPA, the World Bank and the United Nations population division. Geneva: World Health Organization; 2014.
3. WHO, UNICEF, UNFPA, World Bank, United Nations. Trends in Maternal Mortality: 1990 to 2013 Estimates by WHO, UNICEF, UNFPA, The World Bank and the United Nations Population Division. WHO Library Cataloguing-in-Publication Data-20 Avenue Appia, 1211 Geneva 27, Switzerland; 2014.
4. Cleland J, Bernstein S, Ezeh A, Faundes A, Glasier A, Innis J. Family planning: the unfinished agenda. Lancet. 2006;368:1810–27.
5. Upadhyay UD, Gipson JD, Withers M, Lewis S, Ciaraldi EJ, Fraser A, Huchko MJ, Prata N. Women's empowerment and fertility: a review of the literature. Soc Sci Med. 2014;115:111–20.
6. Govindasamy P, Boadi E. A decade of unmet need for contraception in Ghana: Programmatic and policy implications [Internet]. Calverton, Maryland, USA: Macro International; 2000. Available from: https://www.dhsprogram.com/pubs/pdf/FA31/FA31.pdf.
7. Bradley SE., Croft TN, Fishel JD, Westoff CF. Revising unmet need for family planning- DHS analytical studies 25. ICF Int. Calverton Md. USA. 2012;
8. Westoff CF. New estimates for unmet need and demand for family planning; 2006.
9. Bongaarts J. The KAP-gap and the unmet need for contraception. Popul Dev Rev. 1991:293–313.
10. Casterline JB, Sinding SW. Unmet need for family planning in developing countries and implications for population policy. Popul Dev Rev. 2000;26:691–723.
11. Wulifan JK, Brenner S, Jahn A, De Allegri M. A scoping review on determinants of unmet need for family planning among women of reproductive age in low and middle income countries. BMC Womens Health. 2016;16:2.
12. Nortman DL. Measuring the unmet need for contraception to space and limit births. Int Fam Plan Perspect. 1982;8:125–34.
13. Casterline JB, El-Zanatay F, El-Zeini LO. Unmet need and unintended fertility. Longitudinal Evidence From Upper Egypt. Int Fam Plan Perspect. 2003;29:158–66.
14. U.S-Centers for Disease Control and Prevention, UNICEF, Others. Benefits of family planning. Boletn' Asoc Chil Proteccin Fam. 2000;28:3.
15. Ghana Statistical Service. Ghana DHS, 2014 - Final Report-DHS Program, ICF International, Rockville, Maryland, USA. 2015.
16. Palamuleni ME, Adebowale A, Others. Prevalence and determinants of unintended pregnancies in Malawi. Afr Popul Stud 2014;28:551–563.
17. Eliason S, Baiden F, Yankey BA, Awusabo-Asare K. Determinants of unintended pregnancies in rural Ghana. BMC Pregnancy Childbirth. 2014;14:261.
18. Eliason S, Baiden F, Quansah-Asare G, Graham-Hayfron Y, Bonsu D, Phillips J, et al. Factors influencing the intention of women in rural Ghana to adopt postpartum family planning. Reprod Health. 2013;10:34.
19. Horayangkura P. Open working group proposal for sustainable development goals. AU Law J 2015;5:9.
20. Cates W, Abdool Karim Q, El-Sadr W, Haffner DW, Kalema-Zikusoka G, Rogo K, et al. Family planning and the millennium development goals. Science. 2010;329:1603.
21. Government of Ghana. Ghana Demographic and Health Survey, 2008 -statistical service and ICF macro,. Calverton, Maryland, USA; 2008.
22. Korra A. Attitudes toward family planning and reasons for nonuse among women with unmet need for family planning in Ethiopia. ORC Macro Calverton; 2002.
23. Mazalale J, Kambala C, Brenner S, Chinkhumba J, Lohmann J, Mathanga DP, et al. Factors associated with delivery outside a health facility: cross-sectional study in rural Malawi. Trop Med Int Health TM IH. 2015;20:617–26.
24. Imasiku ENS, Odimegwu CO, Adedini SA, Ononokpono DN. Variations in unmet need for contraception in Zambia: does ethnicity play a role? J Biosoc Sci. 2014;46:294–315.
25. Barro RJ, Becker GS. Fertility choice in a model of Economic growth. Econometrica. 1989;57:481–501.

26. Kalemli-Ozcan S. A Stochastic model of mortality, fertility, and Human Capital Investment. J Dev Econ. 2003;70:103–18.
27. Sah RK. The effects of child mortality changes on fertility choice and parental welfare. J Polit Econ. 1991;99:582–606.
28. Tebekaw Y, Aemro B, Teller C. Prevalence and determinants of unintended childbirth in Ethiopia. BMC Pregnancy Childbirth. 2014;14:326.
29. Bhanderi MN, Kannan S. Untreated reproductive morbidities among ever married women of slums of Rajkot City, Gujarat. The role of class, distance, provider attitudes, and perceived quality of care. J Urban health-Bull N Y Acad Med. 2010;87:254–63.
30. Machiyama K, Cleland J. Insights into unmet need in Ghana [internet]. London, UK: London School of Hygiene and Tropical Medicine; 2013. Available from: https://assets.publishing.service.gov.uk/media/57a08a1ce5274a27b2000421/STEP-UP-unmet-FP-need-Ghana.pdf.
31. Kaida A, Kippi W, Hessel P, Konde-Lule J. Male participation in family planning. Results from a qualitative study in Mpigi District, Uganda. J Biosoc Sci. 2005;37:18.
32. Hall MAK, Stephenson RB, Juvekar S. Social and Logistical barriers to the use of reversible contraception among women in a rural Indian Village. J Health Popul Nutr. 2008;26:241–50.
33. Adebowale SA, Palamuleni ME. Determinants of unmet need for modern contraception and reasons for non-use among married women in rural areas of Burkina Faso. Afr Popul Stud. 2014;28:499–514.
34. Karra MV, Stark NN, Wolf J. Male involvement in family planning: a case study spanning five generations of a south Indian family. Stud Fam Plan. 1997;28:24–34.
35. Toure LB. Male Involvement in Family Planning: A Review of Selected Program Initiatives in Africa. SARA; 1996 [cited 2015 Aug 4]. Available from: https://www.popline.org/node/306362.
36. Hailemariam A, Haddis F. Factors affecting unmet need for family planning in southern nations, nationalities and peoples region, Ethiopia. Ethiop J Health Sci. 2011;21:77–89.
37. Wulifan JK, Bagah DA. Male involvement in family planning in Muslem communities in Wa municipality, Ghana. Res Humanit Soc Sci. 2015;5:86–97.
38. Hakim C. A New approach to explaining fertility patterns: preference theory. Popul Dev Rev. 2003;29:349–74.
39. Palamuleni ME. Socio-Economic and Demographic factors affecting contraceptive use in Malawi. Afr J Reprod Health. 2013;17:91–104.
40. Khan S, Bradley SEK, Fishel J, Mishra V. Unmet need and the demand for family planning in Uganda further analysis of the Uganda demographic and health surveys, 1995–2006; 2008.
41. Creanga AA, Gillespie D, Karklins S, Tsui OA. Low use of contraception among poor women in Africa: an equity issue [internet]. Bulletin of the world; 2011. Available from: https://www.who.int/bulletin/volumes/89/4/10-083329/en/.
42. Weldegerima B, Denekew A. Women's knowledge, preferences, and practices of modern contraceptive methods in Woreta, Ethiopia. Res Soc Adm Pharm. 2008;4:302–7.

15

Modern contraceptive utilization and associated factors among married and cohabiting women in Papua New Guinea

Abdul-Aziz Seidu[1,2*], Ebenezer Agbaglo[3], Louis Kobina Dadzie[1], Bright Opoku Ahinkorah[4], Edward Kwabena Ameyaw[4], Justice Kanor Tetteh[1] and Sanni Yaya[5,6]

Abstract

Background: Universal access to family planning has been emphasized by the international development agenda, as evident in the Sustainable Development Goal 3.7. This notwithstanding, the use of modern contraceptives has been minimal in low- and middle-income countries, especially in Papua New Guinea. In view of this, we investigated the factors associated with the use of modern contraceptives and the associated factors among married and cohabiting women in Papua New Guinea.

Methods: The study utilised the Demographic and Health Survey data of 2345 women in sexual unions in Papua New Guinea. We employed a descriptive and binary logistic regression analyses. We presented the results as crude Odds Ratios (COR) and adjusted Odds Ratios (AOR), with 95% confidence intervals (CI) signifying level of precision. Level of statistical significance was set at $p < 0.05$.

Results: We found that 74.4% of the women were using modern contraceptives ranging from injectables (44.5%) to other modern methods (0.23%). Women aged 15–19 [AOR = 7.425, 95% CI = 2.853, 19.32], residents of the Highland region [AOR = 1.521, 95% CI =1.086, 2.131], self-employed women in the agricultural sector [AOR = 1.710, 95% CI = 1.218, 2.400], and women who listened to radio at least once a week [AOR = 1.409, 95% CI = 1.048, 1.895] had higher odds of modern contraceptive usage. However, women in the Islands region [AOR = 0.291, 95% CI = 0.224, 0.377], women whose husbands had higher education [AOR = 0.531,95%CI = 0.318,0.886], women in professional/technical/managerial work [AOR = 0.643, 95% CI = 0.420, 0.986], and those with no child [AOR = 0.213, CI = 0.0498,0.911] had lower odds of modern contraceptive use.

(Continued on next page)

* Correspondence: abdul-aziz.seidu@stu.ucc.edu.gh
[1]Department of Population and Health, University of Cape Coast, Cape Coast, Ghana
[2]College of Public Health, Medical and Veterinary Sciences, James Cook University, Townsville, Queensland, Australia

(Continued from previous page)

Conclusion: Out of the 2345 participants, we found that majority of them were using modern contraceptives and the commonly used modern contraceptive was injectables. Age, region of residence, partner's education, employment, partner's desire for children, and frequency of listening to radio are associated with modern contraceptive usage. Tailored reproductive healthcare should be developed for women who are disadvantaged when it comes to the usage of modern contraceptives in order to boost modern contraceptive use among them. Further investigation is needed to unravel the motivation for the high usage of injectables among married and cohabiting women in Papua New Guinea.

Keywords: Contraceptives, Papua New Guinea, Public health, Global Health, Women

Background

Making access to family planning universal has been an important component of the global development agenda. The International Conference on Population and Development Program of Action, for instance, declared it as a fundamental human right [1–3]. More importantly, the target 3.7 of the Sustainable Development Goals (SDGs) emphasises "the universal access to sexual and reproductive health-care services, including family planning" [4]. In contemporary society, modern contraception is the most preferred option and includes sterilization, intrauterine devices and systems, subdermal implants, oral contraceptives, condoms, injectables, emergency contraceptive pills, patches, diaphragm and cervical caps, spermicidal agents, vaginal rings, and sponge [5]. Utilisation of modern contraception allows couples to determine the number and spacing of their pregnancies. It additionally ensures good health for both mothers and children, by decreasing mortality and morbidity induced by unwanted pregnancies [6–9]. Further, increasing contraceptive use reduces fertility, which indirectly leads to poverty reduction [10].

There has been a flurry of research on modern contraception use all over the world, especially in low- and middle-income countries. Part of such research has focused mainly on reasons for non-use of contraception [11] and factors that positively influence the use of contraception, with others have focused specifically on the influence of social support and parity [12], internal migration, and knowledge of contraceptive use on the use of contraception [13]. In terms of geography, such research has focused on countries such as India [14], twenty-seven sub-Saharan African countries [15], Gambia [16], and Ethiopia [17]. Research by Adebowale et al. [11], for instance, revealed being married more than once and husband's non-approval as barriers to contraception use in Burkina Faso. Women's education [15], parity [17], age, religion, and type of marriage [18] have also been identified as predictors of modern contraceptive use among women.

In the Pacific, previous related studies basically focused on follow-up of a contraceptive outreach program [19], access to contraception and family planning [20], adolescent fertility and family planning [21], and costs and benefits of reducing unmet need for contraception [10]. To be more specific, in Papua New Guinea, previous related studies focused on women's perspective of family planning [22], and impact of the contraceptive implant on maternal and neonatal mortality [23], but failed to reveal the factors associated with modern contraception use. In the present study, we investigated the factors associated with the use of modern contraception in Papua New Guinea. This study is desirable, given that, as previous studies reveal, Papua New Guinea records low use of modern contraceptive, which has led to a high maternal mortality ratio, estimated to be around 57.3% per 100,000 live births [24]. Thus, revealing factors associated with modern contraception use in Papua New Guinea, as this study aims to do, will not only extend the geographical coverage of research of this kind, but also help health intervention programs aimed at reducing maternal mortality due to unintended pregnancies and abortions in the country.

Materials and methods

Data source

The data used for this study forms part of the 2016–2018 Papua New Guinea Demographic and Health Survey (PDHS), which was collected from October 2016 to December 2018. The survey adopted a two-staged stratified sampling technique. Before the sampling, the provinces in the country were apportioned into urban and rural areas, which yielded 43 strata; however, the National Capital District had only urban areas. A two-staged sampling procedure was used to sample census units (CUs) from each stratum. Stage 1 involved the selection of 800 CUs. This was done through probability proportional to CU size. The second stage saw the systematic selection of 24 households from each cluster through probability sampling, and this yielded a total of 19,200 households. For this study, we focused on women in sexual unions, with "sexual union" defined as marriage or cohabitation, and such women numbered 2345, all of which had complete information on the variables the present study is interested in. Details of the methodology, pretesting, training of field workers, the sampling design, and selection are available in the PDHS final report [25] which is also available online at: https://dhsprogram.com/publications/publication-fr364-dhs-final-reports.cfm.

Variables

Outcome variable

The outcome variable was modern contraceptive utilization. A woman was deemed to be a modern contraceptive user if she uses at least one of the following methods: female sterilization, male sterilization, IUD, injectable, implants, pills, male condom, female condom, emergency contraception, and standard days method. On the other hand, non-users are those who resort to the use of traditional methods such as rhythm method, lactation amenorrhea method, and withdrawal or if she had not been using any type of contraception at all [26–28].

Independent variables

Seventeen independent variables that were theoretically and empirically related to contraceptive usage were considered in this study [27–33]. The variables comprised age, occupation, place of residence, region of residence, marital status, education, partner's education, wealth, age at first sex, age at first childbirth, total children ever born, number of living children, husband's desire for children, decision maker on contraception, frequency of listening to radio, frequency of watching television, and frequency of reading newspaper or magazine. Some of these variables were recoded for meaningful and easy interpretation of results. Age at first sex and age at first childbirth were recoded as 1 = < 18, 2 = 18–24, and 3 = 25+. Total children ever born was coded as 1 = 1–2, 2 = 3–4, and 3 = 5 and above. Number of living children was coded as 1 = No Child, 2 = 1–2, 3 = 3–4, and 4 = 5 and above.

Statistical analysis

Both descriptive and inferential analyses were conducted. The descriptive analysis involved the use of frequencies and percentages to describe the study sample and the prevalence of modern contraceptive usage across all the independent variables. After that, two logistic regression models were built and the results were reported as crude and adjusted odds ratios (see Table 2). The model fitness specification was done with the Hosmer-Lemeshow test while multicollinearity was checked using the variance inflation factor (VIF) which showed no evidence of multi-collinearity. We applied sample weight to take care of areas that were under-sampled and also those that were over-sampled. The SVY command was also used to take care of the multi-stage sampling nature of the survey. STATA Version 14.2 for MacOS was used to carry out the analyses, and statistical significance was declared at p-value less than 0.05.

Results

Prevalence of modern contraceptive use among women in union in Papua New Guinea

Findings on the prevalence of modern contraceptive use are presented in Fig. 1. Injectables were the most widely used modern contraceptive, ensued by implants/Norplant, marked by 44.50 and 40.60% respectively. The least reported was other modern methods (0.23%). In all, 74.37% of the women were using modern contraceptives.

Socio-demographic characteristics of women in sexual union in Papua Guinea and modern contraceptives usage

Modern contraceptive use with respect to socio-demographic characteristics have been presented in Table 1. Contraceptive use dominated among women aged 20–24 (83.0%). Nearly 83.3% of women in skilled

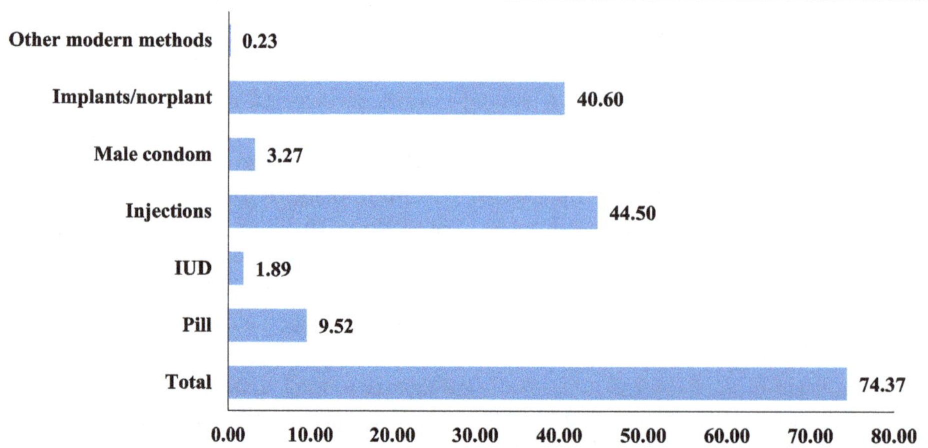

Fig. 1 Prevalence of modern contraceptive use among women in union in Papua New Guinea

Table 1 Socio-demographic characteristics of women in union in Papua New Guinea and modern contraceptives usage ($N = 2345$)

Variable	Weighted N	Weighted %	Modern Contraceptive use	
			No n(%)	Yes n(%)
Age				
15–19	50	2.1	8 (16)	42 (84.0)
20–24	387	16.5	66 (17.1)	321 (83.0)
25–29	581	24.8	107 (18.4)	474 (81.6)
30–34	549	23.4	146 (26.6)	403 (73.4)
35–39	404	17.2	119 (29.5)	285 (70.5)
40–44	249	10.6	93 (37.4)	156 (62.7)
45–49	125	5.3	62 (49.6)	63 (50.4)
Respondent's occupation				
Not working	1398	59.6	375 (26.8)	1023 (73.2)
Professional /technical/managerial	158	6.7	64 (40.5)	94 (59.5)
Clerical	57	2.4	13 (22.8)	44 (77.2)
Sales	128	5.5	30 (23.4)	98 (76.6)
Agricultural- self employed	317	13.5	58 (18.3)	259 (81.7)
Agricultural – employee	42	1.8	12 (28.6)	30 (71.4)
Services	227	9.7	46 (20.3)	181 (79.7)
Skilled manual	18	0.8	3 (16.7)	15 (83.3)
Residence				
Urban	640	27.3	148 (23.1)	492 (76.9)
Rural	1705	72.7	453 (26.6)	1252 (73.4)
Region				
Southern region	751	32.0	149 (19.8)	602 (80.2)
Highlands region	462	19.7	64 (13.9)	398 (86.2)
Momase region	548	23.4	120 (21.9)	428 (78.1)
Islands region	584	24.9	268 (45.9)	316 (54.1)
Current marital status				
Married	2015	85.9	515 (25.6)	1500 (74.4)
Living with partner	330	14.1	86 (26.1)	244 (73.9)
Highest educational level				
No education	389	16.6	99 (25.5)	290 (74.6)
Primary	1141	48.7	282 (24.7)	859 (75.3)
Secondary	698	29.8	175 (25.1)	523 (74.9)
Higher	117	5.0	45 (38.5)	72 (61.5)
Husband/partner's education level				
No education	260	11.1	48 (18.5)	212 (81.5)
Primary	1037	44.2	292 (28.2)	745 (71.8)
Secondary	820	35.0	186 (22.7)	634 (77.3)
Higher	228	9.7	75 (32.9)	153 (67.1)
Wealth index				
Poorest	268	11.4	74 (27.6)	194 (72.4)
Poorer	335	14.3	73 (21.8)	262 (78.2)
Middle	436	18.6	124 (28.4)	312 (71.6)

Table 1 Socio-demographic characteristics of women in union in Papua New Guinea and modern contraceptives usage ($N = 2345$) *(Continued)*

Variable	Weighted N	Weighted %	Modern Contraceptive use	
			No n(%)	Yes n(%)
Richer	637	27.2	158 (24.8)	479 (75.2)
Richest	669	28.5	172 (25.7)	497 (74.3)
Age at first sex				
< 18 yrs	815	34.8	192 (23.6)	623 (76.4)
18–24	1364	58.2	347 (25.4)	1017 (74.6)
25+	166	7.1	62 (37.4)	104 (62.6)
Age at first childbirth				
< 18	419	17.9	91 (21.7)	328 (78.3)
18–24	1539	65.6	376 (24.4)	1163 (75.6)
25+	387	16.5	134 (34.6)	253 (65.4)
Total children ever born				
1–2	925	39.5	218 (23.6)	707 (76.4)
3–4	851	36.3	200 (23.5)	651 (76.5)
5+	569	24.3	183 (32.2)	386 (67.8)
Number of living children				
No child	13	0.6	6 (46.2)	7 (53.8)
1–2	962	41.0	226 (23.5)	736 (76.5)
3–4	857	36.6	206 (24)	651 (76)
5+	513	21.9	163 (31.8)	350 (68.2)
Husband's desire for children				
Both want same	1104	47.1	316 (28.6)	788 (71.4)
Husband wants more	424	18.1	96 (22.6)	328 (77.4)
Husband wants fewer	80	3.4	16 (20)	64 (80)
Don't know	737	31.4	173 (23.5)	564 (76.5)
Frequency of reading newspaper or magazine				
Not at all	1340	57.1	352 (26.3)	988 (73.7)
Less than once a week	551	23.5	137 (24.9)	414 (75.1)
At least once a week	454	19.4	112 (24.7)	342 (75.3)
Frequency of listening to radio				
Not at all	1421	60.6	398 (28)	1023 (72)
Less than once a week	471	20.1	105 (22.3)	366 (77.7)
At least once a week	453	19.3	98 (21.6)	355 (78.4)
Frequency of watching television				
Not at all	1721	73.4	457 (26.6)	1264 (73.4)
Less than once a week	255	10.9	63 (24.7)	192 (75.3)
At least once a week	369	15.7	81 (22)	288 (78)
Decision maker on contraception				
Mainly respondent	659	28.1	146 (22.2)	513 (77.8)
Mainly husband, partner	294	12.5	83 (28.2)	211 (71.8)
Joint decision	1367	58.3	365 (26.7)	1002 (73.3)
Other	25	1.2	7 (28)	18 (72)

Source: 2016–18 PNG DHS

manual labour were using modern contraceptives. Modern contraceptive use was high among urban residents (76.9%). Majority (86.2%) of those in the Highlands region were using modern contraceptives. Modern contraceptives was high among married women (74.4%). Women with primary education dominated in modern contraceptive use (75.3%). Modern contraceptive use was high among women whose partners had no formal education (81.5%). Use of modern contraceptives was high for poorer women (78.2%). Modern contraceptive use stood at 76.4% for those below 18 years. Modern contraceptive use was well pronounced (78.3%) among those under age 18. Modern contraceptive use was high for women with 3–4 births (76.5%). Modern contraceptive use was high among women with 1–2 children living (76.5%). A greater section of the women (47.1%) reported that they and their husbands desired children. Meanwhile, modern contraceptive use was common for women whose husbands alone desired children. We found that modern contraceptive use was commonly reported among those who read at least once a week (75.3%) as well as those who listened to radio at least once a week. Similarly, 78.1% of those who watched television at least once a week made use of modern contraceptives. Most of the women made joint decision on contraceptive with their husbands (58.3%). Nonetheless, 77.9% of those who made solo decisions on contraceptives reported usage.

Predictors of modern contraceptive utilization among women in unions in Papua New Guinea

We present the predictors of modern contraceptive use in Table 2. Relative to women aged 45–49, those aged 15–19 had the highest odds of modern contraceptive use [AOR = 7.425, 95% CI = 2.853, 19.32]. In both models, residents of the Highland region had higher odds of modern contraceptive use, compared to those in the Southern region [AOR = 1.521, 95% CI =1.086, 2.131] but the reverse was the situation for residents of the Islands region [AOR = 0.291, 95% CI = 0.224, 0.377]. Women whose husbands had higher education had less odds of modern contraceptive use, relative to those whose husbands had no formal education [AOR = 0.531, 95% CI = 0.318, 0.886]. Whereas professional/technical/managerial workers had lower odds of modern contraceptive use [AOR = 0.643, 95% CI = 0.420, 0.986], higher odds were noted for women who were self-employed in the agricultural sector, relative to women who were not working [AOR = 1.710, 95% CI = 1.218, 2.400]. Women with no living child were less likely to use modern contraceptives compared to those with five or more children [AOR = 0.213, 95% CI = 0.0498,0.911]. Conversely, women who did not know their partners' desire for children were more likely to use modern contraceptives AOR = 1.286 95% CI = 1.015,1.630].

Discussion

This study investigated the prevalence and drivers of modern contraceptive use in Papua New Guinea, a country with a history of low modern contraceptive use amidst high maternal mortality [34]. In all, we found that at least seven out of ten of the women were using modern contraceptives (74.37%). Injectables were the commonly used modern contraceptives. To a larger extent, modern contraceptive use in Papua New Guinea has levitated at a faster pace. When Marie Stopes [34] started its operations in the country in 2006, contraceptive use was a little above 25% and this seems to have tripled in less than two decades.

The modern contraceptive prevalence observed exceeds modern contraceptive prevalence in the Oceanian region (58%) [35]. The prevalence is analogous to the contraceptive prevalence in Northern America (74%) [35]. Just as observed, the 2006 Demographic and Health Survey of Papua New Guinea noted that injectables were the leading modern contraceptives (36.9%) relative to any other method [36]. A Nigeria-based study that employed time-trend analysis on data ranging between 2000 and 2014 similarly noted that injectables were the leading modern contraceptives (40.7%) [37]. The underlying factors for consistency in preference for injectables in Papua New Guinea are, however, not revealed and a qualitative study will be useful in this regard.

Women aged 15–19 had the highest odds of modern contraceptive use, relative to 45–49 aged women. This finding might rationalize the essence of the ongoing advocacies and initiatives by the Marie Stopes International and its sister organisations. Reporting from a Ugandan population-based study, Rutaremwa et al. [38] also realised a descending trend in modern contraceptive use in relation to age. Since 2006, the Marie Stopes International has focused on making reproductive health services easily accessible to young persons, since this category of people was under-served in the past. In 2018, more than one third of the persons that were served by the organisation (37%) were below 25 years. Practically, institution of a specialised hotline, initiation of youth-friendly services, and collaboration with a revered leading religious institution contributed significantly in achieving this milestone [34].

Residents of the Highland region had higher odds of modern contraceptive use, compared to those in the southern region, but the reverse was the situation for residents of the Islands region. Over the years, several reproductive health policies have been instituted since 1908 [39], the most recent of which are the *National Family Planning Policy (2014), National Youth and Adolescent Health Policy (2014), National Sexual Reproductive Health Policy (2014)*, and the *National Health Sector Gender Policy (2014)* [39]. If in spite of all these, women

Table 2 Predictors of modern contraceptive utilization among women in union in Papua New Guinea ($N = 2345$)

Variable	COR[95%CI]	AOR [95%CI]
Age		
15–19	5.167***[2.245,11.89]	7.425***[2.853,19.32]
20–24	4.786***[3.084,7.428]	6.312***[3.591,11.10]
25–29	4.360***[2.897,6.560]	5.333***[3.281,8.669]
30–34	2.716***[1.824,4.046]	2.803***[1.811,4.338]
35–39	2.357***[1.563,3.554]	2.352***[1.544,3.584]
40–44	1.651*[1.069,2.549]	1.500 [0.966,2.330]
45–49	**Ref**	**Ref**
Marital status		
Married	1.027 [0.787,1.339]	–
Cohabiting	**Ref**	**Ref**
Residence		
Urban	1.203 [0.972,1.488]	–
Rural	**Ref**	**Ref**
Region		
Southern region	**Ref**	**Ref**
Highlands region	1.539** [1.119,2.118]	1.521* [1.086,2.131]
Momase region	0.883 [0.674,1.157]	1.03 [0.773,1.373]
Islands region	0.292***[0.229,0.372]	0.291***[0.224,0.377]
Highest educational level		
No education	**Ref**	**Ref**
Primary	1.04 [0.798,1.355]	1.32 [0.985,1.769]
Secondary	1.02 [0.767,1.357]	1.3 [0.912,1.853]
Higher	0.546** [0.353,0.845]	1.086 [0.577,2.047]
Husband/partner's educational level		
No education	**Ref**	**Ref**
Primary	0.578**[0.411,0.813]	0.737 [0.505,1.076]
Secondary	0.772 [0.542,1.099]	0.881 [0.585,1.325]
Higher	0.462***[0.304,0.701]	0.531* [0.318,0.886]
Wealth status		
Poorest	**Ref**	**Ref**
Poor	1.369 [0.943,1.988]	–
Middle	0.96 [0.684,1.347]	–
Rich	1.156 [0.838,1.597]	–
Richest	1.102 [0.801,1.516]	–
Employment		
Not working	**Ref**	**Ref**
Professional/technical/managerial	0.538***[0.384,0.756]	0.643* [0.420,0.986]
Clerical	1.241 [0.661,2.329]	1.082 [0.519,2.257]
Sales	1.197 [0.782,1.833]	1.299 [0.822,2.054]
Agricultural - self employed	1.637** [1.203,2.228]	1.710**[1.218,2.400]
Agricultural - employee	0.916 [0.464,1.809]	1.246 [0.551,2.817]
Services	1.442*[1.022,2.036]	1.385 [0.944,2.031]
Skilled manual	0.855 [0.220,3.325]	0.646 [0.188,2.223]

Table 2 Predictors of modern contraceptive utilization among women in union in Papua New Guinea ($N = 2345$) *(Continued)*

Variable	COR[95%CI]	AOR [95%CI]
Total children ever born		
1–2	1.538***[1.219,1.940]	1.333 [0.496,3.585]
3–4	1.543***[1.218,1.955]	1.485 [0.788,2.800]
5+	**Ref**	**Ref**
Number of living children		
No child	0.543 [0.180,1.642]	0.213*[0.0498,0.911]
1–2	1.517***[1.195,1.925]	0.469 [0.175,1.257]
3–4	1.472** [1.154,1.877]	0.665 [0.352,1.258]
5+	**Ref**	**Ref**
Age at first sex		
< 18 yrs	1.934***[1.358,2.755]	0.961 [0.616,1.501]
18–24	1.747**[1.247,2.448]	1.158 [0.777,1.727]
25+	**Ref**	**Ref**
Age at first childbirth		
< 18	1.909***[1.396,2.610]	0.892 [0.568,1.401]
18–24	1.638***[1.289,2.082]	0.992 [0.722,1.363]
25+	**Ref**	**Ref**
Partner desire for children		
Both want same	**Ref**	**Ref**
Husband wants more	1.370*[1.054,1.781]	1.318 [0.984,1.765]
Husband wants fewer	1.604 [0.913,2.817]	1.433 [0.764,2.689]
Don't know	1.307*[1.055,1.620]	1.286* [1.015,1.630]
Decision maker for using contraception		
Mainly respondent	1.280*[1.028,1.594]	1.2 [0.934,1.542]
Mainly husband, partner	0.926 [0.699,1.226]	0.923 [0.683,1.247]
Joint decision	**Ref**	**Ref**
Other	0.937 [0.388,2.261]	0.876 [0.333,2.303]
Frequency of listening to radio		
Not at all	**Ref**	**Ref**
Less than once a week	1.356* [1.060,1.734]	1.320*[1.001,1.741]
At least once a week	1.409** [1.096,1.813]	1.409* [1.048,1.895]
Frequency of reading newspaper or magazine		
Not at all	**Ref**	**Ref**
Less than once a week	1.077 [0.857,1.353]	–
At least once a week	1.088 [0.851,1.391]	–
Frequency of watching television		
Not at all	**Ref**	**Ref**
Less than once a week	1.102 [0.813,1.493]	–
At least once a week	1.286 [0.983,1.682]	–
N		2345

Source: 2016–18 PNG DHS
Exponentiated coefficients; 95% confidence intervals in square brackets
* $p < 0.05$
** $p < 0.01$
*** $p < 0.001$
ref. reference, *CI* confidence interval, *COR* Crude Odds Ratio, *AOR* Adjusted Odds Ratios

in some parts of the country exhibit high tendency of modern contraceptive use than others, then the supply or distribution of modern contraceptives should be reconsidered so as to ensure equal access to all women irrespective of geographical location.

Women whose husbands had higher education had less odds of modern contraceptive use, relative to those whose husbands had no formal education. These findings are inconsistent with previous evidence [37, 38, 40]. Education is noted to be a pathway to empowerment over a woman's reproductive health and her holistic wellbeing, and increases awareness of benefits and demerits of contraceptives [38, 41]. These notwithstanding, our finding suggests that highly educated women may be pursuing career and professional objectives and, as such, have limited or no time for contraceptive, relative to low or non-educated women who may not be engaged in highly competitive professions that warrant more commitment.

Whereas professional/technical/managerial workers had lower odds of modern contraceptive use, higher odds were noted for women who were self-employed in the agricultural sector, relative to women who were not working. These variations may be due to preferences of these women. Whilst modern contraceptive is the most preferred [42], some women may prefer either traditional or natural methods for reasons best known to them [43, 44]. We noticed higher odds among women with 3–4 births. However, this observation lost its significance when fitted in the multivariate model variable, which implies that some critical traits of a woman can offset the implication of parity/birth order on her prospects of using modern contraceptives.

Listening to radio at least once a week was associated with higher odds of contraceptive use, compared to not listening at all. Media exposure, such as listening to radio, has similarly been reported to boost modern contraceptive use in Uganda [38]. Some researchers have also contended that mass media enhances demand of services and induces long-term change in behaviour via information, education, and communication initiatives [45].

Strengths and limitations

The study has some limitation worth mentioning. The use of modern contraceptives is subject to social, cultural, and religious interpretations. As a result, a woman may be using contraceptives clandestinely from her partner or family member and may, therefore, not have the courage to report that she uses modern contraceptive [32]. This situation will eventually lead to underreporting of modern contraceptive use. Secondly, since the information on modern contraceptives and the independent variables was gathered concurrently, attribution cannot be made [32]. These notwithstanding, the study has some compelling strengths. It provides current information on the type and prevalence of modern contraceptive use in Papua New Guinea. Additionally, the rigour of the methodological approach and representativeness of the survey render its findings and recommendations generalizable to the country and replicable to other Oceania countries.

Conclusion

We strived to investigate the prevalence of modern contraceptive use and underlying factors in Papua New Guinea, a country in the Oceania region. Of the 2345 participants, we found that the majority of the women were using modern contraceptives, with the commonest method being injectables. Age, region of residence, partners education, employment, partner desire for children, frequency of listening to radio are associated with modern contraceptive usage. Tailored reproductive health care should be developed for women who are disadvantaged when it comes to the use of modern contraceptives in order to boost modern contraceptive use among them. Further investigation is needed to unravel the motivation for injectables among these women.

Abbreviations

COR: Crude Odds Ratio; AOR: Adjusted Odds Ratio; CI: Confidence Interval; PDHS: Papua New Guinea Demographic and Health Survey; NSO: National Statistical Office

Acknowledgments

We are grateful to MEASURE DHS project for giving us for free access to the original data.

Authors' contributions

Conception and design of study: AS; analysis and/or interpretation of data: AS and LKD; drafting the manuscript: AS, EA, LKD, EKA, JKT, and SY; revising the manuscript critically for important intellectual content; AS, EA, LKD, EKA, JKT, and SY; All authors have read and approved the final manuscript.

Author details

[1]Department of Population and Health, University of Cape Coast, Cape Coast, Ghana. [2]College of Public Health, Medical and Veterinary Sciences, James Cook University, Townsville, Queensland, Australia. [3]Department of English, University of Cape Coast, Cape Coast, Ghana. [4]School of Public Health, Faculty of Health, University of Technology Sydney, Sydney, Australia. [5]School of International Development and Global Studies, University of Ottawa, Ottawa, Canada. [6]The George Institute for Global Health, The University of Oxford, Oxford, UK.

References

1. Abrejo FG, Shaikh BT, Saleem S. ICPD to MDGs: missing links and common grounds. Reprod Health. 2008;5(4). https://doi.org/10.1186/1742-4755-5-4.
2. The World Bank. The world bank's reproductive health action plan 2010–2015. Washington DC: The World Bank; 2010.
3. Cleland JG, Ndugwaa RP, Zulu EM. Family planning in sub- Saharan Africa: progress or stagnation? Bull World Health Organ. 2011;89(2):137–43.
4. United Nations, Department of Economic and Social Affair, Population Division. (2019). Family planning and the 2030 agenda for sustainable development: Data booklet. (ST/ESA/SER.A/429). Retrieved from http://creativecommons.org/licenses/by/3.0/igo.

5. Hubacher D, Trusse J. A definition of modern contraceptive methods. Contraception. 2015;92:420–1.
6. Alkema L, Kantorova V, Menozzi C, Biddlecom A. National, regional, and global rates and trends in contraceptive prevalence and unmet need for family planning between 1990 and 2015; a systematic and comprehensive analysis. Lancet. 2013;381:1642–52.
7. Ahmed S, Li Q, Liu L, Tsui A. Maternal deaths averted by contraceptive use: an analysis of 172 countries. Lancet. 2012;380:111–25.
8. Sanga K, Mola G, Wattimena J, et al. Unintended pregnancy amongst women attending antenatal clinics at the post Moresby general hospital. Aust N Z J Obstet Gynaecol. 2014;54:360–5.
9. World Health Organisation. Trends in maternal mortality 1990–2013. Estimates by WHO, UNICEF, UNFPA, the World Bank and the United Nations population division. Geneva: World Health Organisation; 2014.
10. Kennedy EC, Mackesy-Buckley S, Subramaniam S, Demmke A, Latu R, Robertson AS, Tiban K, Tokon A, Luchters S. The case for investing in family planning in the Pacific: costs and benefits of reducing unmet need for contraception in Vanuatu and the Solomon Islands. Reprod Health. 2013; 10(30) http://www.reproductive-health-journal.com/content/10/1/30.
11. Adebowale SA, Palamuleni ME. Determinants of unmet need for modern contraception and reasons for non-use among married women in rural areas of Burkina Faso. Afr Popul Stud. 2014;28(1):499–514.
12. Samandari G, Speizer IS, O'connel K. The role of social support and parity on contraceptive use in Cambodia. Int Perspect Sex Reprod Health. 2010;36(3): 122–31.
13. Lindstrom DP, Hernández CH. Internal migration and contraceptive knowledge and use in Guatemala. Int Fam Plan Perspect. 2006;32:146–53.
14. Chacko E. Women's use of contraception in rural India: a village-level study. Health Place. 2001;7:197–208.
15. Emina JBO, Chirwa T, Kandala N. Trend in the use of modern contraception in sub-Saharan Africa: does women's education matter. Contraception. 2014; 90:154–61.
16. Mace R, Colleran H. Kin influence on the decision to start using modern contraception: a longitudinal study from rural Gambia. Am J Hum Biol. 2009; 21:472–7.
17. Alvergne A, Gibson MA, Gurmu E, Mace R. Social transmission and the spread of modern contraception in rural Ethiopia. PLoS One. 2011;6(7): e22515. https://doi.org/10.1371/journal.pone.0022515.
18. Aliyu AA, Dahiru T, Oyefabi AM, Ladan AM. Knowledge, determinants and use of modern contraceptives among married women in Sabon Gari Zaria-northern Nigeria. J Med Biomed Res. 2015;14(2):13–21.
19. Gupta S, Mola G, Ramsay P, Jenkins G, Stein W, Bolnga J, Black K. Twelve month follow-up of a contraceptive implant outreach service in rural Papua New Guinea. Aust N Z J Obstet Gynaecol. 2017;57:213–8.
20. Thanenthiran S. Access to contraception and family planning in Asia and the Pacific region. Asian-Pacific resource and research center for women; 2019.
21. Kennedy E, Gray N, Azzopardi P, Creati M. Adolescent fertility and family planning in East Asia and the Pacific: a review of DHS reports. Reprod Health. 2011;8:11.
22. Andajani-Sutjahjo S, Tinning ZM, Smith JF. Exploring Women's Perspectives of Family Planning: A Qualitative Study from Rural Papua New Guinea. J Int Womens Studies. 2018;19(6):276–89.
23. Gupta S, Ramsay P, Mola G, McGeechan K, Bolnga J, Kelly-Hanku A, Black KI. Impact of the contraceptive implant on maternal and neonatal morbidity and mortality in rural Papua New Guinea: a retrospective observational cohort study. Contraception. 2019. https://doi.org/https://doi.org/10.1016/j.contraception.2019.03.042.
24. WHO. Summaries of the SDG health and health related targets. 2016.
25. National Statistical Office (NSO) [Papua New Guinea](PNG) and ICF. Papua New Guinea Demographic and Health Survey 2016-2018. National Report. Port Moresby: PNG: National Statistical Office; 2019.
26. Gebre MN, Edossa ZK. Modern contraceptive utilization and associated factors among reproductive-age women in Ethiopia: evidence from 2016 Ethiopia demographic and health survey. BMC Womens Health. 2020;20(1): 1–14.
27. Aviisah PA, Dery S, Atsu BK, Yawson A, Alotaibi RM, Rezk HR, Guure C. Modern contraceptive use among women of reproductive age in Ghana: analysis of the 2003–2014 Ghana demographic and health surveys. BMC Womens Health. 2018;18(1):141.
28. Beson P, Appiah R, Adomah-Afari A. Modern contraceptive use among reproductive-aged women in Ghana: prevalence, predictors, and policy implications. BMC Womens Health. 2018;18(1):157.
29. Seyife A, Fisseha G, Yebyo H, Gidey G, Gerensea H. Utilization of modern contraceptives and predictors among women in Shimelba refugee camp, Northern Ethiopia. PLoS One. 2019;14(3):1–11.
30. Derso T, Biks GA, Yitayal M, Ayele TA, Alemu K, Demissie GD, Kebede A. (2020). Prevalence and determinants of modern contraceptive utilization among rural lactating mothers: findings from the primary health care project in two northwest Ethiopian districts. BMC Womens Health. 2020; 20(1):1–6.
31. Ajayi AI, Adeniyi OV, Akpan W. Use of traditional and modern contraceptives among childbearing women: findings from a mixed methods study in two southwestern Nigerian states. BMC Public Health. 2018;18(1):604.
32. Appiah F, Seidu AA, Ahinkorah BO, Baatiema L, Ameyaw EK. Trends and determinants of contraceptive use among female adolescents in Ghana: analysis of 2003–2014 demographic and health surveys. SSM Popul Health. 2020;10:100554.
33. Asiedu A, Asare BYA, Dwumfour-Asare B, Baafi D, Adam AR, Aryee SE, Ganle JK. Determinants of modern contraceptive use: a cross-sectional study among market women in the Ashiaman municipality of Ghana. Int J Afr Nurs Sci. 2020;12:100184.
34. Marie Stopes International. Marie Stopes Papua New Guinea. 2019 Retrieved from https://www.mariestopes.org/where-we-work/papua-new-guinea/ on April 17, 2020.
35. United Nations, Department of Economic and Social Affairs, Population Division. World family planning 2017 - Highlights (ST/ESA/SER.A/414). 2017.
36. National Statistical Office (NSO). Papua New Guinea Demographic and Health Survey 2006. National Report. Port Moresby: National Statistical Office. p. 2009.
37. Taingson MC, Adze JA, Bature SB, Durosinlorun AM, Caleb M, Amina A, Kana MA, Lydia A. Trend of modern contraceptive uptake and its predictors among women accessing family planning service in a tertiary hospital in northwestern Nigeria, 2000–2014. Trop J Obstet Gynaecol. 2017;34(3):201–6.
38. Rutaremwa G, Kabagenyi A, Wandera SO, Jhamba T, Akiror E, Nviiri HL. Predictors of modern contraceptive use during the postpartum period among women in Uganda: a population-based cross sectional study. BMC Public Health. 2015;15(1):262.
39. World Health Organization. Papua New Guinea: actions for scaling up long-acting reversible contraception. 2017 Retrieved from https://www.google.com/url?sa=t&rct=j&q=&esrc=s&source=web&cd=1&cad=rja&uact=8&ved=2ahUKEwj7ydSv1_LoAhXXSBUIHed4DQQQFjAAegQIAhAB&url=https%3A%2F%2Fapps.who.int%2Firis%2Frest%2Fbitstreams%2F1147870%2Fretrieve&usg=AOvVaw2z1nKP_wVKOCFkGZaQqIoU on April 18, 2020.
40. Creanga AA, Gillespie D, Karklins S, Tsui AO. Low use of contraception among poor women in Africa: an equity issue. Bull World Health Organ. 2011;89:258–66.
41. Mekonnen W, Worku A. Determinants of low family planning use and high unmet need in Butajira District, South Central Ethiopia. Reprod Health. 2011;8:37.
42. WHO (2018). Family planning/Contraception. Retrieved from https://www.who.int/news-room/fact-sheets/detail/family-planning-contraception on April 19, 2020.
43. Desta H, Teklemariam G, Yinager W. Barriers to adherence of optimal birth spacing: a qualitative study among mothers and their husbands in Arba Minch Zuria District, Ethiopia. Am J Health Res. 2014;2(4):188–95.
44. Tobe A, Nahusenay H, Misker D. Factors associated with modern contraceptive service utilization among married reproductive age women in Melo Koza Woreda, southern Ethiopia. J Pregnancy Child Health. 2015;2:128.
45. Wakefield MA, Loken B, Hornik RC. Use of mass media campaigns to change health behaviour. Lancet. 2010;376(9748):1261–71.

16

Prevalence of postpartum family planning utilization and associated factors among postpartum mothers in Arba Minch town, South Ethiopia

Biresaw Wassihun[1*], Kidist Wosen[1], Asmare Getie[1], Kalkidan Belay[1], Rehal Tesfaye[1], Tewodros Tadesse[1], Yosef Alemayehu[1], Manaye Yihune[1], Addis Aklilu[1], Kassahun Gebayehu[2] and Shegaw Zeleke[3]

Abstract

Background: Contraception allows women to realize their human right to decide if and when to have children and helps people to attain their desired family size. Yet 214 million women of a reproductive age in developing countries who want to avoid pregnancy are not using a modern contraceptive method. Women who have recently given birth are among the group with the highest unmet need for contraception. Therefore, this study was aimed to assess the prevalence of postpartum family planning use and associated factors among postpartum women in Southern Ethiopia.

Methods: Institution based cross-sectional study design was conducted. A structured and pretested interviewer-administered questionnaire was used to collect the data from study participants. Study participants were selected using a systematic random sampling technique by allocating proportionally to each health facility. The data was entered using EPI data version 3.1statistical software and exported to Statistical Package for Social Sciences version 22.0 for further analysis. Both bivariate and multivariate logistic regression analyses were performed to identify associated factors. *P* values < 0.05 with 95% confidence level was used to declare statistica significance.

Result: Overall, 44% of postpartum women utilize postpartum family planning. Having an antenatal care visit [adjusted odds ratio (AOR) =1.89(95%CI, 2.42–7.90), having planned pregnancy [adjusted odds ratio (AOR) = 1.17(95%CI, 1.60–2.28)], being married (adjusted odds ratio (AOR) =2.86(1.94–8.73), and having a college and above level educational status (AOR) =1.66(1.28–3.55) were significantly associated with utilization of postpartum family planning.

Conclusion: This study showed that the prevalence of postpartum family planning was 44%. Marital status, educational status of mothers, the status of pregnancy, and having an antenatal care follow-up during pregnancy were some factors associated with postpartum family planning utilization. Therefore, strengthening family planning counselling during antenatal and postnatal care visits, improving utilization of postnatal care services and improving women's educational status are crucial steps to enhance contraceptive use among postpartum women.

Keywords: Postpartum, Family planning, Utilization, Ethiopia

* Correspondence: bireswas@gmail.com
[1]College of Medicine and Health Sciences, Arba Minch University, Arba Minch, Ethiopia

Background

Contraception allows women to realize their human rights, and decide if and when to have children, and also helps women to attain their desired family size. Yet 214 million women of the reproductive age group is in developing countries who want to avoid pregnancy are not using a contraceptive method. Women who have recently given birth are amongst those with the highest unmet need for contraception [1, 2].

Studies show that roughly 95% of women who are 0 to 12 months postpartum want to avoid pregnancy in the next 24 months, but 70% of them are not using contraception. Pregnancies in the postpartum period pose the greatest risk for women, and their infants, and have increased risks of adverse health outcomes [1, 2]. To reduce the risk of adverse maternal, perinatal, and infant outcomes, the World Health Organization (WHO) recommended that the interval between live birth, and an attempt to the next pregnancy should be a minimum of two years [2]. By providing postpartum family planning it is possible to reduce maternal and child mortality [3]. Women need to avoid pregnancy so soon after delivery but due to different reasons, they could not be able to get contraceptives [4]. Postpartum family planning has a dual advantage to reduce maternal mortality and to reduce population growth in low resource countries [5]. The integration of family planning as the part of a comprehensive public health approach is important to achieve sustainable development goals [6]. According to Ethiopian demographic health surveillance (EDHS), 4 and 9% of pregnancies occur within less than six months and less than twelve months respectively after prior delivery [7]. This closely spaced birth interval has a potential effect on the increased risk of maternal death [8]. An increase in contraceptive use during the postpartum period significantly reduces the rates of maternal and infant mortality by averting unplanned and unwanted pregnancies and spacing new pregnancies to at least two years after the previous birth. Moreover, the largest proportion of women with an unmet need for contraception is found amongst those in their first year after childbirth [9, 10]. The finding of the previous study showed that the majority of women would prefer to avoid becoming pregnant within two years after delivery, yet only 40% are using a family planning method worldwide [4]. The majority of maternal and child death in Ethiopia was due to pregnancy and its related complications [11]. One of the goals of the ministry of health of Ethiopia, concerning improving maternal and child health, is to raise the contraceptive prevalence rate to 66% by 2015. Currently, overall family planning coverage and modern contraceptive uses that are the key indicator of maternal and child health remain low in the country 29 and 27%, respectively [12]. Despite the accepted demand for postpartum contraception, many postpartum women do not have access to family planning information or service that they need to delay or prevent consequent pregnancy [13]. A previous study, which was conducted in Ethiopia, showed that the prevalence of postpartum family planning was low as compared to other countries. There is no study conducted in our study area on the utilization of postpartum family planning and associated factors so this study fills this gap.

Methods

Study area and period

This study was conducted in public health facilities in Arba Minch town, which is the administrative town of the Gamo zone in South Ethiopia. Gamo zone is among the 15 zones found in the Southern Nations, Nationalities, and Peoples Region. Arba Minch town is located at a distance of 495 km from Addis Ababa and 275 km from Hawassa, the capital of Southern Nations, Nationalities, and Peoples Region in the South direction. There is one Governmental hospital (Arba Minch general hospital) and two public health centers. The study was conducted in all health facilities between October 2018 and January 2019.

Study design

Health facility-based cross-sectional study was conducted.

Study population

The study participants were postpartum women who came for postnatal care (after six weeks of.

Postpartum).

Sampling criteria

Inclusion criteria

Those postpartum women who delivered at least before six weeks were included in the study.

Exclusion criteria

Mothers who were critically ill and unable to communicate during the data collection period.

Sample size determination

The sample size required for this study was calculated based on a single population proportions formula with the following assumptions: n is a sample size, Z is standard normal distribution corresponding to significance level at $\alpha = 0.05$, d is a margin of error assumed to be 5%, P is anticipated proportion of women who had used post-partum family planning 41% taken from the previous study. With the above inputs, the minimum sample size required for the study is 371 taking a 10% non-response rate the final sample size was 408.

Sampling procedure

There is one public hospital (Arba Minch General Hospital) and two public health centers (Sikela and Shecha Health centers) in Arbaminch town and all the health institutions were included in the study. The average number of children who received Vaccination in Arbaminch hospital, Sikela health center, and Shecha health center is 400, 174, and 158 respectively. To include 408 in the study, the proportional allocation method was done which means 222 women from the Arba Minch hospital, 96 women from the Sikela health center, and 88 women from Shecha health center. Data collector use systematic sampling technique to interview the respondents by considering the assumption of **N** (the average number of children who received Vaccination three months period in the health institutions which is 732, and **n** (required minimum sample size = 408 which gives a k of 2): K = N/n = > 732/408 = 1.8 ≈ 2 (Fig. 1).

Data collection tool

Data were collected by face-to-face interviews using a structured questionnaire adapted from the different literature. The questionnaire was used to assess the postpartum family planning utilization and associated factors. The entire questioner was checked for completeness and accuracy before and after the period of data collection. Four BSc Midwifery students who were fluent in speaking the local language were involved in the data collection. The principal investigator supervised the data collection process.

Data quality control

A structured interviewer-administered questionnaire was first prepared in English and then translated into local languages, then back to English by independent language experts to ensure its consistency. The explanation was given to data collectors about techniques of data collection and briefed on each question included in the data collection tool by principal investigators. After that, a pre-test was conducted on 5% of the sample size outside the study area before 15 days of actual data collection to ensure the validity of the tool, then correction was made accordingly.

Data processing and analysis

The collected data were checked visually by the investigators, then data were coded, entered, and cleaned using Epi-Data version 3.1 software and finally exported into SPSS version 22 for analysis. Descriptive statistical analysis such as simple frequencies, measures of central tendency, and measures of variability was used to describe the characteristics of participants. Then the information was presented using frequencies, summary measures, tables, and figures (charts). Bivariate analysis, COR with 95% CI, was used to see the association between each independent variable and the outcome variable by using binary logistic regression. Independent variables with a p-value of ≤0.25, significant in previous st.

Table 1 Socio-demographic characteristics of respondents in Arba Minch town public health facility, South, Ethiopia, 2019 (n = 408)

Variables	Frequencies	Percent
Age		
15–20	55	13.5
21–25	260	63.7
26–30	59	14.5
31 and above	34	8.3
Marital status		
Married	345	84.6
Divorced	15	3.7
Widowed	19	4.7
Single	29	7.1
Ethnicity		
Gamo	201	49.5
Gofa	73	17.9
Amhara	61	15.0
Waleyta	56	13.7
Others	17	4.2
Educational status of mothers		
No formal education	39	9.6
Primary	104	25.5
Secondary	148	36.3
College and above	117	28.7
Respondents religion		
Orthodox	206	50.5
Muslim	58	14.2
Catholic	2	0.5
Protestant	142	34.8
Mothers residency		
Urban	348	85.3
Rural	60	14.7
Mothers occupation		
Housewife	177	43.4
Private employee	46	11.3
Government employee	93	22.8
Merchants	78	19.1
Daily workers	14	3.4
Family monthly income		
≤ 107USD	244	59.8
> 107USD	164	40.2

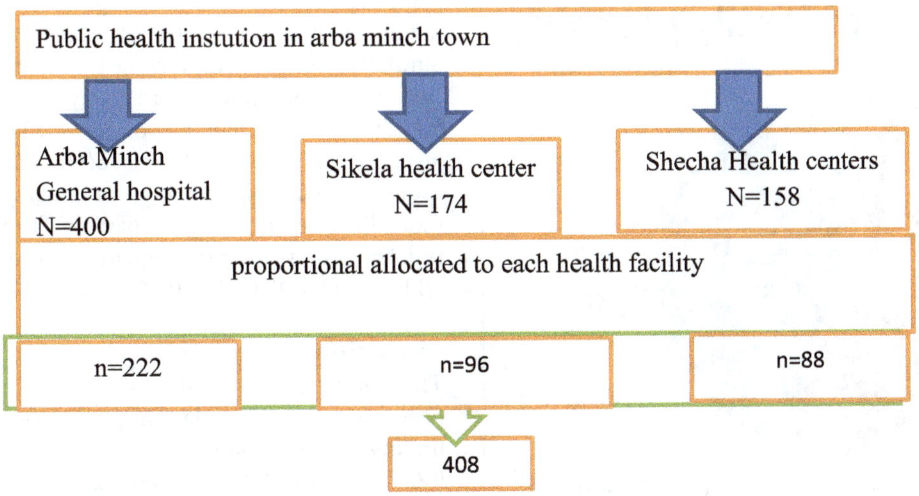

Fig. 1 Flow chart indicating the sampling procedure of postpartum family planning utilization in Arba Minch Tow

udies, and based on the context were included in the multivariable analysis. Multi-collinearity was checked to see the linear correlation among the independent variables by using the variance inflation factor and standard error. Variables with variance inflation factor > 10 and standard error of > 2 were dropped from the multivariable analysis. AOR with 95% CI was estimated to identify the factors associated with post-partum family planning using multivariable logistic regression analysis. The level of statistical significance was declared at p-value ≤0.05.

Table 2 Obstetric characteristics of respondents in Arba Minch town public health facility, South, Ethiopia, 2019 ($n = 408$)

Variables	Frequencies	Percent
ANC		
Yes	365	89.5
No	43	10.5
Institutional delivery history		
Yes	356	87.3
No	52	12.7
Parity		
One	172	42.2
Two	139	34.1
Three and above	97	23.8
Status of pregnancy		
planned	349	85.5
Un planned	59	14.5
History of abortion		
Yes	74	18.1
No	334	81.8
History of stillbirth		
Yes	58	14.3
No	349	85.5

Result

Socio-demographic characteristics of mothers

From a total of 408 respondents who were invited for an interview, all consented to participate in the study giving a response rate of (100%). The mean age of the respondents was 26.8 (SD ± 5.5) years with a minimum and maximum age of 16 and 42 respectively. Almost half of the study participants 201 (49.4%) were from the Gamo ethnic group and 206 (50.5%) were Orthodox Christianity religious followers. Regarding their marital status, 345 (84.6%) of them were married. Out of the total respondents, 244 (59.8%) of them had a monthly family income less than or equal to 107 USD. And the majority of mothers, 148(36.3%) had secondary education followed by 117(28.7%) college and above (Table 1).

Obstetric history of respondents

Out of 408 respondents, 365 (89.5%) had a history of antenatal care follow up. The majority of 257 (72%) of the respondents were multigravida and 236 (57.9%) were multipara. From the total of respondents, 349 (85.5%) of the pregnancy was planned and supported and almost all of the respondents 334 (81.8%) of the respondents had no previous history of abortion and also 349 (85.5%) of the respondents had no history of stillbirth (Table 2).

Utilization of family planning

From the total of 408 respondents, 181(44.4%) use postpartum family planning whereas 227(55.6%) didn't use postpartum family planning, majority of 70(38%) use implant as post-partum family planning followed by oral

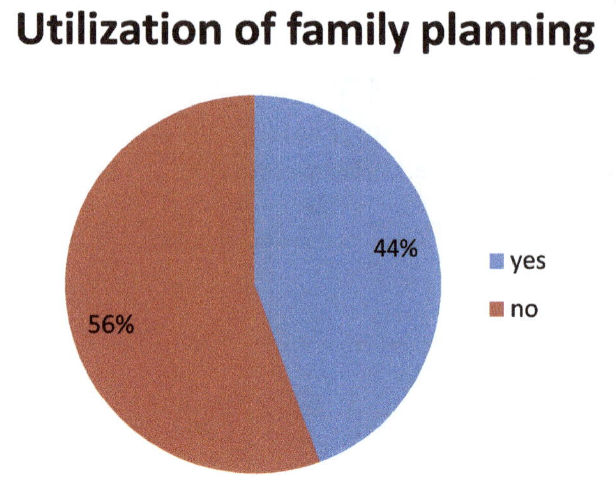

Fig. 2 Overall current utilization of postpartum family planning in Arba Minch town Southern Ethiopia, 2019 ($n = 408$)

pill 47(25%) and 24(13.2%) of the respondents use injection(depo) (Fig. 2 and Table 3).

Source of information for postpartum family planning

Out of 408 respondents, 394(96.5%) heard information about post-partum family planning. Of those who heard family planning information majority of 327 were heard from health institution, 11 from family, 45 from friend and relatives, and 11 from mass media of those who heard family planning majority of them heard oral contraceptives as a family planning 242(59.7%), IUCD 19(4.8%), injections 43(10.9%), (Table 4).

Factors associated with family planning utilization

The result of multiple logistic regression analysis showed that respondent educational status, marital status. Having antenatal care follow up and status of pregnancy were some of the factors associated with post-partum family planning utilization at P-value < 0.05. Respondents who have had the educational status of college and above were 1.66 times more likely to utilize family planning than respondents who had no formal education [adjusted odds ratio (AOR) = 1.66(95%CI; 1.28,3.55)]. Similarly, respondents having the marital status of married were 2.86 times more likely to utilize postpartum family planning than respondents who had single [adjusted odds ratio (AOR) = 2.86(95%CI; 1.94, 8.73)]. Respondents who had planned pregnancy were 1.17 times more likely to utilize post-partum family planning than respondents who had unplanned pregnancy [adjusted odds ratio (AOR) = 1.17(95%CI; 1.60,2.28)] (Table 5).

Table 3 Utilization of family planning methods in Arba Minch town Southern Ethiopia, 2019($n = 408$)

Variable	Frequencies	Percent
Currently, the use of family planning	181	44.4
Family planning method used		
Oral pill	47	25.9
Emergency pill	11	6.1
Condom	8	4.4
IUCD	21	11.6
Implant	70	38.7
Injection	24	13.3

Discussion

The finding of this study revealed that the prevalence of post-partum family planning utilization was 44%. This finding is lower than a study conducted in Burkina Faso (56%), Malawi (75.5%), and Kenya (52.1%) [3, 14, 15]. The discrepancy might be due to socio-economic and cultural differences. On the other hand, the finding was higher than studies that were done in Burundi (20%), Uganda (28%), Kebribeyah Town Ethiopia (12.3%), and Butajira District South Central Ethiopia, 25% [16–19]. The discrepancy might be due to differences in sample size because the previous study used a large sample size. Besides, it might be due to the differences in socio-demographic characteristics and types of data used in which the former studies used secondary data but the data for our study was primary. The finding of this study was consistent with a study conducted at Gondar town, Ethiopia (48.4%) [20].

Respondent educational status, marital status. Having antenatal care follow up and status of pregnancy were some of the factors associated with post-partum family planning utilization at P-value < 0.05.

In this study, married mothers were 2.8 times more likely to use postpartum modern contraceptives. This is

Table 4 Source of information towards Postpartum contraceptive in Arbaminch town, Southern Ethiopia 2019($n =$ 408)

Variables	Frequencies	Percent
Heard of contraceptive	394	96.5
Source of information		
From health institution	327	82.9
From family	11	2.79
Friend	45	11.4
Mass media	11	2.79
Which method do you know		
Oral pill	242	59
Emergence pill	21	7.8
Condom	69	17.5
IUCD	19	4.8
Injection	43	10.9

Table 5 Bivariate and multivariate logistic regression analysis with its predictor variables in Arbaminch town, Southern Ethiopia, 2019($n = 408$)

Variable	Family planning utilization		Crud odds ratio COR (95%CI)	Adjusted odds ratio AOR(95%CI)
	Yes	No		
Residence				
Urban	159	189	1.	1
Rural	22	38	1.45 (0.82–2.55)	0.84 (0.45–1.58)
Marital status				
Marred	161	184	3.35 (1.33–8.44)*	2.86 (1.94–8.73)*
Divorced	6	9	1.31 (0.45–3.76)	1.23 (0.41–3.69)
Widowed	8	11	1.20 (0.47–3.06)	1.15 (0.42–3.12)
Single	6	23	1	1
Educational status of mothers				
No formal education	14	25	1	1
Primary	39	65	0.93 (0.43–2.55)	0.98 (0.43–2.22)
Secondary	71	77	0.58 (0.29–1.26)	0.67 (0.30–1.53)
College and above	57	60	1.58 (1.27–3.24)*	1.66 (1.28–3.55)*
Educational status of Husband				
No formal education	9	21	2.22 (1.97–5.04)*	1.58 (0.60–4.11)
Primary	26	32	1.17 (0.65–2.08)	0.87 (0.44–1.73)
Secondary	29	47	1.54 (0.90–2.61)	1.41 (0.80–2.49)
College and above	116	187	1	1
Type of pregnancy				
Planned	162	187	1.82 (1.01–3.27)*	1.17 (1.60–2.28)*
Un planned	19	40	1	1
History of ANC				
Yes	166	199	1.55 (1.80–3.01)*	1.89 (2.42–7.90)**
No	15	28	1	1
Income				
< 107USD			1.05 (0.70–1.56)	0.84 (0.53–1.32)
≥ 107USD			1	`1

* indicates $p < 0.05$
** indicates $P \leq 0.01$

in line with the study done at Addis Ababa [11]. This might be due to since married women living with their husbands, might start regular sexual intercourse earlier than the non-married couples that may necessitate the utilization of PPFP to program the birth of the next child.

ANC utilization was the other important variable affecting contraceptive use. Women who had antenatal care follow up during pregnancy were 1.89 times more likely to use postpartum family planning than others. The possible explanation is women who attend antenatal care are more likely to get information about contraceptive use. This is consistent with a prospective study done in Kenya and Zambia [20, 21].

In this study, respondents who have had the educational status of college and above were 1.66 times as likely to utilize FP methods as illiterate participants were. This finding implies a significant role in the education status of participants in utilizing available health care services. Education status was reported as a predictor of the use of family planning methods by a few other studies as well [22, 23]. Similarly higher education level attainment invariably gives postpartum women a better understanding of the available modern contraceptive methods and the benefits of fertility regulation and hence the need for contraception during the postpartum period. Besides, higher education increases awareness of the side effects of contraceptive methods and preference for the most convenient ones [16]. The finding of this study showed that mothers who had planned pregnancies were 1.17

times more likely to use postpartum family planning than others. This finding was similar to other study done in Ethiopia [16, 19].

Conclusions

The finding of this study showed that the prevalence of post-partum family planning utilization was low as compared to others' study and some of the identified factors associated with post-partum family planning utilization were being married, higher education level, having antenatal car follow up, and having planned pregnancy. Providing health education is an important step to improve post-partum family planning utilization in collaboration with various family planning stakeholders. Mothers should be addressed not only during antenatal care checkup days but also in immunization clinics, mother group meetings, and during home visits by health extension workers. Incorporation of family planning services with maternal and child health (MCH) should continue highly strengthened is recommended to increase contraceptive use in the post-partum period in Ethiopia. Mobilization of the community is also important because the responsibility to reduce maternal & infant mortality through the promotion of family planning lies not only in the medical profession alone but also on the social and political leaders.

Limitation of the study

- The limitation of this study includes; the present study focused on mothers only but

better to include institutions delivering service, health care providers, and male partners to identify factors influencing utilization of postpartum contraception

- lack of qualitative study to dig out psychosocial factors that hindering the utilization of family planning.
- This study was conducted in selected government hospitals; hence the findings might not adequately reflect the entire population.

Abbreviations

ANC: Antenatal care; AOR: Adjusted odds ratio; CI: Confidence interval; PPFP: Postpartum family planning

Acknowledgments

The authors are grateful for the data collectors and study participants.

Authors' contributions

BW, KW YA, KB.AA, TT. KG, AG, and RT conceived the study and undertook the statistical analysis. BW, SZ, MY, and KW supervised the study design and statistical analysis. All contributed to the writing of the manuscript and approved the submitted version of the manuscript.

Author details

[1]College of Medicine and Health Sciences, Arba Minch University, Arba Minch, Ethiopia. [2]Department of Nursing, College of Medicine and Health Sciences, University of Gondar, Gondar, Ethiopia. [3]Colleges of Medicine and Health Sciences, Debre Tabor University, Debre Tabor, Ethiopia.

References

1. Organization WH. Programming strategies for postpartum family planning. 2013.
2. Gaffield ME, Egan S, Temmerman M. It's about time: WHO and partners release programming strategies for postpartum family planning. Global Health: Science and Practice. 2014;2(1):4–9.
3. Hounton S, Winfrey W, Barros AJ, Askew I. Patterns and trends of postpartum family planning in Ethiopia, Malawi, and Nigeria: evidence of missed opportunities for integration. Glob Health Action. 2015;8(1):29738.
4. Ross JA, Winfrey WL. Contraceptive use, intention to use and unmet need during the extended postpartum period. Int Fam Plan Perspect. 2001:20–7.
5. Cleland J, Ali MM, Shah I. Trends in protective behavior among single vs. married young women in sub-Saharan Africa: the big picture. Reproductive health matters. 2006;14(28):17–22.
6. Prata N. Making family planning accessible in resource-poor settings. Philosophical Transactions of the Royal Society B: Biological Sciences. 2009; 364(1532):3093–9.
7. Csa I. Central statistical agency (CSA) [Ethiopia] and ICF. Ethiopia demographic and health survey. Addis Ababa, Ethiopia and Calverton, Maryland, USA. 2016.
8. Ndugwa RP, Cleland J, Madise NJ, Fotso J-C, Zulu EM. Menstrual pattern, sexual behaviors, and contraceptive use among postpartum women in Nairobi urban slums. J Urban Health. 2011;88(2):341–55.
9. Do M, Hotchkiss D. Relationships between antenatal and postnatal care and post-partum modern contraceptive use: evidence from population surveys in Kenya and Zambia. BMC Health Serv Res. 2013;13(1):6.
10. Gebreselassie T, Rutstein SO, Mishra V. Contraceptive use breastfeeding amenorrhea and abstinence during the postpartum period: an analysis of four countries; 2008.
11. Gebremedhin AY, Kebede Y, Gelagay AA, Habitu YA. Family planning use and its associated factors among women in the extended postpartum period in Addis Ababa, Ethiopia. Contraception Reprod Med. 2018;3(1):1.
12. Ahmed S, Li Q, Liu L, Tsui AO. Maternal deaths averted by contraceptive use: an analysis of 172 countries. Lancet. 2012;380(9837):111–25.
13. Eliason S, Baiden F, Quansah-Asare G, Graham-Hayfron Y, Bonsu D, Phillips J, et al. Factors influencing the intention of women in rural Ghana to adopt postpartum family planning. Reprod Health. 2013;10(1):34.
14. Tran NT, Yameogo WME, Langwana F, Gaffield ME, Seuc A, Cuzin-Kihl A, et al. Participatory action research to identify a package of interventions to promote postpartum family planning in Burkina Faso and the Democratic Republic of Congo. BMC Womens Health. 2018;18(1):122.
15. Jalang'o R, Thuita F, Barasa SO, Njoroge P. Determinants of contraceptive use among postpartum women in a county hospital in rural KENYA. BMC Public Health. 2017;17(1):604.
16. Mekonnen W, Worku A. Determinants of low family planning use and high unmet need in Butajira District. South Central Ethiopia Reproductive Health. 2011;8(1):37.
17. Rutaremwa G, Kabagenyi A. Postpartum family planning utilization in Burundi and Rwanda: a comparative analysis of population-based cross-sectional data. Pan African Medical Journal. 2018;30(1).
18. Rutaremwa G, Kabagenyi A, Wandera SO, Jhamba T, Akiror E, Nviiri HL. Predictors of modern contraceptive use during the postpartum period among women in Uganda: a population-based cross-sectional study. BMC Public Health. 2015;15(1):262.
19. Nigussie A, Girma D, Tura G. Postpartum family planning utilization and associated factors among women who gave birth in the past 12 months, Kebribeyah town, Somali region. Eastern Ethiopia J Women's Health Care. 2016;5(340):2167–0420.1000340.

20. Abera Y, Mengesha ZB, Tessema GA. Postpartum contraceptive use in Gondar town, Northwest Ethiopia: a community-based cross-sectional study. BMC Womens Health. 2015;15(1):19.
21. Mai D, David H. Relationship between antenatal and postnatal care and postpartum modern contraceptive method. BMC Health Service Res. 2013; 13:6.
22. Nattabi B, Li J, Thompson SC, Orach CG, Earnest J. Family planning among people living with HIV in post-conflict northern Uganda: a mixed-methods study. Confl Heal. 2011;5(1):18.
23. Muyindike W, Fatch R, Steinfield R, Matthews LT, Musinguzi N, Emenyonu NI, Martin JN, Hahn JA. Contraceptive use and associated factors among women enrolling into HIV care in southwestern Uganda. Infect Dis Obstet Gynecol. 2012;2012.

17

Desire for and barriers to obtaining effective contraception among women experiencing homelessness

Elizabeth Corey*, Stephanie Frazin, Samantha Heywood and Sadia Haider

Abstract

Background: Homelessness is a significant and growing problem in the United States. Women experiencing homelessness face unique challenges as they have high rates of unintended pregnancy. They often face significant barriers to obtaining effective contraception. This study aimed to explore the contraceptive preferences, desire for, and barriers to obtaining effective contraception among women experiencing homelessness.

Study design: In this cross-sectional study, 54 women experiencing homelessness in Chicago who were at risk for unintended pregnancy were surveyed.

Results: While 94% of the women experiencing homelessness surveyed desired avoiding pregnancy, most were using the least effective contraceptive methods. Among participants, 80% had health insurance, 75% had a high school diploma, and 90% knew where to obtain birth control. Despite these factors, participants faced barriers to obtaining contraception. One significant barrier was lack of comprehensive contraceptive counseling as 62% report a physician had never counseled them on LARC methods. Approximately half of participants desired or would consider using a LARC in the future.

Conclusions: Women experiencing homelessness in our study demonstrate significant unmet needs for effective contraception. Women experiencing homelessness would benefit from comprehensive contraceptive counseling and improved access to effective forms of contraception.

Keywords: Contraception, Long-acting reversible contraceptives, Unplanned pregnancy, Homeless

A homeless individual is defined as one who lacks a fixed, regular and adequate nighttime residence [1]. In the United States, homelessness remains a substantial and increasing problem. The odds of becoming homeless are 1:194, and over a half a million individuals are homeless each night [1]. Overall, women and children remain one of the fastest growing segments of the homeless population. Women comprise 37% of homeless individuals, while families comprise up to 50% of the homeless population. In the vast majority of homeless families, women lead the household as single parents [1].

Nearly 75% of pregnancies among women experiencing homelessness are unintended compared to 45% nationally [2]. A limited number of studies have explored risk of unintended pregnancy among women experiencing homelessness [3, 4]. Women experiencing homelessness have unique reproductive health needs given that having mistimed or unintended children can further perpetuate the cycle of poverty and homelessness. Approximately 13% of women experiencing homelessness are pregnant at any given time. This rate is more than double the rate of pregnancy among all American women and

* Correspondence: lizcorey@gmail.com
Department of Obstetrics and Gynecology, University of Illinois at Chicago, 820 South Wood Street, Chicago, IL 60612, USA

significantly higher than the 5% of housed low-income women who are currently pregnant [3]. In addition, women experiencing homelessness who become pregnant have an increased rate of complications.

Although previous research has shown that many women experiencing homelessness want to prevent pregnancy, they face significant barriers to obtaining effective contraception [4–6]. Previously cited barriers to contraceptives include fear of side effects, partner barriers, cost, storage, and lack of services on site [7]. Compared to the general population, women experiencing homelessness have decreased use of contraception and higher use of less effective contraceptive methods [2, 4, 6]. A survey of women experiencing homelessness in Los Angeles found that one-third of women experiencing homelessness used contraception rarely or never in the past year. Another study reported that 92% of women experiencing homelessness relied primarily on condoms and among those women only 32% reported condom use with every sexual encounter [4].

A potential solution to the increased rate of unintended pregnancies among women experiencing homelessness is ensuring access to comprehensive contraception counseling and to all methods of contraception including long-acting reversible contraceptives (LARC) if desired. Among women experiencing homelessness, other contraceptives may have higher failure rates than anticipated due to the daily challenges faced by women experiencing homelessness. There is little information on LARC use among women experiencing homelessness and LARC-specific barriers. One study explored the provider barriers to administering LARCs to women experiencing homelessness [8]. The survey suggested extremely limited access to LARCs among women experiencing homelessness. Only one-third of the organizations that provide healthcare services to women experiencing homelessness surveyed directly provided either intrauterine devices (IUDs) or the contraceptive implant to their patients. The significant barriers identified include lack of provider training, lack of resources for placement, costs, lack of insertion equipment, and concerns about complications [8]. A second study used mixed methodology to explore barriers to LARC use among homeless youth. Barriers identified included distrust of healthcare personnel who provide contraceptive counseling and misconceptions such as the inability to remove LARCs at the users' discretion [9]. This study was a preliminary study, had a small sample size, and the results were not intended to be generalized. To our knowledge, no other study has focused on barriers to LARC use among women experiencing homelessness. Therefore, our study adds current knowledge to this topic as it assesses desire for and personal barriers to effective contraception, including LARCs, among women experiencing homelessness. Our hypothesis is that women experiencing homelessness have a strong desire for contraception, but are not regularly accessing reproductive health services.

Methods

The Institutional Review Board (IRB) at the University of Illinois Chicago approved this study. After IRB approval was obtained, homeless shelters that serve women of reproductive age in Chicago were recruited to participate in our study through recruitment letters and phone calls. Researchers spent time developing long-term and trusting relationships with the local partners. The three Chicago-based homeless shelters that were chosen to participate in our study include New Moms, Sarah's Circle, and The Night Ministry. The participants were recruited using a convenience sampling method and included both sheltered women and unsheltered women recruited through outreach services. Research personnel introduced our study at various programming events at New Moms. In addition, posters were placed throughout the shelter, and participants were asked to sign up at the front desk if interested. At Sarah's Circle, research personnel and staff members were present during various hours at their day shelter in order to approach and recruit interested women. At The Night Ministry, participants were recruited at three of their homeless shelters that house women of reproductive age. Staff explained the study and asked women to sign up if they were interested. Research personnel also participated in their street outreach programs to recruit women currently living without shelter. The research was conducted from January 2016 to June 2017. In total, 54 women participated in the study.

To be eligible to participate, women had to be aged 18 to 45 years old and had to have spent at least one night in the past month in a homeless shelter, transitional shelter, public space, or vehicle. In addition, eligible participants were sexually active with at least one male partner in the last year. Participants were excluded if they were currently pregnant, unable to consent, if they had a tubal ligation or their primary partner had a vasectomy. The inclusion and exclusion criteria were designed to capture women experiencing homelessness who were currently at risk for unintended pregnancy. Among the participants who were identified and who met the inclusion and exclusion criteria, the response rate was 90%.

Participants were screened by research personnel in a private area of the shelter or mobile van in the case of the outreach programs in order to protect confidentiality. Care was taken to minimize coercion and undue influence by training research staff in informed consent, ethical considerations while working with vulnerable population, and study details. Therefore, research personnel provided written informed consent with the opportunity to ask questions for all participants.

After written consent was obtained, participants completed an online survey through REDCap on an iPad equipped with internet access. REDCap is a secure web application used to collect data. Although most women filled out the survey on their own, researchers were available to assist women by reading the questions and potential answers out loud if requested. It was suggested that these women move the iPad out of view from the researcher in order to continue to answer the question privately.

The survey contained approximately 60 question sets that focused on demographic information, homelessness, obstetric history, and experiences with contraceptives. The survey took approximately 30 min to complete. The survey was developed based on previous research questionnaires that were obtained [3, 6, 7]. Previously validated research questions were obtained from the National Survey of Family Growth and Pregnancy Risk Assessment and Monitoring [10, 11]. In addition, unique questions were created that were specific to women experiencing homelessness and LARC use, as standardized questions were not available. Participants were asked a series of closed-ended questions regarding desire for and barriers to both IUD use and contraceptive implant use. The surveys were translated into Spanish and a research personnel who was fluent in Spanish was available throughout the study. However, all participants in this study requested the English version.

Participants received a post-survey counseling session focused on either contraception education or preparing for a healthy pregnancy depending on their pregnancy desire. For women who desired avoiding pregnancy, this counseling session included a map with locations of Title X clinics in their neighborhood with details of which contraceptives were available at each location. All women received a $10 gift card to a local food store and two public transportation passes in order to provide transportation to visit the healthcare clinics if desired.

Statistical Package for the Social Sciences (SPSS) was used to calculate descriptive statistical analysis. Bivariate analysis was also performed utilizing the chi-square test and ANOVA. In regards to missed data, two individuals ended the survey early. The data associated with these participants was omitted from analysis. All other individuals completed the survey without missed data.

Results

The participants' demographic information is listed in Table 1. The mean age of participants was 28 years old. Among participants, 79% identified as black, 13% as white, and 4% as Hispanic. Approximately one quarter of participants were employed. Among the participants who were unemployed, the majority (73%) were looking for work. Eighty-three percent of participants described themselves as single without having been married. A high percentage of participants (68%) described themselves as chronically homeless, meaning they had been continuously homeless for one year or on 4 separate occasions in the past 3 years.

Table 1 Demographic Information of Participants

Demographic Variable	% Sample ($n = 54$)
Ethnicity	
Black	79
White	13
Hispanic	4
Asian	0
Other	0
Education	
None	2
1-4th grade	0
5-8th grade	0
Some high school	26
High school graduate	26
Some college	33
Technical, vocational	2
College degree	7
Masters or doctorate	4
Marital Status	
Married	2
Widowed	0
Divorced or annulled	11
Separated	4
Single, never been married	83
Employment Status	
Employed for wages	20
Self-employed	6
Out of work but looking for work	46
Out of work but not currently looking for work	17
Homemaker	2
Student	6
Military	0
Retired	0
Health Insurance	
None	20
State health insurance	74
Private health insurance	8

A large majority of participants desired to prevent pregnancy within the next year. When asked if they intended to avoid pregnancy in the next year regardless of housing status, 81% stated that they would like to avoid or would not mind avoiding pregnancy. If they

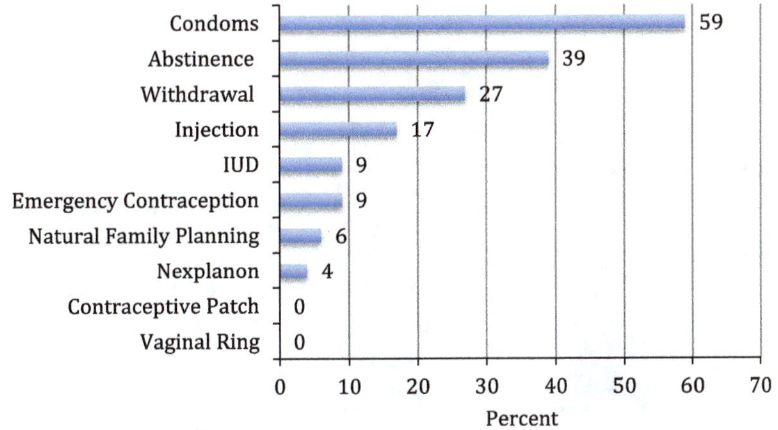

Fig. 1 Current use contraception including all methods used among women experiencing homelessness in Chicago (n = 54)

remain homeless in the next year, 94% stated they would like to avoid pregnancy or would not mind avoiding pregnancy.

Despite a desire to avoid pregnancy, the women experiencing homelessness surveyed were using the least effective methods in preventing pregnancy (Fig. 1). The most commonly reported methods selected when women were able to multi-select their current contraceptive use were condoms (58%), abstinence (38%), and withdrawal (27%). Figure 2 shows current contraceptive use filtering for the most effective method used for each woman. The most used method remains condoms with 35% of women using condoms as their most effective method of contraception (Fig. 2). Contraceptive methods were being used inconsistently with only 30% of participants stating that they had used contraceptives all the time in the past 6 months.

The participants had many assets that can be leveraged to assist them in obtaining contraception. Many participants had high levels of formal education with 72% completing high school or higher. Nearly 80% of participants had health insurance. The vast majority (90%) of participants knew where to go to access contraception and 83% were confident that they could consistently use birth control with every sexual encounter in the next 6 months.

Participants were also asked about their desire for effective contraception, in particular their desire for LARCs. Approximately 43% of participants desired an IUD or desired more information about an IUD. One-third of participants desired a nexplanon or more information about a nexplanon (Fig. 3). In total, over half of participants desired a LARC or more information about LARCs. Women experiencing homelessness who had been pregnant previously were more likely to have heard of LARCs ($p < .01$) and women experiencing homelessness who had health insurance were significantly more likely to be using a LARC ($p = .04$). Age, race, education, and length of time women were homeless were not associated with current use or future desire for LARCs.

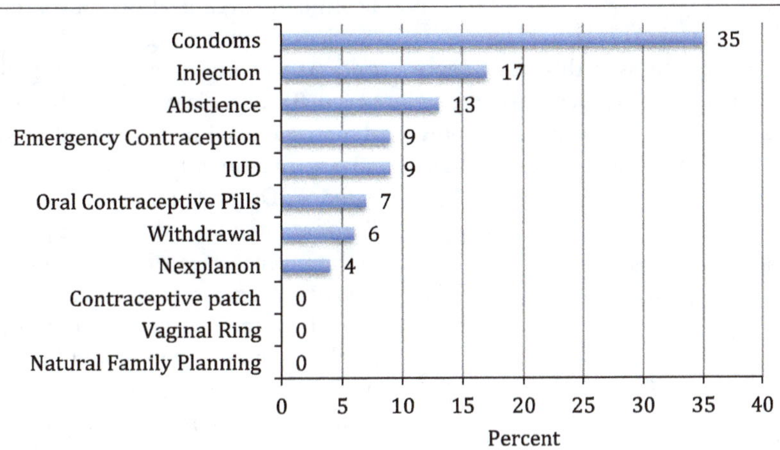

Fig. 2 Current use contraception showing only the most effective method used among women experiencing homelessness in Chicago ($n = 54$)

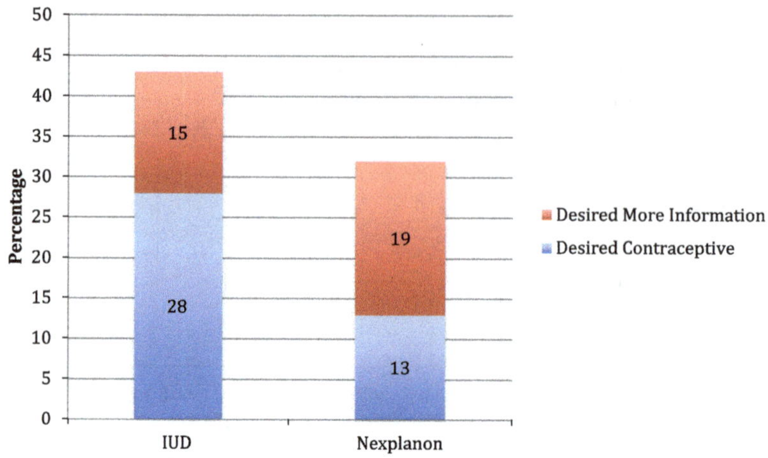

Fig. 3 Desire for long-acting reversible contraceptives among women experiencing homelessness in Chicago

Participants expressed many concerns and barriers to obtaining effective contraception (Table 2). The most commonly cited barriers to contraception in general were concerns regarding side effects and the potential for birth control to negatively influence their health. In particular, among participants who did not desire LARCs, they cited a variety of reasons why they avoided LARC use (Table 3). The women were most commonly concerned about a foreign body being inserted into their body and complications with insertion.

One important barrier to LARC use identified in this study is the lack of comprehensive contraceptive counseling by their healthcare provider. Seventy percent of participants reported that their main source of information about effective contraceptives is their healthcare provider. Most participants receive care at community health clinics (51%) or the hospital outpatient clinic (30%). However, the majority of participants (62%) report that they have not been counseled regarding LARCs by their healthcare provider.

Discussion

The women experiencing homelessness in this study demonstrated a significant unmet need for comprehensive contraception counseling and access to contraception. Overall, women experiencing homelessness are at high-risk for unintended pregnancy. In our study, 94% of women experiencing homelessness surveyed would like to avoid pregnancy in the next year if they remain homeless. Yet, women in our study were more likely to be using the least effective contraceptive methods. This may help to explain previous research that found young women experiencing homelessness have a significantly higher pregnancy rate compared to young women in the general population [12]. Nearly 75% of pregnancies among women experiencing homelessness are unintended compared to 45% nationally [2, 4, 13].

Table 2 Most common concerns about birth control cited by women experiencing homelessness in Chicago

I am worried about the side effects of birth control	47%
I fear that birth control is harmful to my health	40%
My husband or partner does not like to use birth control, such as condoms	34%
Using birth control is uncomfortable	30%
I know what type of birth control to use	25%

We hypothesized that women experiencing homelessness did not have access to effective contraception because they were not regularly accessing reproductive healthcare services. However, our results indicate that women experiencing homelessness are seeking reproductive healthcare. The unexpected barrier we found is that the healthcare providers are not counseling women on the full spectrum of contraceptive options available.

Barriers exist both at the level of the provider and the healthcare organization. Saver et al. explored provider barriers to providing the full spectrum of contraceptive options to women experiencing homelessness. They surveyed 31 organizations in the national Health Care for the Homeless Practice-Based Research Network. Of the 17 organizations that provide contraceptives only 6 provided IUDs and 2 provided the contraceptive implant. Barriers cited include lack of provider training, resources and concerns regarding complications [8].

Where contraceptive services are available, healthcare providers need to employ comprehensive counseling for all their patients who would like to prevent pregnancy. A model involving shared decision making and patient-centered counseling should be employed. A chart or a graphic depicting all contraceptive can be utilized. For example, www.bedsider.org can be used as a resource to

Table 3 Most common concerns about LARC use cited by women experiencing homelessness in Chicago

I do not like the idea of something inside my body	81%
I worry there will be a complication with insertion	67%
I fear that the insertion of the device will be painful	62%
I worry about getting an infection from the device	57%
I worry about how these methods would change my bleeding pattern	43%
I fear that the device will cause infertility	40%
They are too expensive	27%

assist patients in finding and utilizing a method of birth control that best suits their needs.

If all contraceptive options are not available, healthcare providers should still counsel women on their options with referrals to other locations if desired. Providers should be aware that there is a tendency to counsel less effectively on methods that are unavailable at their location. Providers should counter this tendency by exploring all contraceptive methods with their patients and making referrals as necessary. Since the majority of women in our study received care at community health clinics, efforts should first be focused on these clinics to help ensure they offer the full spectrum of contraceptive options and counseling.

While counseling women experiencing homelessness, however, care should be taken to avoid coercion by the healthcare providers as women experiencing homelessness remain a vulnerable population. The counseling should therefore be patient-centered with the goal of enhancing informed choice through a shared-decision making framework. Future studies could be performed to assess the women's perception of coercion and informed choice while receiving contraceptive counseling.

Many women in our study desired, but were not accessing long-acting reversible contraceptives. Participant-identified barriers should be addressed in comprehensive contraceptive counseling. Patients should be counseled on risks of insertion and side effect profiles. Providers should facilitate access and provision of LARCs when desired in an evidence-based fashion. For example, care should be taken to remove barriers, such as requiring two visits for a LARC insertion [14].

Furthermore, one quarter of participants cited money as a barrier to LARC use. As demonstrated in the Contraceptive CHOICE research project, when money was removed as a barrier, 75% of the women chose a LARC and the continuation rates were high [15]. Women experiencing homelessness who desire LARC use should be counseled on clinics that offer free LARCs through Title X funding or other avenues for subsidized contraceptive services.

The women experiencing homelessness in our study exhibited many assets that could be leveraged to assist the women in obtaining the full spectrum of reproductive healthcare. These include high levels of formal education, possession of health insurance, knowledge of where to access contraception, and confidence in ability to use birth control. As women experiencing homelessness are a heterogeneous group, the goals and assets of each individual should be evaluated and used to help empower her to meet her reproductive health goals.

Our study provides new information regarding limitations in contraception counseling and barriers to accessing effective contraceptive methods among women experiencing homelessness. However, some limitations should be considered. Our study is limited by a small sample size and a convenience sample that limits generalizability. Future studies are needed to further elucidate barriers that women experiencing homelessness face in accessing reproductive health care and barriers that healthcare personnel face in providing the full spectrum of contraceptive options. In addition, future studies should explore novel approaches aimed at increasing access to contraception for women experiencing homelessness with patient-centered approaches.

Implications

Additional efforts by healthcare providers are needed to ensure women experiencing homelessness receive full contraceptive counseling while taking care to avoid coercion in this vulnerable population. Additional research should explore the most effective ways to deliver reproductive health services to women experiencing homelessness with subsequent programming initiated to apply the findings.

Conclusion

This article adds to already existing literature as it demonstrated that the women experiencing homelessness in our study have a significant unmet need for effective forms of contraception. Approximately half of women experiencing homelessness surveyed desired a LARC or wanted additional information on LARCs. However, most women were not receiving comprehensive contraception counseling from their healthcare providers. Additional research and programming must be instituted in order to ensure that the reproductive needs of this vulnerable population are being met.

Acknowledgements
Jennifer Grage, Chelsie Carlton, Mamatha Challa, Ellen Barry, and Chandler Farris for helping to recruit and interview women experiencing homelessness. We would also like to acknowledge our community partners for recruiting women and providing a private space for interviews.

Authors' contributions
All authors contributed substantially to the final manuscript. It was approved and reviewed by all authors.

References

1. US Department of Housing and Urban Development. The 2016 Annual homeless assessment report (AHAR) to congress, 2016. Accessed https://www.hudexchange.info/resources/documents/2016-AHAR-Part-1.pdf.
2. Gelberg L, Lu MC, Leake BD, Andersen RM, Morgenstern H, Nyamathi AM. Homeless women: who is really at risk for unintended pregnancy? Matern Child Health J. 2008;12:52–60.
3. Bassuk E, Weinreb L, Buckner J, Browne A, Salomon A, Bussuk S. The characteristics and needs of sheltered homeless and low-income housed mothers. JAMA. 1996;276:640–6.
4. Gelberg L, Leake BD, Lu MC, Andersen RM, Wenzel SL, Morgenstern H, et al. Use of contraceptive methods among homeless women for protection against unwanted pregnancies and sexually transmitted diseases: prior use and willingness to use in the future. Contraception. 2001;63:277–81.
5. Kennedy S, Grewal M, Roberts EM, Steinauer J, Dehlendorf C. A qualitative study of pregnancy intention and the use of contraception among homeless women with children. J Health Care Poor Underserved. 2014;25: 757–70.
6. Gelberg L, Browner CH, Lejano E, Arangua L. Access to women's health care: a qualitative study of barriers perceived by homeless women. Women Health. 2004;40:87–100.
7. Gelberg L, Leake B, Lu MC, Andersen R, Nyamathi AM, Morgenstern H, et al. Chronically homeless women's perceived deterrents to contraception. Perspect Sex Reprod Health. 2002;34:278–85.
8. Saver BG, Weinreb L, Gelberg L, Zerger S. Provision of contraceptive services to homeless women: results of a survey of health care for the homeless providers. Women Health. 2012;52:151–61.
9. Dasari M, Borrero S, Akers AY, Sucato GS, Dick R, Hicks A, et al. Barriers to long-acting reversible contraceptive (LARC) uptake among homeless young women. J Pediatr Adolesc Gynecol. 2016;29:104–10.
10. Centers for Disease Control and Prevention. National Survey for Family Growth. https://www.cdc.gov/nchs/nsfg/index.htm. Accessed 8/2015.
11. Centers for Disease Control and Prevention. Pregnancy Risk Assessment Monitoring System. https://www.cdc.gov/prams/index.htm. Accessed 8/2015.
12. Crawford DM, et al. Pregnancy and Mental Health of Young Homeless Women. Am J Orthopsychiatry. 2011;81:173–83.
13. Finer LB, Zolna MR. Declines in unintended pregnancy in the United States, 2008-2011. N Engl J Med. 2016;374:843.
14. Bergin A, Tristan S, Terplan M, Gilliam ML, Whitaker AK. A missed opportunity for care: two-visit IUD insertion protocols inhibit placement. Contraception. 2012;86:694–7.
15. Peipert JF, Madden T, Allsworth JE, Secura GM. Preventing unintended pregnancies by providing no-cost contraception. Obstet Gynecol. 2012;120: 1291–7.

18

Men's involvement in family planning service utilization among married men in Kondala district, western Ethiopia

Lemessa Assefa[1], Zemenu Shasho[2], Habtamu Kebebe Kasaye[3], Edao Tesa[4], Ebisa Turi[1] and Ginenus Fekadu[5,6*]

Abstract

Background: Men involvement is one of the important factors in family planning (FP) service utilization. Their limitation in the family planning program causes a decrease in service utilization as well as the discontinuation of the method which eventually leads to failure of the program. Family planning uptake is low but there is no enough study conducted on the parameters of husband involvement in Ethiopia. Hence, this study focused to assess men's involvement in family planning service utilization in Kondala district, western Ethiopia.

Methods: Community based comparative cross-sectional study design was employed in urban and rural kebeles of kondala district using quantitative and qualitative data collection tools. The multi-stage sampling method was employed to select 370 participants from each of the four urban and eight rural kebeles. Logistic regression analysis was used to identify variables that affect husbands' involvement in FP service utilization. Statistical significance was declared at *p*-value of < 0.05 with 95% confidence interval (CI) and strength of association was reported by odds ratio (OR).

Results: The study showed that 203(55.6%) men from urban and 178(48.8%) from rural were involved in FP service utilization. The median age of the respondents was 36± 8.5 years (IQR: 27.5–44.5) in urban and 35 years (IQR: 25–45) in rural parts. Respondents who had four and above current children (AOR = 3.25, 95%CI = 1.51–7.02) in urban and (AOR = 4.20, 95%CI = 1.80–9.79) in rural were positively associated with men's involvement in FP service utilization. In the urban setting, being government employee (AOR = 2.58, 95%CI = 1.25–5.33), wishing less than two children (AOR = 3.08, 95%CI = 1.80–5.24) and having a better attitude towards FP methods (AOR = 1.86, 95%CI = 1.16–2.99) were positively associated with FP service utilization. While good educational background (AOR = 2.13, 95%CI = 1.02–4.44), short distance from home to health facility (AOR = 2.29, 95%CI = 1.24–4.19) and having better knowledge (AOR = 4.49, 95%CI = 2.72–7.38) were positively associated with men involvement in FP service utilization in the rural area.

(Continued on next page)

* Correspondence: take828pharm@gmail.com
[5]Department of Pharmacy, Institute of Health Sciences, Wollega University, P.O Box:395, Nekemte, Oromia, Ethiopia
[6]School of Pharmacy, Faculty of Medicine, The Chinese University of Hong Kong, Shatin, New territory, Hong Kong

(Continued from previous page)
Conclusion: Low involvement of men in family planning service utilization was reported in both settings. Factors associated with husbands' involvement were varied between the two setups, except for the current number of children. Future FP program should incorporate infrastructure associated with the health facility, knowledge, and attitudinal factors.

Keywords: Men's involvement, Family planning, Service utilization, Ethiopia

Background

Men involvement in family planning (FP) means that those participated by using family methods by themselves or made discussion with their wives on family planning, support and approve its utilization [1–5]. The most efficacious means of controlling population growth were pursued to turn the family planning reasoning on its head rather than looking to women's adoption of family planning as the source of social change [6–8]. Traditionally the concept of reproductive health was more overemphasized on the females. However, from the day International Conference on population and Development (ICPD) made paradigm shift, men's started to share responsibility and promote their active participation in liable parenthood, sexual and reproductive behavior including family planning [9, 10].

Family planning programs have paid attention primarily on women, though some studies suggest that involving males and obtaining their support and encouragement to family planning is of crucial importance, especially in developing countries where decision making are influenced by the men [7, 11–13].

Women are denied the use of contraceptives by her husband when tried to point out the involvement of the husband especially in decision making in reproductive health like in family planning [14, 15]. On the other hand, even if the wife wants to use family planning, she may not be able to use it or maybe forced to discontinue the method without the involvement of the males on the service [16]. A number of pocket research articles revealed that joint decision making and communications with partners in family planning issues will not only improve contraceptive utilization but also plays paramount role in averting discontinuation of the methods [14, 17, 18]. Men's health status and behavior affect women's health and reproductive health [6, 19]. Involving them increases their awareness, acceptance and support to their partners' needs, choices and rights [6, 8]. Men's involvement is also crucial to the success of family planning programs including the use of modern contraceptives [18–21]. They play this role by actively participating in family planning by using the method and discussion, decision making, support and approval of the service utilization by their wives, relatives and friends [7, 16, 22].

In many developing countries, several studies showed that men's involvement brought a significant change in FP utilization. However, their involvement is still low in the patronage of family planning services [11, 15, 16, 23]. In Ethiopia, several studies have conducted in different parts of the country which concerned male involvement in reproductive health as well as in the utilization of family planning [4, 12, 14, 24, 25]. In this country, the husband has a great role in approving/disapproving the utilization of family planning services by their wives based on several barriers among these religions and cultures are stated to play negative influence on them [7, 24]. This is because in many developing countries like Ethiopia males often dominate in taking important decisions in the family including contraceptive use by their wives [18, 24].

Men as a decision-maker need to inform their wives to use FP and the discussion between the couples also play an important role in family planning. What was known by several studies as major factors to male involvement in family planning services utilization includes influence of culture and religion, perception towards family planning as women's issue, lack of education of husband, sex preference for inheritance and fear of partner sexual promiscuity [19, 26, 27] . The presence of culture considers the husband as a decision-maker related to reproductive health, more specifically FP and it impeded the progress of service over the period despite the efforts being implemented to raise the utilization of FP services [19, 26]. These make low participation of the husband which has negative effects on the effectiveness of FP program as shown by studies conducted in several towns [19, 24, 27].

In Ethiopia even though the family planning uptake is low [28], most of the studies conducted on the parameters of male involvement and its determinants are conducted in the urban areas [29]. Little is known regarding male involvement in family planning utilization in the rural areas including the Kondala district. This study result creates an opportunity for couples to know about factors associated with husband involvement in family planning service utilization and can be used to revise the existing strategies and to design new ones to solve the problem associated with the program. Hence, the study aimed to explore the male involvement in family planning service utilization and associated factors in kondala district, Western Ethiopia.

Methods

Study area, period and design

Community based comparative cross-sectional study design was employed in urban and rural kebeles of kondala district from April to May 2019. Kondala district is found in the West Wollega zone, Oromia regional state, Ethiopia located 633 km away from Addis Ababa. The total population living in this district is about 1, 32,655 of whom 67,008 are males and 27,636 households. The district comprises a total of 36 kebeles, 32 rural and 4 urban kebeles. The major economic activities of the district are traditional farming and few of them are engaged in trading. The healthcare delivery within the district is carried out through 4 health centers, 33 health posts and 30 private clinics of different levels and one drug store. Family planning services are mainly obtained from public health institutions [30].

Eligibility criteria

Inclusion criteria

- Men who were living together with their wives.
- Men who lived with their wives for at least in the past one year.
- Participants were expected to spend at least the past six months in the study area.

Exclusion criteria

- Men who were living in semi-urban kebele.

Study variables

Dependent variable

Male involvement in family planning service utilization.

Independent variables

- Socio-demographic characteristics: Age, family size, religion, ethnicity, residence, educational status, occupation, and family income
- Reproductive health characteristics: Marriage duration, number of living children, knowledge regarding FP methods, the ideal number of children, attitude toward FP methods, health concern (fear of side effect, infertility, and low libido)

Sample size determination and sampling techniques

The sample size was determined using a formula for estimation of double population proportion considering the following assumptions: level of significance (0.05), power (0.80), the proportion of husband who supports their wives to use contraceptive in urban (60%), and proportion of husband who supports their wives to use contraceptive in rural women (44.9%) [21]. The design effect and non-response rate were considered.

$$n = \left(Z_{\alpha/2} + Z_{\beta}\right)^2{}_{*} \left(p_1(1-p_1)_{+} p_2(1-p_2)\right)/(p_1-p_2)^2;$$

Where; -.

$Z\alpha$ = the z-score corresponding to the 95% confidence level which is 1.96.

$Z_{\beta\,=}$ is the critical value of the normal distribution at β which is 0.84

$$n = \frac{(\mathbf{1.96 + 0.84)2{*}0.60(1-0.060) + 0.449(1-0.449))}}{\mathbf{(0.60-0.449)2.}} = \mathbf{168}$$

By consideration of the design effect of 2 and the non-response rate of 10%, the total sample sizes were 370 from urban and 370 from rural kebeles.

The multi-stage sampling method was used in the sampling technique. Out of 32 rural kebeles, 8 kebeles were taken by simple random sampling and 4 urban kebeles were taken purposively. Households were sampled by a systematic random sampling method and the husband was asked from the household. The first households were selected by using the lottery method and the sample was taken every other K^{th} household until the required numbers of eligible husbands were recruited in the kebele. The K factor was derived from the formula K = N/n, where N is the total number of households in the kebele which were taken from district health office and n = sample size assigned for each kebele. Sample sizes for each rural and urban kebeles were allocated proportionally. If the husband has more than one partner/wife in one household, the husbands were asked for one partner taken by lottery method. In the case where the respondents were not found at the time of the study, a repeat visit was made for at least three times.

Data collection process

Data was collected using quantitative and qualitative data collection tools. Quantitative data was collected using interviewer-administered structured questionnaires. The questionnaire was developed by the investigators after extensive review of literatures [19, 29, 31–33]. The questionnaire included socio-demographic characteristics, knowledge on family planning methods, the attitude of the husband towards family planning and husband involvement in family planning service utilization. Three health officers were assigned as research supervisors and six clinical nurses were trained and undertook the overall data collection activities under the immediate supervision of the principal investigator.

Focus group discussion (FGD) was conducted among purposively selected groups of key informants of the kebele to collect qualitative information on male involvement and factors associated with husband participation in family planning in the study area. The qualitative data was used to support the quantitative findings and it was carried out by the principal investigator. Three focus group discussions from urban kebeles and four from rural kebeles were conducted.

The groups were assigned according to their age; 18–39 years and 40 years or more. Each focus group comprised of 6 to 8 persons. The interviews and discussions were held in Afan Oromo language. The interview guide included questions on knowledge and attitude toward family planning, as well as factors towards male involvement in family planning. The principal investigator took data from FGDs by sound recording using mobile phone and notes.

Data quality control and management

Questionnaires were translated to the regional language and then back translated to English to maintain its consistency. The training was given for data collectors and pretest was made on 5% of the study subjects in Gimbi district that have similar socio-demographic characteristics with the people of the study area before the actual data collection. The supervisors and principal investigators were performed immediate supervision daily. Every completed questionnaire was checked for its completeness and consistency.

Measurement

Men involvement in family planning service utilization

Based on the summative score of questions designed to assess husband involvement in FP services utilization, husband those who score 60% and above were considered as having better involvement in FP services and those who score less than 60% were categorized as not involved [19].

Men's attitude towards FP service utilization

To assess husband's attitude towards involvement in F/P service utilization and they asked to answer five attitude related questions, which were a three points Likert's scale. Based on the statements assessing attitude, the mean score of the distribution was considered as having positive attitude and those who score less than the mean value were categorized as negative attitudes towards family planning service utilization [19].

Knowledge about family planning methods

Refers to the husband's knowledge of different family planning methods, which is based on knowledge question. Based on the summative score of questions designed to assess knowledge, men with above the mean of the distribution was considered as having adequate knowledge and those who score less than the mean value were categorized as not having adequate knowledge [19].

Data processing, and analysis

The collected data were coded and entered into EPI info version 7.2.2.6 before the analysis. Then, data were exported and analyzed using Statistical Package for Social Sciences (SPSS) version 25. Mean and standard deviation as well as the median and interquartile range (IQR) was calculated for continuous variables, whereas frequency and proportion were calculated for categorical variables. The result was summarized and presented by statements, tables and graphs. Furthermore, binary logistic regression analysis was used to identify factors that affect husband involvement in family planning.

Variables having 0.25 and less p-value in bi-variable logistic regression model were candidates for multi-variable logistic regression model. The multi-variable logistic regression model was used to control the effect of confounding variables and the strength of association of predictor variables was assessed using odds ratio (OR) and significance of variables was reported at p-values $<$ 0.05 using 95% CI. Model fitness was assessed by Hosmer and Lemeshow goodness of fit test (accepted with $p > 0.05$) and multicollinearity was assessed by variance inflation factor (VIF). Histogram and skewness were used for the normality check. Qualitative data were transcribed and back translated to English version, by senior experts, and the ideas rearranged according to their thematic area manually. Lastly, information linked and analyzed to its congruence with data obtained through interviewer-administered structured questionnaires.

Results

Socio-demographic characteristics of the study participants

A total of 365(98.6%) participants from urban and 364 (98.4%) from rural have participated in the study with a response rate of 729(98.5%). The median age of the respondents was 36 years (IQR: 27.5–44.5) in urban and 35 years (IQR: 25–45) in rural parts. Most husbands in urban 128(35.1%) attended secondary school and 120(33%) of rural areas attended primary school. Up on Chi-square ($\chi 2$) test, there is significant difference between urban and rural in terms of educational status, ethnicity, occupation and length of time spent to reach the family planning clinic (Table 1)

Reproductive health characteristics of the respondents

Most of the respondents in both settings had duration of $\geq$5 years of marriage [319(87.4%) in urban and 285(84.3%) in rural areas]. The median age at first marriage of the respondents was 24 (IQR: 18–30) among urban and 20 (IQR: 14–26) among rural participants. The mean (±SD) number of current children per husband was 3.44 ± 2.2 in urban setting and 3.6 ± 2.4 in rural settings (Table 2).

Knowledge of husbands towards family planning methods

Overall, knowledge about family planning service utilization was 233(63.8%) in urban and 199(54.7%) in rural areas. In both settings, most of the husbands have ever heard about the family planning methods [361(98.9%) in urban and 352(96.7%) in rural areas]. Out of total study participants, 309(84.7%) in urban and 305(83.8%) in rural have heard about family planning methods from television and radio, respectively (Table 3). The benefit of family planning methods was mentioned mostly as birth spacing among 294(80.5% in urban and 282(77.5%) in rural participants (Fig. 1).

The most reported family planning method was injectable both in urban 334(91.5%), and rural area 323(88.7%) (Fig. 2)

Most of the respondents [330(90.4%) in urban and 320(87.9%) in rural areas mentioned injectable as safest family planning method for females. About 299(81.9%) in urban and 264(72.5%) in rural area reported condoms as safest family planning method for men. Around 245(67.1%) of husband in urban and 243(66.8%) in rural area knew safe method of family planning as injectable (Fig. 3).

Family planning methods available for utilization identified during the study was injectable both in urban 260(71.2%) and rural areas 240(65.9%). According to their responses, most of the respondents were going to health center to use family planning, 295(80.8%) and 279(76.6%) in urban and rural, respectively. More than half of the participants in both rural and urban faced challenges to be engaged in family planning. About 74(20.3%) in urban and 129(35.4%) in rural of the respondents reported that negative community participation is among the most common challenges faced by the husbands to engage in family planning (Table 3).

The attitudes of husbands towards the involvement of family planning service utilization were assessed whether they had an interest to involve or not in the services. Husband's opinions about their roles in FP service utilization were assessed on a five-tier scale of strongly agree, agree, neutral, disagree and strongly disagree. Accordingly, about half 188(51.5%) of respondents from urban disagreed that FP issue should concern only women and 135(37.1%) of husband from rural strongly disagreed. In FGD majority of the participants stated, *"By nature men cannot give birth; it is the women who give birth, so they should use family planning and not husband" (FGD community 1 from urban).* However; some participants raised *"It is not only women who face problems when the children lack what to eat, wear and materials for education so the family planning issue also concerns the men" (FGD community 3 from the urban).*

The study showed that about 159(43.6%) husbands from urban agreed that spouses can seek FP services without permission from husband but 117(32.1%) from rural strongly disagreed. About 158(43.3%) of husband from urban and 52(14.3%) from rural areas agreed that FP practice reduces confidence between husband and wife.

About 128(35.1%) of respondents from urban indicated neutral to discussion of FP issue with women as it is taboo and 133(36.5%) from rural strongly disagreed. About 91(24.9%) from urban strongly agreed that it is only women who are promiscuous that use FP without their husband consent and 72(31.6%) from rural indicated as they were strongly agreed. Generally, 204(55.9%) of urban and 102(28%) of rural husbands had a positive attitude towards contraceptive methods (Table 4).

Involvement of husbands in family planning service utilization

The study revealed that out of study participants, 203(55.6%) with 95%CI (50.5–60.7) in urban and 178(48.9%) with 95%CI (44–54) in rural were involved in family planning service utilization by using or by encouraging their wives. About 135(37%) and 94(25.8%) of husbands in urban and rural have ever used condoms, respectively (Table 5). In FGD some participants stated that *"The perception of our community is not good and makes you not to use and support women on family planning usage, you perceived as you are jobless if you support your wife by accompanying her to health facility"(FGD community 4 from rural). "Using condom is not comfortable, I remember last two years I used after Dr. ordered me to use condom as not to transmitted to my wife when I become ill with sexual transmitted disease" (FGD community 2 from urban). "Using family planning is seen as acting opposite of Allah. Creator blessed human being as reproduce and fill the earth" (FGD community 4 from rural).* Similar responses were given in other group discussions.

According to participants responses, 272(74.5%) from urban and 212(58.2%) from rural married men discussed family planning with their partner in the last 1 year. Of those who discussed about family planning 214(58.6%) from urban and 136(37.4%) from rural husbands were initiated the discussion on family planning issues (Table 5). In FGD some participants stated; *"The current situation in terms of economic hardship cannot be explained and this factor ordered you to limit the number of children this was why we ordered to discuss with our wife*

Table 1 Socio-demographic variables of husbands in urban and rural kebele of Kondala district, Western Wollega, Ethiopia, 2019

Socio-demographic variables		Urban (= 365)	Rural (=364)	p-value
Age (years)	20–30	78(21.4%)	98(26.9%)	0.14
	31–40	196(53.7%)	184(50.5%)	
	41–50	80(21.9%)	62(17%)	
	> 50	11(3%)	15(4.1%)	
Educational status	No formal education	55(15.1%)	120(33%)	< 0.001*
	Primary school	87(23.5%)	120(33%)	
	Secondary school	128(35.1%)	67(18.4%)	
	Diploma and above	95(26%)	57(15.7%)	
Ethnicity	Oromo	340(93.2%)	277(76.1%)	< 0.001*
	Amhara	11(3.0%)	9(2.47%)	
	Tigre	5 (1.37%)	4 (1.1%	
	Mao	9(2.5%)	74(20.3%)	
Religion	Protestant	74(20.3%)	41(11.3%)	0.001*
	Orthodox	71(19.5%)	58(15.9%)	
	Muslim	220(60.3%)	265(72.8%)	
Occupation	Merchant	106(29%)	28(7.7%)	< 0.001*
	Government employee	97(26.6%)	32(8.8%)	
	Farmer	93(25.5%)	287(78.8%)	
	Daily worker	69(18.9%)	17(4.7%)	
Length of time spent to reach the family planning clinic	< 30 min	340(93.2%)	112(30.8%)	< 0.001*
	30–60 min	25(6.8%)	137(37.6%)	
	≥ 60 min	–	115(31.6%)	

Note: *Statistically significant at p < 0.05

Table 2 Reproductive health characteristics of the study participants, in Urban and rural kebele of Kondala district, West Wollega, Ethiopia, 2019

Reproductive health characteristics		Urban, n (%)	Rural, n (%)	p-value
Duration of marriage (years)	0–5	46(12.6%)	79(21.7%)	0.002*
	≥ 5	319(87.4%)	285(78.3%)	
Age at first marriage	15–19	50(13.7%)	95(26.1%)	< 0.001*
	20–24	160(43.8%)	166(45.6%)	
	25–29	114(31.2%)	73(20.1%)	
	≥ 30	41(11.2%)	30(8.2%)	
Current number of children	None	60(16.4%)	58(15.9%)	0.81
	1–3	117(32.1%)	110(30.2%)	
	≥ 4	188(51.5%)	196(53.8%)	
Desired number of children	1–2	11(3%)	22(6%)	0.007*
	3–4	152(41.6%)	116(31.9%)	
	≥ 5	202(55.3%)	226(62.1%)	
Birth interval (years)	> 2	124(33.8%)	140(38.5%)	0.32
	3–4	123(33.7%)	105(28.8%)	
	3–4	83(22.7%)	76(20.9%)	
	> 4	35(9.6%)	43(11.8%)	

Note: *Statistically significant at p < 0.05

Table 3 Knowledge of study participant towards family planning in urban and rural kebele of Kondala district, West Wollega, western Ethiopia, 2019

Knowledge of study participant towards family planning		Urban, n (%)	Rural, n (%)
Ever heard about FP	Yes	361(98.9%)	352(96.7%)
	No	4(1.1%)	12(3.3%)
Source of information	Radio	212(58.1%)	305(83.8%)
	TV	309(84.7%)	130(35.7%)
	Health professional	267(73%)	280(76.9%)
	Neighbor	162(44.4%)	152(41.8%)
	Friends	194(53.2%)	176(47.4%)
	Wife	226(61.9%)	214(58.8%)
	Poster	205(56.2%)	191(58.8%)
	Other	54(14.8%)	22(6%)
Know side effect of FP	Yes	261(71.5%)	254(69.8%)
	No	100(27.4%)	98(26.9%)
side effect of FP experienced by their partner	Vomiting	108(29.6%)	95(26.9%)
	Abnormal menstrual	264(72.3%)	225(61.8%)
	Unwanted weight gain	152(41.6%)	139(38.2%)
	Headache	181(48.6%)	193(53%)
FP used by their partner	Pills	309(84.7%)	312(85.7%)
	Injectable	330(90.4%)	320(87.9%)
	Implant	255(69.9%)	236(64.8%)
	Loop	220(60.3%)	183(50.3%)
	Condom	119(32.6%)	99(27.2%)
	Calendar	136(37.6%)	127(34.9%)
	Permanent	197(54%)	167(45.9%)
	Breast feeding	208(57%)	178(48.9%)
FP for male	Condom	299(81.9%)	264(72.5%)
	Permanent	204(55.9%)	180(49.5%)
	Withdrawal	185(50.7%)	160(44%)
	Periodic Abstinence	189(51.8%)	156(42.9%)
	I don't know	37(10.1%)	53(14.6%)
FP available for utilization	Pills	225(61.6%)	212(58.2%)
	Injectable	260(71.2%)	240(65.9%)
	Implant	146(40%)	120(33%)
	Loop	107(29.3%)	75(20.6%)
	Condom	211(57.8%)	196(53.8%)
	I don't know	14(3.8%)	22(6%)
Where FP can be got	Hospital	107(28.9%)	87(23.9%)
	Health center	298(80.5%)	279(76.6%)
	Health post	145(39.2%)	161(44.2%)
	Private clinic	208(57%)	164(45.1%)
	Other	21(5.8%)	18(4.9%)
FP clinic arrangements special for male	Yes	177(48.5%)	162(44.5%)
	No	184(50.4%)	190(52.2%)
Any challenge to be involved in FP	Yes	194(53.2%)	190(52.2%)

Table 3 Knowledge of study participant towards family planning in urban and rural kebele of Kondala district, West Wollega, western Ethiopia, 2019 *(Continued)*

Knowledge of study participant towards family planning		Urban, n (%)	Rural, n (%)
	No	167(45.8%)	162(44.5%)
Challenges faced by Men's to be involved in FP	Inadequate awareness of existing FP	34(9.3%)	63(17.3%)
	Religious prohibition	50(13.7%)	99(27.2%)
	Culture	58(15.9%)	83(22.8%)
	Shyness	70(19.2%)	123(33.8%)
	Negative community participation	74(20.3%)	129(35.4%)
	Lack of male FP service providers	31(8.5%)	60(16.5%)
	Fewer contraceptive choices for men	43(11.8%)	66(18.1%)

and told her she had used family planning so that we can take good care for ourselves and our children"(FGD Community 2 from Urban). "Allah who gives you a child will not ignore you on their growth no need of discussion on this matter" (FGD community 3 from rural). "Sometimes children can be counted as an asset; they will support you when you become old. There was a person who die without any care and buried without respect like other animals because he has no child, therefore the discussion that inhibits childbirth is not goods" (FGD Community 4 from rural).

About 212(58.1%) and 144(39.6%) of the husbands from the urban and rural, respectively approved the use of family planning methods (both the male and female method). The main reasons for disproval were desire to have more children in both urban 105(28.8%) and rural 107(29.4%) parts of the respondents (Table 5). In qualitative part (FGD) participants stated that; – *"The type of our occupation makes us have more children; let God show you if the children limited to 3 or 4 who can act as housekeeper, shepherd, who should help the father at farming place and who should help the mother at home this is why family planning usage can be disapproved" (FGD community 1 from Rural). "Ahh .... Women cannot be obeyed if they not caught at least by two to three years with birth-giving" (FGD community 3 from rural).*

About 222 (60.8%) from urban and 178(48.9%) from rural husbands' partners were used family planning and the most preferred contraceptive method in urban was implant 220(60.3%) and injectable 182(50%) in rural area. The main reason reported for utilization of family planning method was for child spacing in both setting 196(53.7%) and 138(37.9%) in urban and rural respectively. The study also revealed that around 266(72.9%) of urban and 193(53%) of rural husbands have supported their wives. About 257(70.4%) of husbands in urban supported by accompanying their wives to health facility and 190(52.2%) from rural supported by financial. About 67.7% from urban and 52.2% from the rural support their wives psychologically.

In FGD, most participants they stated that;-*"In the past 3 three years my wife bleeds profusely on delivery*

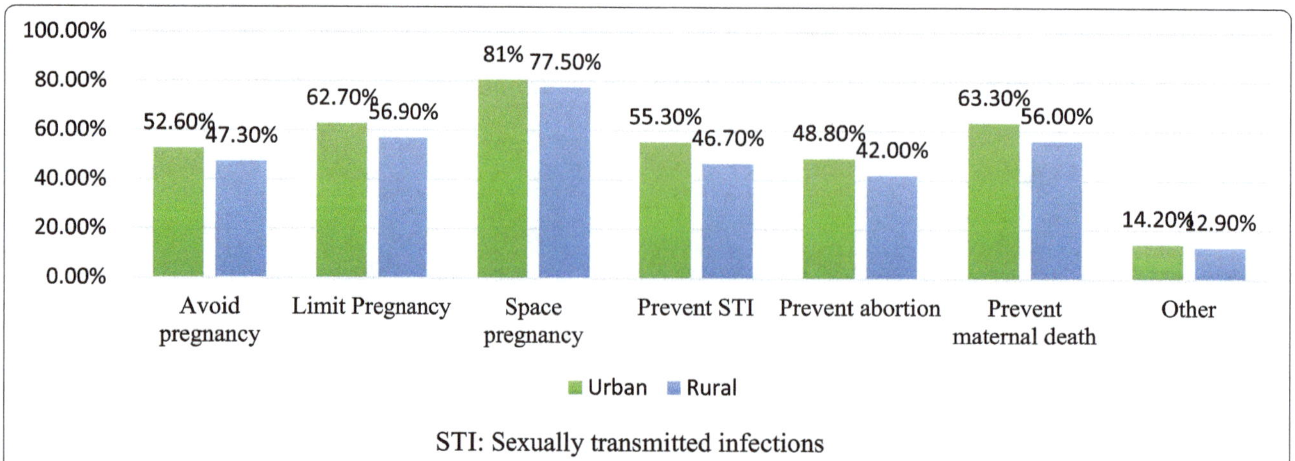

Fig. 1 Knowledge of the study participants about the benefit of FP methods, in urban and rural kebele of Kondala district, West Wollega, Ethiopia, 2019

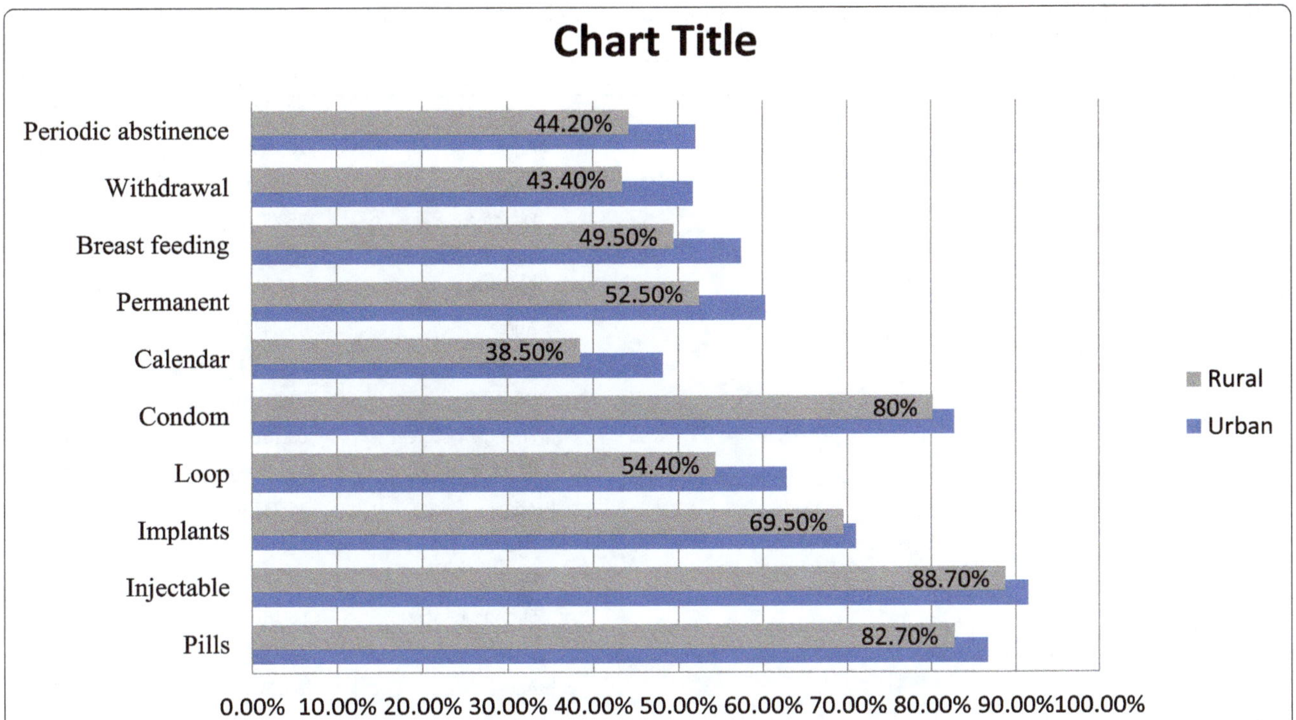

Fig. 2 Most known FP among study participants, in urban and rural kebele of Kondala district, West Wollega, Oromia regional state, 2019

and it was only God intervention that safe my wife after that we have decided to use family planning and my support was never stopped starting from that occasion even I am going with her the health center" (FGD community 2 from rural). "It is good to support partners in family planning usage because the women can forget the appointment and unwanted childbearing might have happened" (FGD community 1 from urban). Other participants did not see its importance and they stated, *"It feels you shy to accompany women for family planning services to health facility. It is good if men with men and women with women" (FGD community 2 from rural).*

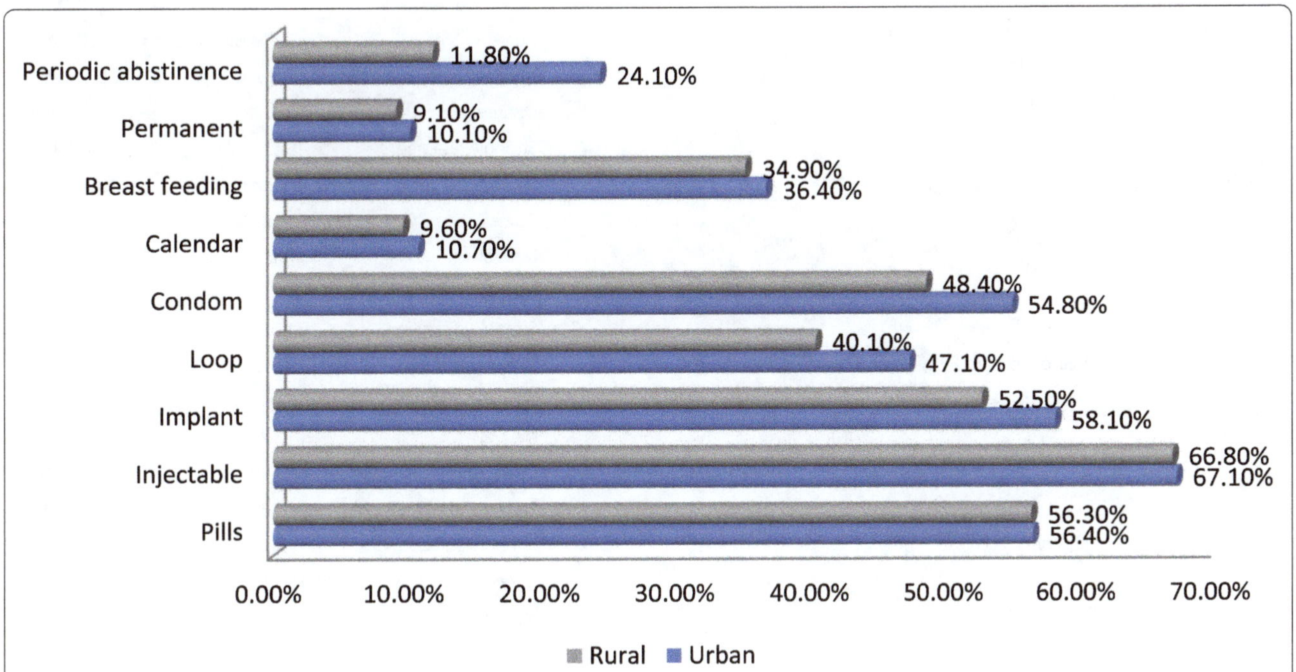

Fig. 3 Safe method reported by participants, in urban and rural kebele of Kondala district, West Wollega, Oromia regional state, 2019

Table 4 Attitude of husbands concerning family planning service utilization in urban and rural kebele of Kondala district, West Wollega, western Ethiopia, 2019

Attitude of husbands		Urban, n (%)	Rural, n (%)
FP issue should concern only women	Strongly agree	8(2.19%)	39(10.7%)
	Agree	26(7.1%)	43(11.8%)
	Neutral	59(16.2%)	52(14.3%)
	Disagree	188(51.5%)	83(22.8%)
	Strongly disagree	80(21.9%)	135(37.1%)
Spouse can seek FP services without permission from husband	Strongly agree	23(6.3%)	22(6%)
	Agree	159(43.6%)	52(14.3%)
	Neutral	19(5.2%)	77(21.2%)
	Disagree	92(25.2%)	84(23.1%)
	Strongly disagree	68(18.6%)	117(32.1)
FP practice reduces confidence b/n husband and wife	Strongly agree	39(10.7%)	26(7.1%)
	Agree	158(43.3%)	52(14.3%)
	Neutral	34(9.3%)	74(20.3%)
	Disagree	62(17%)	74(20.3%)
	Strongly disagree	68(18.6%)	126(34.6%)
Its taboo for men to discuss with women about FP	Strongly agree	28(7.7%)	22(6%)
	Agree	24(6.6%)	43(11.8%)
	Neutral	128(35.1%)	71(19.5%)
	Disagree	118(32.3%)	83(22.8%)
	Strongly disagree	63(17.3%)	133(36.5%)
It is only women who are promiscuous that use FP without their husband consent	Strongly agree	91(24.9%)	115(31.6%)
	Agree	53(14.5%)	39(10.7%)
	Neutral	86(23.6%)	72(19.8%)
	Disagree	88(24.1%)	67(18.4%)
	Strongly disagree	43(11.8%)	59(16.2%)
Only men need to decide on family planning	Strongly agree	54(14.8%)	25(6.9%)
	Agree	49(13.4%)	39(10.7%)
	Neutral	86(23.6%)	93(25.5%)
	Disagree	124(34%)	88(24.2%)
	Strongly disagree	48(13.2%)	107(29.4%)
FP methods decrease sexual urge	Strongly agree	46(12.6%)	29(8.0%)
	Agree	68(18.6%)	42(11.5%)
	Neutral	106(29%)	120(33%)
	Disagree	117(32.1%)	77(21.2%)
	Strongly disagree	24(6.6%)	84(23.1%)
Men should accompany their partners to FP clinics	Strongly agree	158(43.3%)	151(41.5%)
	Agree	159(43.6%)	66(18.1%)
	Neutral	14(3.8%)	31(8.5%)
	Disagree	16(4.4%)	57(15.7%)
	Strongly disagree	14(3.8%)	47(12.9%)
Husband involvement is important in FP	Strongly agree	158(43.3%)	113(31%)
	Agree	159(43.6%)	153(42%)
	Neutral	14(3.8%)	42(11.5%)
	Disagree	16(4.4%)	34(9.3%)
	Strongly disagree	14(3.8%)	10(2.7%)

Table 5 Involvement of husbands concerning family planning service utilization planning in urban and rural kebele of Kondala district, West Wollega, western Ethiopia, 2019

Involvement of husbands concerning family planning service utilization		Urban, n (%)	Rural, n (%)
Attended FP clinic	Yes	167(45.8%)	158(43.4%)
	No	194(53.2%)	200(53.3%)
How many times did you attended	Once	41(11.2%)	40(11%)
	Twice	54(14.8%)	51(14%)
	Many times	57(15.6%)	51(14%)
	I don't remember	13(3.6%)	18(4.9%)
Method used by husband	Condom	135(37%)	94(25.8%)
	Permanent	6	7
Discussed with your wife on FP	Yes	272(74.5%)	212(58.2%)
	No	89(24.4%)	140(38.5%)
Frequency of discussion	Once	57(15.6%)	43(11.8%)
	Twice	44(12.1%)	45(12.4%)
	Many times	125(34.2%)	88(24.2%)
	I don't remember	51(14%)	39(10.7%)
Initiated the discussion	Yes	214(58.6%)	136(37.4%)
	No	147(40.3%)	216(59.3%)
Approved FP for wife	Yes	212(58.1%)	144(39.6%)
	No	149(40.81%)	208(57.1%)
Reason for disapproval	Desire to have more child	105(28.8%)	107(29.4%)
	Fear of side effect	99(27.1%)	90(24.7%)
	Religious prohibition	89(24.4%)	73(20.1%)
	Fear of promiscuity	94(25.8%)	74(20.3%)
	Other	32(8.8%)	34(9.3%)
FP used by partner	Pills	214(58.6%)	177(48.6%)
	Injectable	216(59.2%)	182(50%)
	Implant	220(60.2%)	179(49.2%)
	Loop	201(55.1%)	176(48.4%)
	Permanent	39(10.7%)	34(9.3%)
	Calendar	198(54.2%)	176(48.4%)
	Breast feeding	190(51.1%)	169(46.4%)
Reason for utilization	For birth spacing	196(53.7%)	138(37.9%)
	For birth limiting	27(7.4%)	42(11.5%)

"There is no favorable option for husbands like women to use FP so how men can support his partner so she should uses as given for her from God" (FGD community 3 from urban).

About 263(72.1%) in urban and 227(62.4%) in rural respondents were discussed with their friends on family planning issues. About 251(68.8%) from urban and 221(60.7%) from rural encouraged their friends in family planning service utilization. Out of the respondents about half [203(55.6%) from urban and 168(46.2%) from rural] had participated in community mobilization in family planning service utilization issues. During the group discussion, some participants stated that; *"As you know there is no method of choice for men if you tied yourself you will not able to have sexual intercourse again and with condom, you cannot enjoy sex so I have no reason to encourage my friend to family planning" (FGD community 1 from urban). "We had accessed to similar source of information, but I have encouraged my friends who had many children because he discontinued his wife FP usage fearing its side effect" (FGD community 1 from urban).* Similar suggestions were obtained from the rest FGD discussions

Factors that influence husband involvement in FP service utilization

Bi-variable logistic regression analysis with selected variables

On bi-variable logistic regression, out of fifteen independent variables, six variables from urban and five variables from rural had an association with the outcome variable at p-value of 0.25. Based up on this husbands with educational level of diploma and above were nearly three times more likely to be involved in FP utilization in rural (COR = 2.89; 95% CI: 1.46–5.73) and urban COR = 2.42; 95%CI 1.19, 4.88) respectively. Regarding occupational status, government employee are about two times (COR = 2.07(1.09, 3.90) more likely to be involved in FP utilization in urban. Husbands who walk less than 30 min from health facility are about 2.29 times more likely to be involved in FP utilization than those who walkt for > 60 min (COR = 2.29; 95% CI: 1.34,3.92) in the rural. Those husbands who have been together for morethan five years since married are about three times (COR = 3.29, 95%CI: 1.68–6.44) in urban and about 1.7 times (COR = 17; 95%CI: 1.02–2.85) in rural to be involved in the FP utilization. Those couples who have four and above children are about four times (COR = 4.69; 95%CI: 2.4–9.16) in rural and about three times (COR = 3.50; 95%CI:1.89–6.47) in urban to be involved in FP. For urban husbands, those who have desire to have 3–4 children are about two times (COR = 2.12; 95%CI: 1.37–3.29) more likely to be involved in FP utilization. For rural respondents, those who have adequate knowledge are nearly five times (COR = 4.58, 95%CI: 2.91,7.21) more likely to be involved in FP utilization than those who have inadequate knowledge. For urban husbands, those who have positive attitude towards FP service utilization are about two times 2.02(1.32,3.08) more likely to be involved in FP utilization (Table 6).

Multi-variable logistic analysis of husband involvement with associated factors

Out of six from urban and five from rural variables which were candidate for multi-variable logistic regression analysis, 4 variables both in urban and rural were statistically significant with the husbands' involvement in FP service utilization at $p < 0.05$. In Urban areas, husbands who participated in government employees were about 2.5 times more likely to be involved in family planning service utilization than other types of occupational status (AOR = 2.58,95%CI = 1.25–5.33, $p = 0.01$). Respondents who had four and above or a greater number of current children were 3.25 times more likely to be involved in family planning service utilization than those who had less than four children. (AOR = 3.25, 95%CI = 1.51–7.02, $p = 0.003$). Husbands who had desired number of children less than two were 3 times more likely to be involved in family planning service utilization than husbands who had desired number of children more than two (AOR = 3.07, 95%CI = 1.80–5.24, $p =$ 0.003. Finally, husbands who had positive attitude towards family planning methods were 1.86 times more likely to be involved than those who had negative attitude in family planning service utilization (AOR = 1.86, 95%CI = 1.15–2.99. p = 0.01).

In rural setting, husbands who had diploma and above were about two times more likely to be involved in family planning service utilization than those who had below educational background (AOR = 2.13, 95%CI = 1.02–4.44, $p = 0.05$). Husband who goes less than 30 min to reach health facility to get service were 2.28 times more likely to be involved in family planning service utilization than those who traveled more than 30 min (AOR = 2.28, 95%CI = 1.24–4.19, $p = 0.008$). Participants who had four and above number of current children were about 4 times more likely to be involved in family planning service utilization than those who had less than four children. (AOR = 4.27, 95%CI = 1.88, 9.73, $p = 0.001$). Lastly, husbands who were knowledgeable to family planning methods were 4.48 times more likely to be involved than husbands who were not knowledgeable in family planning service utilization (AOR = 4.48,95%CI = 2.72–7.38, $p < 0.001$) (Table 7)

Discussion

The finding of the study revealed that more than half (55.6%) from urban and (44.9%) from rural husbands were involved in family planning service utilization in the district. This was low when compared with world health organization (WHO) attention towards male involvement in reproductive health including family planning service utilization [34]. The reasons for this low finding might be due to low provision of information on service utilization, low service targeting men within the health facilities and low attention to satisfied users to promote the usage of the methods. The involvement in service utilization was higher in urban compared to the rural areas. This might be because in rural areas negative community perception on husbands supporting ladies, health facility setup and the distance from home to health facility negatively influenced husbands' involvement in family planning service utilization. However, the service utilization was higher than the study results in west Shoa (36%) [27] and in India 22% in urban and 17% in rural [35]. The discrepancy may be due to the improvement of the health facilities on the provision of the family planning service with time variation.

However, the current study on husbands' involvement in family planning service utilization was lower than similar studies conducted in Gedeo zone, (70.9%) in

Table 6 Bi-variable analysis of factors contributing to husbands' involvement in family planning service utilization in urban and rural kebele of Kondala district, West Wollega, western Ethiopia, 2019

Variable	Category	Husband Involvement in FP				OR (95%CI)	
		Urban		Rural		Urban	Rural
		Involved (%)	Not involved (%)	Involved (%)	Not involved (%)		
Educational status	No Formal education	29(53.7)	2546.29)	54(46.95)	61(53.04)	1	1
	Primary school	41(48.23)	44(51.76)	51(44.35)	64(55.65)	0.80(0.40, 1.59)	0.90(0.54, 1.51)
	Secondary school	63(49.6)	64(50.3)	32(49.23)	33(50.76)	0.85(0.45, 1.60)	1.09(0.59, 2.01)
	Diploma & above	70(73.68)	25(26.3)	41(71.92)	16(28.07)	2.42(1.19, 4.88)*	2.89(1.46, 5.73)*
Occupational status	Merchant	58(55.76)	46(44.23)	**	**	1.23(0.66, 2.25)	**
	Government employee	66(68.04)	31(31.95)			2.07(1.09, 3.90)*	
	Farmer	44(48.35)	47(51.64)			0.90(0.48, 1.70)	
	Daily Worker	35(50.72)	34(49.27)			1	
Distance to HF (min)	< 30	**	**	66(61.11)	42(38.89)	**	2.29(1.34,3.92)*
	30–60			66(50.38)	65(49.61)		1.48(0.89,2.45)
	> 60			46(40.7)	67(59.29)		
Duration of marriage (years)	0–5	14(31.11)	31(68.88)	31(40.25)	46(59.74)	1	1
	> 5	189(59.81)	127(40.18)	147(53.45)	128(46.54)	3.29(1.68,6.44)*	1.70(1.02,2.85)*
Current number of children	None	21(35.59)	38(64.40)	14(24.13)	44(75.86)	1	1
	1–3	60(51.28)	57(48.71)	52(48.59)	55(51.41)	1.90(1.00,3.63)*	2.97(1.46,6.05)*
	≥4	122(65.94)	63(34.06)	112(59.89)	75(40.11)	3.50(1.89,6.47)*	4.69(2.40,9.16)*
Desired number of children	1–2	4(36.36)	7(63.63)	**	**	0.59(0.16,2.09)	**
	3–4	102(67.10)	50(32.89)			2.12(1.37,3.29)*	
	≥5	97(48.89)	101(51.01)			1	
Knowledge about FP	Not Knowledgeable	**	**	46(30.06)	107(69.93)	**	1
	Knowledgeable			132(66.33)	67(33.66)		4.58(2.91,7.21)*
Attitude Towards FP	Negative attitude	73(46.49)	84(53.51)	**	**	1	**
	Positive attitude	130(63.72)	74(36.27)			2.02(1.32,3.08)*	

* Variables which are significant at 95%CI with p-value < 0.05, ** Data which are not included in the model, 1: reference category
COR Crudes Odds Ratio; *FP* Family planning; *HF* Health facility

urban and (63.4%) in rural areas [21], Agaro town 74.4%) [7], Asosa (70%) [26], urban part of Nigeria (80%) [11] and in rural areas of India (West Bengal) (74.4%) [36]. This discrepancy perhaps be due to most of the indicated studies are conducted in the urban areas [7, 26] where majority of them are supposed to be literate and have access to information and services.

This study also attempted to identify factors associated with husband involvement in family planning service utilization. Socio-economic status, husband's reproductive characteristics, Knowledge and attitudes towards FP service utilization were among factors associated with the involvement of males in FP services utilization.

It revealed that there is positive association of husband's FP knowledge with the involvement in FP service utilization, especially in rural parts. The finding complements to other studies done in Tigray, Debremarkos, Gedeo zone, Bahir Dar and Afar [4, 5, 14, 19, 21]. This is because knowledge is pre-request to be involved in family planning service utilization. Additionally, husband's having positive attitude towards FP were 1.86 times more likely to be involved family planning service utilization than those having negative attitude in urban setting. This is supported by the previous study conducted in Nigeria, India and Gedeo zone [21, 35, 37].

In Urban areas, husbands who were government employees were nearly three times more likely to be involved in family planning service utilization than other types of occupational status. This finding is supported by similar studies conducted in Ethiopia; Angecha woreda [12], Bahirdar town [29]. This is due to the fact that most of government employees in Ethiopia are educated and this in turn associated with the statement that the more a husband is educated, the more he will accept

Table 7 Multi-variable logistic analysis of husband involvement in family planning service utilization with associated factors in urban and rural kebele of Kondala district, West Wollega, western Ethiopia, 2019

Variable	Category	Urban areas		Rural areas	
		AOR (95%CI)	p-value	AOR (95%CI)	p-value
Educational status	No Formal education	1	1	1	1
	Primary school	0.851(0.39, 1.82)	0.676	0.928(0.52, 1.66)	0.802
	Secondary school	0.806(0.39, 1.65)	0.556	1.198(0.60, 2.38)	0.606
	Diploma and above	2.193(0.99, 4.83)	0.051	2.126(1.02, 4.44)	0.045*
Occupational status	Merchant	1.378(0.70, 2.69)	0.349	**	**
	Government employee	2.585(1.25, 5.33)	0.010*		
	Farmer	0.828(0.41, 1.66)	0.595		
	Daily Worker	1	1		
Distance from home to HF	< 30 min	**	**	2.283(1.24, 4.19)	0.008*
	30–60 min			1.251(0.70, 2.23)	0.447
	> 60 min			1	1
Duration of marriage	0–5 years	1	1	1	1
	> 5 years	2.114(0.94, 4.75)	0.070	1.088(0.54, 2.18)	0.812
Current number of children	None	1	1	1	1
	1–3	1.304(0.61, 2.78)	0.493	4.275(1.88, 9.73)	0.001
	> 4	3.255(1.51, 7.02)	0.003*	4.204(1.80, 9.79)	0.001*
Desired number of children	1–2	2.217(0.55, 8.93)	0.263*	**	**
	3–4	3.076(1.80, 5.24)	< 0.001*		
	> 5	1	1	1	1
Knowledge about FP	Not Knowledgeable	**	**	1	1
	Knowledgeable			4.478(2.72, 7.38)	< 0.001*
Attitude Towards FP	Negative attitude	1	1	**	**
	Positive attitude	1.863(1.15, 2.99)	0.010*		

* Variables which are significant at 95% CI with p-value of < 0.05, ** Data which are not included in the model, 1 reference category
AOR Adjusted odds ratio; *HF* Health facility

gender equality and believe in equal participation in decision making [38].

This indicated that the more educated respondents are more familiar with family planning methods and utilizes it to give special care for their having children. Respondents who had a greater number of current children were about 3 times in urban and 4 times in rural more likely to be involved in family planning service utilization compared to individuals who had no more children. This finding was in line with the studies conducted in Asosa town, North Shoa and Loka Abay district [18, 20, 26]. However, the finding was contrary to study conducted in urban area (Bahir Dar) where involvement in family planning was higher among individuals who had no or less children than who had more children [14]. The reason for the discrepancy in the current study might be because the current living expense was becoming difficult to have more children related to the current economic hardship in the country.

From this study husbands who do not want to have any more children were more likely to be involved in family planning service utilization than husbands who want to have more children. This finding was supported by the study conducted in Kembata Tembaro zone [12]. However, educational status and duration of marriage did not show association with husband involvement in family planning service after confounding was controlled in urban setting.

According to the findings of this study educational status was one significant predictor of husbands' involvement on family planning in rural areas. It showed as the educational status of respondents increases, there showed an evidence of husbands' involvement in family planning service utilization. This was supported by previous studies conducted in different areas and countries where education was significantly affected family planning service utilization [14, 18, 25, 39]. The study also revealed that husband who goes less than 30 min from home to health facility to get service were about 2 times more likely to be involved in family planning service utilization than those who traveled more than 30 min. However, duration of marriage toward family planning did not show strong association with husband involvement following controlling confounder in rural areas.

The study assessed through qualitative way also identified husbands' perception towards involvement in family planning service utilization. Most of the husbands in urban area perceived that they believe in the involvement of males in FP issue as it was not the only issue of the women. In rural areas the participants' perception was not far from the answer to quantitative questions. Culturally perceived reproductive issues as the women business, desire of more children, fear of side effects of family planning and fear of community perception determined them as not to be involved as much like in urban areas. Generally, husbands living in urban areas were more likely to be involved than their rural counterparts. This finding was in line with the study conducted in Kembata Tembaro zone and India [12, 35]. The discrepancy could be due to in urban areas relatively good income, easily access to health facilities, educational facilities, broadcasting facilities and other services are more accessible than rural counterpart.

As strength, qualitative method was used to supplement the result and to explore factors that were not addressed by quantitative survey. Our study is not without some limitations. The result of this study totally relied on self-report and willingness of the participants to give real information and thus does not provide an objective measure of husbands' involvement in family planning.

Conclusion

The finding of the study showed the proportion of husbands' involvement in family planning utilization in urban and rural areas was low. Factors associated with the involvement varied between the two setups, except the current number of children. Being government employee, wishing less than two children and having a better attitude towards family planning methods in urban and good educational background, less distance from home to health facility and having better knowledge were factors associated with husband involvement in family planning utilization in rural areas. In the qualitative study, most husbands in rural areas were not experienced good perception like urban areas in the involvement of FP service utilization due to different Socio-cultural factors.

Hence the governmental (the district and zonal health office) and non-governmental organizations working on the family planning issues should address socio-cultural, infrastructure associated with health facility, knowledge and attitudinal factors in future family planning programs. Besides family planning service utilization interventions in the area need to be promoted, awareness creation should be made, and health extension worker should enhance health education especially in rural part in family planning service utilization.

Abbreviations

AOR: Adjusted Odd Ratio; CI: Confidence Interval; FGD: Focused Group Discussion; FP: Family Planning; IQR: Inter Quartile Range; IUCD: Intra Uterine Contraceptive Device; MOH: Ministry of Health; NGO: Non-Governmental Organizations; OC: Oral Contraceptive; OR: Odds Ratios; RH: Reproductive Health; SPSSS: Statistical Package for Social Sciences; WHO: World Health Organization

Acknowledgements

We thank Wollega University, Institute of health sciences for logistic support. We are grateful to Kondala district administration, kebele administration, data collectors and study participants for their cooperation in the success of this study.

Authors' contributions

LA and ZS contributed to the design of the study, analysis, interpretation and writes up of the manuscript. HK, ET and GF contributed to the design of the study, data analysis, drafting and edition of the manuscript. All authors critically revised the manuscript and have approved the final manuscript.

Author details

[1]Department of Public health, Institute of Health Sciences, Wollega University, Nekemte, Ethiopia. [2]Deputy of the health center, Gimbi Health Center, Western Wollega Zone, Gimbi, Ethiopia. [3]Department of Midwifery, Institute of Health Sciences, Wollega University, Nekemte, Ethiopia. [4]Department of Public Health, College of Medical and Health Sciences, Madda Walabu University, Goba Referral Hospital, Goba, Ethiopia. [5]Department of Pharmacy, Institute of Health Sciences, Wollega University, P.O Box:395, Nekemte, Oromia, Ethiopia. [6]School of Pharmacy, Faculty of Medicine, The Chinese University of Hong Kong, Shatin, New territory, Hong Kong.

References

1. Sternberg P, Hubley J. Evaluating men's involvement as a strategy in sexual and reproductive health promotion. Health Promot Int. 2004;19(3):389–96. https://doi.org/10.1093/heapro/dah312.
2. Family planning in Kenya. A review of national district policies and budgets [http://www.dsw.org/en/wp-content/uploads/2017/01/DSW_Kenya-Budget-Study_30062014.pdf]. Accessed 5 Mar 2019.
3. Dudgeon MR, Inhorn MC. Men's influences on women's reproductive health: medical anthropological perspectives. Soc Sci Med. 2004;59(7):1379–95. https://doi.org/10.1016/j.socscimed.2003.11.035.
4. Chekole MK, Kahsay ZH, Medhanyie AA, Gebreslassie MA, Bezabh AM. Husbands' involvement in family planning use and its associated factors in pastoralist communities of Afar, Ethiopia. Reprod Health. 2019;16(1):33. https://doi.org/10.1186/s12978-019-0697-6.
5. Bayray A. Assessment of male involvement in family planning use among men in south eastern zone of Tigray, Ethiopia. Scholar J Med. 2012;2(2):1–10.
6. Kakaire O, Kaye DK, Osinde MO. Male involvement in birth preparedness and complication readiness for emergency obstetric referrals in rural Uganda. Reprod Health. 2011;8(1):12. https://doi.org/10.1186/1742-4755-8-12.
7. Girum T, Shegaze M, Tariku Y. The role of currently married men in family planning and its associated factors in Agaro Town, South West Ethiopia. Ann Med Health Sci Res. 2017;7(6):119–24.
8. Bishwajit G, Tang S, Yaya S, Ide S, Fu H, Wang M, et al. Factors associated with male involvement in reproductive care in Bangladesh. BMC Public Health. 2017;17(1):3. https://doi.org/10.1186/s12889-016-3915-y.

9. International Planned Parenthood Federation (2011). Male involvement in family planning utilization. In.
10. Cohen SA, Richards CL. The Cairo consensus: population, development and women. Fam Plan Perspect. 1994;26(6):272–7. https://doi.org/10.2307/2135895.
11. Ijadunola MY, Abiona TC, Ijadunola KT, Afolabi OT, Esimai OA, FM OO. Male involvement in family planning decision making in Ile-Ife, Osun State, Nigeria. Afr J Reprod Health. 2010;14(4):43–50.
12. Helamo D, Tessema F, Doyore F. Assessment of husband-wife communication and practice of contraceptives in Angecha Woreda, Kembata Tembaro zone, South Ethiopia: a cross sectional study. Reprod Syst Sex Disord. 2014;3(134):2.
13. Char A. Male involvement in family planning and reproductive health in rural Central India: Tampere University press; 2011.
14. Walle Y, Alamrew Z. The current states of male involvement on family planning and factors correlated with among male FactoryWorkers in Bahir Dar City. Am J Public Health Res. 2014;2(5):188–97. https://doi.org/10.12691/ajphr-2-5-2.
15. Mattebo M, Sharma B, Dahlkvist E, Molinder E, Erlandsson K. Perceptions of the role of the man in family planning, during pregnancy and childbirth: a qualitative study with fifteen Nepali men. J Asian Midwiv (JAM). 2016;3(1):31–45.
16. Shisoka J, Litali G. Male involvement in family planning services for population development. J Emerg Trends Econ Manag Sci. 2015;6(7):237–43.
17. Yasir BC. Male Involvement in Reproductive Health in District Khairpur, Sindh. Pakistan: The David Lucile & Packard Foundation; 2011.
18. Bifato B. Assessment of male involvement in family planning use in Loka Abaya District, Southern Ethiopia: Cross-Sectional Study; 2016.
19. Kassa M, Abajobir AA, Gedefaw M. Level of male involvement and associated factors in family planning services utilization among married men in Debremarkos town, Northwest Ethiopia. BMC Int Health Hum Rights. 2014;14(1):33. https://doi.org/10.1186/s12914-014-0033-8.
20. Mohammed A, Woldeyohannes D, Feleke A, Megabiaw B. Determinants of modern contraceptive utilization among married women of reproductive age group in north Shoa zone, Amhara region, Ethiopia. Reprod Health. 2014;11(1):13. https://doi.org/10.1186/1742-4755-11-13.
21. Eshete A, Adissu Y. Women's joint decision on contraceptive use in Gedeo zone, Southern Ethiopia: A Community Based Comparative Cross-Sectional Study. Int J Fam Med. 2017;2017(9389072):9. https://doi.org/10.1155/2017/9389072.
22. Rekha T, Unnikrishnan B, Prasanna PM, Nithin Kumar RH, Vishal Raina HH. Married men's involvement in family planning–a study from coastal southern India. J Clin Diagn Res. 2015;9(4):LC04.
23. Catherine GK. Barriers to male involvement in family planning in Kiambu County, Central Kenya. University of Nairobi Research Archive: Master s thesis). 2016. Retrieved from http://erepository.uonbi.ac.ke/handle/11295/99341. Accessed 20 June 2019.
24. Tamiso A, Admasu T, Henok B, Zale Z, Admasu D. Barriers to male involvement in family planning services in Arba Minch town, southern Ethiopia: qualitative case study. Int J Public Health Serv. 2016;5(1):46–50.
25. Adera A, Belete T, Gebru A, Hagos A, Gebregziabher W. Assessment of the role of men in family planning utilization at Edaga-Hamuse town, Tigray, North Ethiopia. Am J Nurs Sci. 2015;4(4):174–81. https://doi.org/10.11648/j.ajns.20150404.15.
26. Tessema ZK. Husband-wife communication about family planning in Assosa town (Ethiopia); 2002.
27. Demissie DB, Tilahun A, Arga A, Kurke A, Awel A, Oljira K. Male involvement in family planning and associated factors among Marriedin Malegedo town west Shoa zone, Oromia, Ethiopia. J Culture Soc Develop. 2016;15:12–8.
28. ICF. CSACEa: Ethiopia Demographic and Health Survey 2016. Addis Ababa, and Rockville: CSA and ICF. In; 2016.
29. Belay AD, Mengesha ZB, Woldegebriel MK, Gelaw YA. Married women's decision making power on family planning use and associated factors in Mizan-Aman, South Ethiopia: a cross sectional study. BMC Womens Health. 2016;16(1):12. https://doi.org/10.1186/s12905-016-0290-x.
30. Kondala Woreda Health Office: Background of kondala district. In.; 2019.
31. Vouking MZ, Evina CD, Tadenfok CN. Male involvement in family planning decision making in sub-Saharan Africa- what the evidence suggests. Pan Af Med J. 2014;19:349.
32. Berhane A, Biadgilign S, Berhane A, Memiah P. Male involvement in family planning program in northern Ethiopia: an application of the Transtheoretical model. Patient Educ Couns. 2015;98(4):469–75. https://doi.org/10.1016/j.pec.2014.12.012.
33. Bogale B, Wondafrash M, Tilahun T, Girma E. Married women's decision making power on modern contraceptive use in urban and rural southern Ethiopia. BMC Public Health. 2011;11(1):342. https://doi.org/10.1186/1471-2458-11-342.
34. World health Organization. WHO recommendation on interventions to promote the involvement of men during pregnancy, childbirth and after birth (2015). WHO reproductive health library. Geneva: World Health Organization. In; 2015.
35. Dhingra R, Manhas S, Kohli N, Mushtaq A. Attitude of couples towards family planning. J Hum Ecol. 2010;30(1):63–70. https://doi.org/10.1080/09709274.2010.11906273.
36. Basu A, Das D, Singh R, Chatterjee S, Bhattacharya S, Dutta M. Perception and role of husbands about family planning in a rural area of West Bengal. IOSR J Dental Med Sci. 2015;14(10):37–9.
37. Adelekan A, Omoregie P, Edoni E. Male involvement in family planning: challenges and way forward. Int J Population Res. 2014;2014:1–9. https://doi.org/10.1155/2014/416457.
38. Alemayehu M, Meskele M. Health care decision making autonomy of women from rural districts of southern Ethiopia: a community based cross-sectional study. Int J Women's Health. 2017;9:213–21. https://doi.org/10.2147/IJWH.S131139.
39. Ouma S, Turyasima M, Acca H, Nabbale F, Obita K, Rama M, et al. Obstacles to family planning use among rural women in Atiak health center IV, Amuru District, northern Uganda. East Afr Med J. 2015;92(8):394–400.

19

Characteristics and contraceptive outcomes of women seeking medical or surgical abortion in reproductive health clinics in Cambodia

Chris Smith[1,2*], Rachel H. Scott[2], Caroline Free[2] and Tansy Edwards[3]

Abstract

Background: Since the approval of medical abortion in Cambodia in 2010, the proportion of women reporting an abortion has increased. We describe the characteristics and contraceptive outcomes of women seeking medical abortion compared to surgical abortion at four reproductive health clinics in Cambodia.

Methods: Secondary data analysis using data collected in the MObile Technology for Improved Family Planning (MOTIF) trial, a single blind, randomized trial of a personalized, mobile phone-based intervention designed to support post-abortion family planning in Cambodia. Baseline interviews were conducted after women had received post-abortion family planning counselling at the clinic, and follow-up interviews were conducted at 4 and 12 months. We used multivariable logistic regression to assess associations between abortion type and baseline characteristics, contraceptive uptake, repeat pregnancy and repeat abortion. We conducted an exploratory analysis to compare the timing of initiation of long-acting (LA) contraception between women having medical versus surgical abortion over the four-month post-abortion period.

Results: Of the 500 women who participated in the trial, 41% had a medical abortion. In multivariate analyses, women undergoing medical abortion were more likely to be urban residents, have a higher level of education, be undecided or not intending to use family planning, and be undecided or intending to have another child. There was no association between type of abortion and contraceptive uptake, repeat pregnancy or repeat abortion. Women who had medical abortion initiated LA contraception post abortion later than women who had surgical abortion.

Conclusions: Our results suggest women having a medical abortion in Cambodia have different baseline characteristics and had delayed uptake of contraception compared to women having a surgical abortion. However, we cannot draw conclusions on the direction of associations and causality. Further research is recommended to explore reasons for the observed findings with view to increasing access to abortion and post-abortion contraception.

Keywords: Contraception, Post-abortion family planning, Post-abortion contraception, Medical abortion, Surgical abortion

* Correspondence: christopher.smith@lshtm.ac.uk
[1]Graduate School of Tropical Medicine and Global Health, Nagasaki University, Nagasaki, Japan
[2]Department of Population Health, London School of Hygiene & Tropical Medicine, London, UK

Introduction

It is estimated that globally around 25% of pregnancies resulted in induced surgical or medical abortion during the period 2010–2014, equating to an annual abortion rate of 35 per 1000 women aged 15–44. [1] In Cambodia in response to high maternal mortality, estimated at 900/100,000 live births, abortion laws were reformed in 1997 to allow abortion on request until the 12th week of pregnancy, and in certain circumstances during the second trimester. [2]. According to the 1997 law, abortions can only be provided by medical doctors, medical practitioners or midwives authorized by the Ministry of Health and only carried out in a hospital, health center, health clinic or maternity ward. [3] The medical abortion pack 'Medabon' containing mifepristone and misoprostol was approved by the Cambodia Ministry of Health in 2010 and made available in a restricted number of health facilities and pharmacies. [2] Medical abortion is available in clinic settings and from pharmacies and medical abortion packs have been distributed in Cambodia via social marketing and franchising programmes by non-governmental organisations such as Population Services Khmer. [4] Cambodian women also use other pharmaceutical products to induce an abortion, purchased from pharmacists, markets and drug sellers; typically unregistered combinations of mifepristone and misoprostol, sometimes described as "Chinese pills" [4, 5].

Sequential demographic and health surveys in Cambodia indicate that the proportion of women reporting having had an induced abortion in the previous 5 years increased from 4% in 2005 to 7% in 2014. [3, 6, 7] Following the approval of medical abortion in 2010, the proportion of women having medical rather than surgical abortion increased: from 31% in 2010 to 47% in 2014. [3, 7]

Women seeking abortion services often have an unmet need for family planning. Post-abortion family planning (PAFP) can reduce subsequent unplanned pregnancies and repeat abortion and was identified as a high-impact practice in family planning by a USAID technical advisory group in 2012. [8] Women are at risk of pregnancy soon after abortion; studies that have examined return to ovulation post-abortion show that this can occur around 2–3 weeks following the abortion, but earlier among some women. [9, 10] All contraceptive methods are safe to use in the immediate post-abortion period to reduce the risk of pregnancy, with the exception of the intra-uterine device (IUD), which can be inserted at the time of surgical abortion but in the case of medical abortion should be delayed until after the abortion is complete. [11–13] The type of abortion obtained may therefore affect uptake of post-abortion contraception or the contraceptive method chosen.

We describe characteristics and contraceptive outcomes of women seeking medical abortion vs. surgical abortion, using data collected in the MObile Technology for Improved Family Planning (MOTIF) trial. [14] The specific objectives are to compare: (1) baseline characteristics amongst women seeking medical versus surgical abortion in the MOTIF trial; (2) outcomes: contraception use, repeat pregnancy and abortion amongst women seeking medical versus surgical abortion in the trial; and (3) the timing of initiation of long-acting contraception between women having medical versus surgical abortion over the four-month post-abortion period.

Methods

We analysed data collected during the MOTIF trial. The trial protocol, results and process evaluation are reported in separate manuscripts. [15, 16] In brief, the MOTIF trial was a single blind, randomized trial of a personalized, mobile phone-based intervention designed to support post-abortion contraception. Women were recruited by research assistants from four clinics in Cambodia during May to September 2013. The clinics in Phnom Penh (2), Battambang and Siem Reap served clients from urban and rural areas. On recruitment, women were asked whether they considered their residence to be urban or rural. Women were eligible for inclusion if they were aged 18 or older, attending for an induced abortion at the MSI clinic (either surgical or medical, using licensed medication), had a mobile phone primarily for their own use, reported not wanting to become pregnant and were willing to receive automated messages about contraception. Baseline interviews were conducted after women had received post-abortion family planning counselling at the clinic for the abortion visit, and follow-up interviews were conducted at 4 and 12 months. Follow-up was 86% at 4 months and 66% at 12 months. There was no evidence of differential loss to follow-up between women receiving medical compared to surgical abortion at four or 12 months. [17]

Analysis

First, factors associated with medical versus surgical abortion in univariable analyses were identified, based on a likelihood ratio test (LRT) p-value< 0.1. A multivariable model was obtained from a stepwise model building process, whereby covariates were added to the multivariable model in turn, and the goodness of fit of the model with the additional parameter was compared to the previous model using a LRT. Covariates were retained in the multivariable model if the LRT p-value $<$ 0.1. Covariates were removed if not associated with the outcome after adjustment for other covariates during this process.

Table 1 Characteristics of the study sample

	N	%
Type of abortion		
Medical	207	41
Surgical	293	59
Age group		
Age > 25	343	69
Age < 25	157	31
Residence		
Rural	321	64
Urban	179	36
Socio-economic status		
No access to motorised transport	65	13
Access to motorised transport	435	87
Level of Education		
None or primary	196	39
Some secondary or above	304	61
Marital status		
Never married or living together	29	6
Married/living together	464	93
Divorced/separated	7	1
# living children		
1 or more	353	71
0	147	29
# previous abortions		
0	299	60
1 or more	201	40
Previous contraception use		
Yes	299	60
No	201	40
Occupation		
Housewife	102	20
Factory worker	76	15
Entertainment worker	27	5
Farmer	32	6
Employed	99	20
Self-employed/own business	134	27
Casual work/casual labour	3	1
Student	17	3
Unemployed	9	2
vOther	1	0
Contraception decision-making[a]		
Mainly woman	96	21
Mainly husband/partner	78	17
Joint decision	290	63
Phone sharing		
Shares	241	48
Never shares	259	52
Disclosure of abortion to others[b]		
Yes	204	85
No	37	15
PAFP intentions		
Yes	187	37
No	42	8
Undecided	271	54
Fertility plans		
No more/none	139	28
Have a/another child	308	62
Undecided	53	11
Phone credit		
Sometimes	193	39
Usually	128	26
Always	179	36
Randomisation		
Intervention	249	50
Control	251	50

[a]36 missing values [b]259 missing values

Secondly, we assessed crude and adjusted associations between abortion method and effective contraceptive use, repeat pregnancy and abortion at 4 and 12-months using logistic regression. We define effective modern methods to be those associated with < 10% 12-month pregnancy rates, as commonly used: Oral Contraceptive (OC), injectable, implant, IUD, or permanent methods [18]. A participant was considered to be using an effective method if she reported that she: (i) was currently using the implant or IUD; (ii) had received the injectable within the previous 3 months; (iii) was sterilized (or partner was sterilized); or (iv) had taken an OC within 24 h of the interview or according to instructions. Long acting methods were defined as the IUD, implant or a permanent method. The pre-specified approach was to adjust for age, socio-economic status and residence a priori, as well whether the participant was allocated to receive the intervention or not. Access to motorised transport was used as a measure of socio-economic status, similar to the assessment of household wealth in the Cambodia DHS survey. [3] Age cut offs above and below 25 were selected to be consistent with MSI definitions of young women and our previous publications. [19] All participants who were allocated to the intervention and could be contacted received the intervention messages. Those who could not be

Table 2 Associations with type of abortion

	Surgical N = 293	Medical N = 207	Crude OR	LRT *p* value	Adjusted OR[a]	LRT *p* value
Age group						
Age > 25	213 (62%)	130 (38%)	1.00			
Age < 25	80 (51%)	77 (49%)	1.58 (1.08–2.31)	0.019		
Residence						
Rural	216 (67%)	105 (33%)	1.00			
Urban	77 (43%)	102 (57%)	2.73 (1.87–3.97)	< 0.001	2.18 (1.46–3.25)	< 0.001
Socio-economic status						
No access to motorised transport	45 (69%)	20 (31%)	1.00			
Access to motorised transport	248 (57%)	187 (43%)	1.70 (0.97–2.97)	0.058		
Level of Education						
None or primary	130 (66%)	66 (34%)	1.00			
Some secondary or above	163 (54%)	141 (46%)	1.70 (1.17–2.47)	0.005	1.45 (0.97–2.17)	0.068
Marital status						
Never married or living together	18 (62%)	11 (38%)	1.00			
Married/living together	271 (58%)	193 (42%)	1.17 (0.54–2.52)	0.924		
Divorced/separated	4 (57%)	3 (43%)	1.23 (0.23–6.55)			
# living children						
1 or more	223 (63%)	130 (37%)	1.00			
0	70 (48%)	77 (52%)	1.89 (1.28–2.78)	0.001		
# previous abortions						
0	171 (57%)	128 (43%)	1.00			
1 or more	122 (61%)	79 (39%)	0.87 (0.60–1.25)	0.435		
Previous contraception use						
Yes	180 (60%)	119 (40%)	1.00			
No	113 (56%)	88 (44%)	1.18 (0.82–1.69)	0.376		
Occupation						
Housewife	67 (66%)	35 (34%)	1.00			
Factory worker	35 (46%)	41 (54%)	2.24 (1.22–4.12)	< 0.001		
Entertainment worker	15 (56%)	12 (44%)	1.53 (0.65–3.63)			
Farmer	29 (91%)	3 (9%)	0.20 (0.06–0.70)			
Employed	57 (58%)	42 (42%)	1.41 (0.80–2.50)			
Self-employed/own business	78 (58%)	56 (42%)	1.37 (0.81–2.34)			
Casual work/casual labour	2 (67%)	1 (33%)	0.96 (0.08–10.93)			
Student	5 (29%)	12 (71%)	4.59 (1.50–14.09)			
Unemployed	4 (44%)	5 (56%)	2.39 (0.60–9.48)			
Other	1 (100%)	0 (0%)	1.00 (-.)			
Contraception decision-making						
Mainly woman	71 (74%)	25 (26%)	1.00			
Mainly husband/partner	47 (60%)	31 (40%)	1.87 (0.98–3.56)	0.001		
Joint decision	154 (53%)	136 (47%)	2.51 (1.50–4.18)			
Phone sharing						
Shares	142 (59%)	99 (41%)	1.00			
Never shares	151 (58%)	108 (42%)	1.03 (0.72–1.46)	0.888		

Table 2 Associations with type of abortion *(Continued)*

	Surgical N = 293	Medical N = 207	Crude OR	LRT *p* value	Adjusted OR[a]	LRT *p* value
Disclosure of abortion to others						
Yes	122 (60%)	82 (40%)	1.00			
No	20 (54%)	17 (46%)	1.26 (0.63–2.56)	0.515		
PAFP intentions						
Yes	135 (72%)	52 (28%)	1.00			
No	22 (52%)	20 (48%)	2.36 (1.19–4.68)	< 0.001	2.08 (1.02–4.23)	0.001
Undecided	136 (50%)	135 (50%)	2.58 (1.73–3.84)		2.18 (1.44–3.31)	
Fertility plans						
No more/none	105 (76%)	34 (24%)	1.00			
Have a/another child	162 (53%)	146 (47%)	2.78 (1.78–4.35)	< 0.001	2.07 (1.29–3.32)	0.007
Undecided	26 (49%)	27 (51%)	3.21 (1.65–6.22)		2.08 (1.03–4.18)	
Phone credit						
Sometimes	123 (64%)	70 (36%)	1.00			
Usually	67 (52%)	61 (48%)	1.60 (1.02–2.52)	0.120		
Always	103 (58%)	76 (42%)	1.30 (0.85–1.97)			

[a]Adjusted for factors included in the final model

contacted were considered lost to follow up and excluded from the analyses on contraceptive use, repeat pregnancy and repeat abortion.

Thirdly, we conducted an exploratory analysis to compare the timing of initiation of long-acting contraception between women having medical versus surgical abortion over the four-month post-abortion period. This analysis used data on weekly contraceptive use was obtained retrospectively at four-month follow-up.

Ethical approval for the MOTIF study was obtained from ethics committees at the London School of Hygiene and Tropical Medicine and Marie Stopes International and from the Cambodia Human Research ethics committee. All analyses were conducted using Stata, Version 15.

Results

Of the 500 women who participated in the trial 41% had a medical abortion. Over two thirds of the sample were aged over 25, almost two thirds lived in rural areas, and the majority had access to motorized transport. Almost two thirds had secondary level education or above, and nearly all were married or living together. The full description of the sample is shown in Table 1. Table 2 shows the characteristics of women attending for medical versus surgical abortion. Univariable analyses suggested that younger age ($p = 0.019$), urban versus rural area of residence ($p < 0.001$), access to motorized transport ($p = 0.058$), higher level of education ($p = 0.005$), having no living children ($p = 0.001$), having mainly joint or mainly partner decision-making about contraception ($p = 0.001$), not intending or undecided about PAFP ($p < 0.001$), plans to have another child or undecided about more children ($p < 0.001$), were associated with increased odds of medical versus surgical abortion. Occupation was associated with type of abortion ($p < 0.001$). During development of a final multivariable model, age was included first, then factors identified in univariable analyses were added and evaluated for association with abortion type after adjustment in turn, first looking at socio-economic factors and then fertility and contraceptive related factors. The final model included level of education, PAPF intentions, fertility plans and area of residence. Age and number of children were no longer associated with type of abortion after adjustment for contraceptive and fertility plans. After adjustment for factors included in the final model, medical versus surgical abortion was more likely amongst those with more education, those without plans for or undecided about PAFP, those undecided or desiring a child in future and those living in urban areas. Whether contraceptive decisions were mainly made by a husband/partner or made jointly was only asked to those who were currently married. Of this group of 464 women, joint or partner contraceptive decision making was not strongly associated with type of abortion after adjustment for other factors in the final model for all women ($p = 0.085$). After adjustment for the other variables in the final model, occupation was not associated with abortion type (LRT $p = 0.289$).

Table 3 shows associations between abortion method and subsequent contraceptive use, repeat pregnancy and repeat abortion. Surgical abortion was associated with increased odds of using effective contraception at 4 months compared to medical abortion but this

Table 3 Associations between abortion method and subsequent contraception use, repeat pregnancy and abortion

	Four month follow-up						12 month follow-up					
	No	Yes	Crude OR	P value	Adjusted OR*	P value	No	Yes	Crude OR	P value	Adjusted OR*	P value
Effective contraception use												
Medical	93 (52%)	85 (48%)	1.00				75 (54%)	63 (46%)	1.00			
Surgical	102 (40%)	151 (60%)	1.62 (1.10–2.38)	0.015	1.44 (0.95–2.18)	0.084	101 (53%)	89 (47%)	1.05 (0.68–1.63)	0.831	0.87 (0.55–1.39)	0.563
Long-acting contraception use												
Medical	146 (82%)	32 (18%)	1.00				113 (82%)	25 (18%)	1.00			
Surgical	205 (81%)	48 (19%)	1.07 (0.65–1.75)	0.794	0.87 (0.51–1.49)	0.611	154 (81%)	36 (19%)	1.06 (0.60–1.86)	0.848	0.84 (0.46–1.54)	0.573
Repeat pregnancy												
Medical	171 (97%)	6 (3%)	1.00				116 (84%)	22 (16%)	1.00			
Surgical	248 (98%)	5 (2%)	0.57 (0.17–1.91)	0.367	0.82 (0.23–2.86)	0.750	162 (85%)	28 (15%)	0.91 (0.50–1.67)	0.764	0.97 (0.51–1.84)	0.924
Repeat abortion												
Medical	176 (99%)	1 (1%)	1.00				127 (92%)	11 (8%)	1.00			
Surgical	251 (99%)	2 (1%)	1.40 (0.13–15.59)	0.783	2.04 (0.17–24.22)	0.572	182 (96%)	8 (4%)	0.51 (0.20–1.30)	0.157	0.50 (0.19–1.35)	0.172

*Adjusted for age, residence, socio-economic status and whether randomised

association did not remain after adjusting for confounding variables (aOR 1.44; 95%CI 0.95–2.18). There were no statistically significant differences in contraceptive use, repeat pregnancy or repeat abortion comparing women having medical versus surgical abortion, but it is acknowledged that power was low for these analyses.

Figure 1 shows the timing of initiation of long-acting contraception over the four-month post-abortion period. Women having surgical abortion appear more likely to initiate long-acting contraception sooner compared to women having medical abortion; 50 women reported initiating long-acting contraceptive after surgical abortion, of whom 34 (68%) started during the first week. 29 women reported initiating long-acting contraception use after medical abortion, of whom nine (31%) started during the first week ($p = 0.001$). Of the 34 women who had a surgical abortion and started using long-acting contraception during the first week, 14 (41%) started using an IUD and 20 started using the implant. Of the nine women who had a medical abortion and started using long-acting contraception during the first week, two (22%) started using an IUD and seven started using the implant.

Discussion

Summary of main results

In this observational study using randomized controlled trial data, women having a medical abortion were more likely than those having a surgical abortion to be of urban residence, more educated, not planning to use or undecided about PAFP, and be planning to have another child or undecided. There was no association between type of abortion (medical vs. surgical) and use of effective contraception at 4 months, repeat pregnancy, or repeat abortion. Initiation of long-acting contraception within the first week was less likely with medical than surgical abortion.

Strengths and weaknesses

To our knowledge, this is the first quantitative study reporting differences in characteristics of medical versus surgical abortion clients attending non-governmental health facilities in Cambodia, and complements trends in medical abortion use observed in the Demographic and Health Survey and previous qualitative studies in Cambodia and neighbouring Vietnam. [2, 5, 20] The study benefits from a sample size of 500 and a follow-up period of 12 months with good follow-up rates.

A key limitation of the study is the potential for residual and unmeasured confounding. It would have been particularly useful to have data on pregnancy duration. The 2014 Cambodian Demographic and Health Survey reported that use of surgical abortion increased with age and pregnancy duration [3, 7]. We also do not have information on provider behaviors – it is possible that providers may show bias in the type of abortion that they offer or recommend. Furthermore, we cannot draw

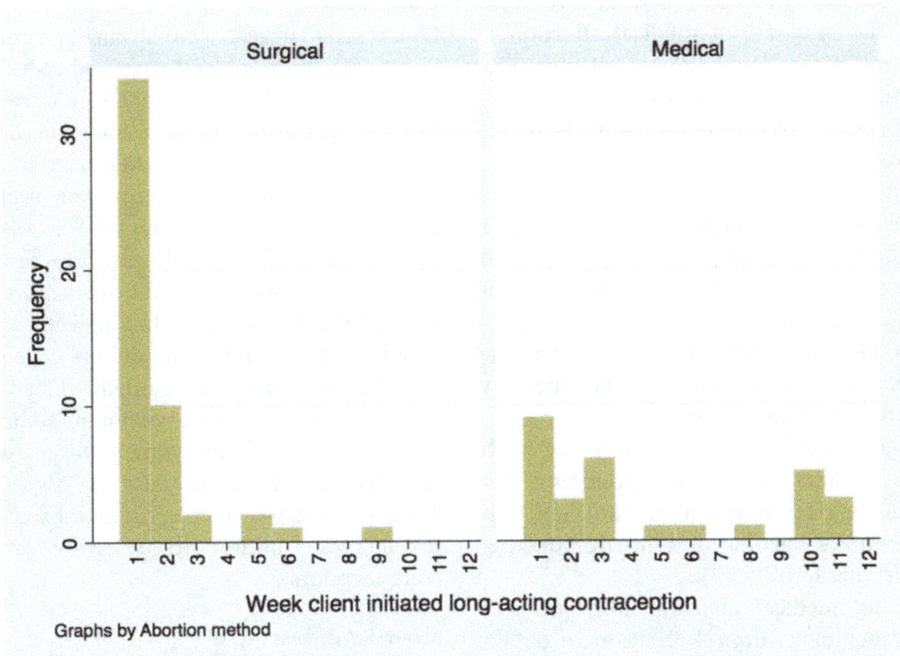

Fig. 1 Initiation of long-acting contraception (IUD or implant) over 4-month post-abortion period *data obtained retrospectively at 4months asking participants about weekly contraceptive use. 50 women reported initiating long-acting contraceptive after surgical abortion, of whom 34 (68%) started during the first week. 29 women reported initiating long-acting contraception use after medical abortion, of whom 9 (31%) started during the first week

conclusions on the direction of associations and causality.

A further limitation concerns the generalizability of the findings. These results reflect the NGO clinic population and may be different in public and private health facilities, and among women obtaining medical abortion from pharmacies. However, the proportions obtaining medical abortion are similar to 2013 data from MSI Cambodia. [14] In addition, the sample was restricted to women who had access to a mobile phone, although in Cambodia over 90% of women are estimated to own a mobile phone [21]. Future research should examine the needs of women using MA outside of the formal heath sector (e.g. from drug sellers) in terms of follow-up and PAFP. Further qualitative research could also consider how fertility intentions and provider biases might influence both the type of abortion that a woman has and subsequent use of PAFP.

Finally, the study was underpowered to examine differences in contraceptive and reproductive outcomes between women having medical and surgical abortions – although we found no evidence of a difference in PAFP uptake, repeat pregnancy or repeat abortion in this sample, a larger study may do.

Discussion of the findings in context of existing research

Previous research has shown that a wide range of socio demographic variables as well as knowledge of abortion methods influence the uptake of medical abortion rather than surgical abortion. Our finding that rural women were less likely to choose MA are consistent with findings from Ethiopia, India, and Nepal but not Vietnam [22–25]. Our finding that educated women were more likely to use MA are in keeping with study findings in the USA and Nepal, but studies in Ethiopia and Vietnam did not find such an association [24–26]. To our knowledge no previous studies have reported the association between choice of MA and uncertainty about future contraceptive and fertility plans.

Access to a clinic is a barrier to obtaining abortion services and poor geographic access has been shown to be a barrier to women seeking other maternal health services in rural areas of Cambodia [27, 28]. Our finding that women living in rural areas are more likely to opt for surgical abortion rather than medical abortion could be due to the distance to clinic and the desire for greater certainty about the abortion being complete at the time of the clinic visit. It may also be that greater difficulties in access result in rural women attending later for medical abortion.

In this setting, women were offered a follow-up visit to check for post-abortion complications or a continuing pregnancy after both medical and surgical abortion as per national guidelines, [13] although routine data show that many women do not attend. [29] MSI Cambodia reports a 97.3% success rate for medical abortion. Self-assessment of the outcome of medical abortion is accurate, feasible and safe in low-resource settings. [30, 31] Enabling women to self-manage follow-up, as recommended in the WHO guidelines, [32] is likely to reduce barriers to medical abortion in urban and rural low-resource settings. [33].

Women with more education might be more confident in using medical abortion as it might be easier for them to read any written instructions provided and contact the clinic in case of a problem.

The associations between abortion type and contraception and fertility intentions could be explained by concerns about future fertility. Women who were undecided or planning on having more children (i.e. birth spacers rather than limiters) may have a preference for medical abortion if surgical abortion or contraception use is perceived as more harmful, potentially affecting the uterus and impacting fertility. [4]

Women undergoing medical abortion were no less likely than those undergoing surgical abortion to obtain post-abortion family planning (PAFP), including long-acting reversible contraception (LARC). All participants received standard care at the clinic prior to randomization, which included contraceptive counselling and the choice of a range of methods (e.g. pill, injectable and implant), all of which could be obtained on the day. It is unsurprising that women obtaining MA have lower uptake of IUD than women having surgical abortion as women could have an IUD inserted during surgical procedure, while women undergoing medical abortion have to attend and appointment for fitting 2 weeks later. It is perhaps surprising that women undergoing surgical abortion were not more likely to use LARC given the convenience of IUD insertion during the procedure, versus a repeat visit following medical abortion. However, LARC use is relatively low in Cambodia; roughly 2% of married women use the implant and 4% use the IUD compared to 9% who use the injectable, and 18% who use the contraceptive pill [3]. In contexts with a different baseline method mix, there might be greater differences in uptake of LARC between those undergoing medical and surgical abortion.

The findings did show that among women who started LARC methods post-abortion, women who obtained a medical abortion had a more delayed initiation. This may reflect the delay required between the procedure and the insertion of an IUD following medical abortion. This is supported by the finding that, among those who started LARC in the first week, the proportion starting to use an IUD (rather than implant) was higher among women who had a surgical abortion. Additionally, women having a medical abortion may have wished to have confirmation that the abortion was complete before starting to use the implant.

Conclusion

Our results suggest women having a medical abortion in Cambodia are more likely to be educated and live in urban areas and had delayed uptake of contraception compared to women having a surgical abortion, although there was not strong evidence for a difference in contraceptive use at four or 12 month follow up. Our findings suggest there is a continuing need to improve access to abortion services, particularly in rural areas, as well as to take into account the factors influencing women's choice of abortion method during the consultation. They also raise questions about whether routine follow-up is required after abortion. Enabling self-management of medical abortion follow up may increase women's choice around the procedure by enabling women who would prefer medical abortion but cannot because of loss of earnings or distance barriers to do so Further research is recommended to increase access to abortion and post-abortion contraception.

Acknowledgements

We thank all clients and clinic staff who participated in the study; Channe Suy at the InSTEDD iLab South East Asia; and Uk Vannak, Ly Sokhey, Sieklot Chinn, Melissa Cockcroft, Nicky Jurgens, Michelle Phillips, Sras Thorng, Stefanie Wallach and Amy Williamson at Marie Stopes International.

Authors' contributions

CS conceived of the current study, CS, RS and TE analysed and interpreted the data. CS and RS wrote successive drafts. CF commented on some of the drafts. All authors reviewed, contributed to and approved the final version for publication.

Author details

[1]Graduate School of Tropical Medicine and Global Health, Nagasaki University, Nagasaki, Japan. [2]Department of Population Health, London School of Hygiene & Tropical Medicine, London, UK. [3]MRC Tropical Epidemiology Group, London School of Hygiene & Tropical Medicine, London, UK.

References

1. Sedgh G, Singh S, Hussain R. Intended and unintended pregnancies worldwide in 2012 and recent trends. Stud Fam Plan. 2014;45:301–14. https://doi.org/10.1111/j.1728-4465.2014.00393.x.
2. Petitet PH, Ith L, Cockroft M, Delvaux T. Towards safe abortion access: an exploratory study of medical abortion in Cambodia. Reprod Health Matters. 2015;22:47–55. https://doi.org/10.1016/S0968-8080(14)43826-6.
3. National Institute of Statistics: Directorate General for Health and ICF International. Cambodia Demographic and Health Survey 2014 [Internet]. 2015. Available from: https://dhsprogram.com/pubs/pdf/FR312/FR312.pdf.
4. Hemmings J, Rolfe B. Abortion in cambodia [Internet]. Options; 2008. Available from: www.options.co.uk.
5. Petitet P, Desclaux A. Reproductive health and HIV in Cambodia: from anthropology to public health. Aix Marseille III (France): Groupe de Recherche cultures, Santé, Sociétés, Paul Cézanne Université; 2011.
6. National Institute of Public Health: National Institute of Statistics and ORC Macro. Cambodia Demographic and Health Survey 2005. 2006;487. Available from: https://dhsprogram.com/pubs/pdf/FR185/FR185%5BApril-27-2011%5D.pdf.
7. National Institute of Statistics: Directorate General for Health and ORC Macro. Cambodia Demographic and Health Survey 2010 [Internet]. 2010. Available from: http://www.measuredhs.com/pubs/pdf/FR249/FR249.pdf.
8. USAID. High Impact Practices in Family Planning (HIP). Postabortion family planning: strengthening the family planning component of postabortion care. Washington DC: USAID; 2012.

9. Stoddard A, Eisenberg DL. Controversies in family planning : timing of ovulation after abortion and the conundrum of postabortion intrauterine device insertion. Contraception. 2011;84:119–21. https://doi.org/10.1016/j.contraception.2010.12.010.
10. USAID. Post-Abortion family planning: a key component of Post abortion care. 2013.
11. World Health Organization. Medical eligibility criteria for contraceptive use; 2015. https://doi.org/10.2165/00128413-200112870-00010.
12. Cameron S. Postabortal and postpartum contraception. Best Pract Res Clin Obstet Gynaecol. 2014;28:871–80. https://doi.org/10.1016/j.bpobgyn.2014.05.007.
13. Cambodia Ministry of Health. National Protocol Cambodia: comprehensive abortion care 2010.
14. Smith C, Ngo T, Gold J, Edwards P, Vannak U, Sokhey L, et al. Effect of a mobile phone-based intervention on post-abortion contraception: a randomized controlled trial in Cambodia. Bull World Health Organ. 2015;93: 842–50. https://doi.org/10.2471/BLT.15.160267.
15. Smith C, Ly S, Uk V, Edwards P, Warnock R, Free C. Process evaluation of a mobile phone based intervention to support post-abortion contraception in Cambodia. Contracept Reprod Med. 2017;16. https://doi.org/10.1186/s12978-017-0329-y.
16. Smith C, Vannak U, Sokhey L, Ngo TD, Gold J, Khut K, et al. MObile Technology for Improved Family Planning services (MOTIF): study protocol for a randomised controlled trial. Trials. 2013;14(427):1–9.
17. Smith C, Jarvis C, Free C. Assessing loss to follow-up in the MObile Technology for Improved Family Planning (MOTIF) randomised controlled trial. Trials. 2017;18:577. https://doi.org/10.1186/s13063-017-2316-6.
18. World Health Organization. Family planning: a global handbook for providers. 2011.
19. Maries Stopes International. Young people [Internet]. Available from: https://mariestopes.org/who-we-serve/young-people/. [cited 2019 Jan 15].
20. Ngo TD, Free C, Le HT, Edwards P, Pham KHT, Nguyen YBT, et al. Women's perspectives on termination service delivery in Vietnam: a cross-sectional survey in three provinces. Int J Women's Health. 2014;6:927–33. https://doi.org/10.2147/IJWH.S72343.
21. Kimchhoy P, Sola J. Mobile Phones in Cambodia 2014 [Internet]. 2014. Available from: https://asiafoundation.org/resources/pdfs/MobilephonesinCB.pdf.
22. Tamang A, Tuladhar S, Tamang J, Ganatra B, Dulal B. Factors associated with choice of medical or surgical abortion among women in Nepal. Int J Gynecol Obstet. 2012;118:52–6. https://doi.org/10.1016/j.ijgo.2012.05.011.
23. Das V. Evaluation of newer methods of early pregnancy termination. J Obs Gynecol India. 2005;55:454–6.
24. Woldetsadik MA, Sendekie TY, White MT, Zegeye DT. Client preferences and acceptability for medical abortion and MVA as early pregnancy termination method in Northwest Ethiopia. Reprod Health. 2011;9:4–8.
25. Ngo TD, Free C, Le HT, Edwards P, Pham KHT, Nguyen YBT, et al. Service users' attributes associated with the uptake of medical versus surgical abortion at public health facilities in Vietnam. Int J Gynecol Obstet. 2014; 125:247–52.
26. Clark S. Is medical abortion acceptable to all American women: the impact of sociodemographic characteristics on the acceptability of mifepristone-misoprostol abortion. J Am Med Womens Assoc. 2012;5:177–82.
27. Matsuoka S, Aiga H, Chan L, Rathavy T, Okitsu A. Perceived barriers to utilization of maternal health services in rural Cambodia. Health Policy. 2010; 95:255–63. https://doi.org/10.1016/j.healthpol.2009.12.011.
28. Yanagisawa S, Oum S, Wakai S. Determinants of skilled birth attendance in rural Cambodia. Trop Med Int Heal. 2006;11:238–51. https://doi.org/10.1111/j.1365-3156.2005.01547.x.
29. Smith C, Vannak U, Sokhey L, Ngo TD, Gold J, Free C. Mobile Technology for Improved Family Planning (MOTIF): the development of a mobile phone-based (mHealth) intervention to support post-abortion family planning (PAFP) in Cambodia. Reprod Health. 2016;13:1–8. https://doi.org/10.1186/s12978-015-0112-x.
30. Blum J, Sheldon WR, Ngoc NTN, Winikoff B, Nga NTB, Martin R, et al. Randomized trial assessing home use of two pregnancy tests for determining early medical abortion outcomes at 3, 7 and 14 days after mifepristone. Contraception. 2016;94(2):115–21. https://doi.org/10.1016/j.contraception.2016.04.001.
31. Iyengar K, Paul M, Iyengar SD, Klingberg-Allvin M, Essén B, Bring J, et al. Self-assessment of the outcome of early medical abortion versus clinic follow-up in India: a randomised, controlled, non-inferiority trial. Lancet Glob Heal. 2015;3:e537–45. https://doi.org/10.1016/S2214-109X(15)00150-3.
32. WHO. Clinical practice handbook for safe abortion. 2014.
33. Sheldon WR. Home use of urine pregnancy tests for medical abortion follow-up. Lancet Glob Heal. 2015;3:e504–5. https://doi.org/10.1016/S2214-109X(15)00153-9.

Factors affecting men's support for the use of the contraceptive implant by their female intimate partners

Kim Jonas[1,2*], Moira Kalichman[3], Seth Kalichman[3], Chelsea Morroni[4,5,6] and Catherine Mathews[1,2]

Abstract

Background: Family planning services have been available at no cost in the public health settings of South Africa since 1994, and now include the long-acting reversible contraceptives (LARCs) namely, the contraceptive implant and intra-uterine device (IUD). However, the uptake of LARCs has been declining in the recent years and little is known about the cause of the decline. In many relationships, men may influence their female intimate partner's contraceptive choices. Thus, men's involvement in reproductive health decisions and family programming may improve their support for contraceptive use, including the LARC use by their female intimate partners. This study investigated factors affecting men's support for the use of contraceptive implant by their female intimate partners.

Methods: A quantitative, cross-sectional survey was conducted among adult men attending a public, primary health clinic in Cape Town, South Africa. Using a structured questionnaire, we measured men's knowledge, awareness and support of, and attitudes towards use of the contraceptive implant by their female intimate partners. Data were analyzed using SPSS version 25.

Results: The sample included 65 men with a mean age of 31.2 years. Most (76.6%) believed that both men and women should be responsible for family planning. Support for general contraception use by their female intimate partners was prevalent at 80.0%, but only 33.9% reported that they would like their partners to use the implant in the future, while 35.6% were unsure and 30.5% did not support their partner's use of the implant. Factors significantly associated with men's support of their partner's future use of the contraceptive implant included men's reports that their partner wished to have another child in future, knowledge that the implant is safe for use by women who have not had children, knowledge that the implant can effectively prevent pregnancy for 3 years, and a positive attitude towards the implant's long-lasting effectiveness.

Conclusion: Improving men's knowledge of, and attitudes toward the contraceptive implant might increase their support for their partner's use of the implant, which in turn might promote uptake of the implant among women. The findings of our study suggest the importance of actively engaging men in reproductive health and family planning programs.

Keywords: Long-acting reversible contraceptives (LARCs), Contraceptive implant, Implant, Implanon, Implanon NXT, Family planning, Men's support, Men

* Correspondence: kim.jonas@mrc.ac.za
[1]Health Systems Research Unit, South African Medical Research Council, Cape Town, South Africa
[2]Adolescent Health Research Unit, Department of Psychiatry and Mental Health, University of Cape Town, Cape Town, South Africa

Introduction

Family planning services have been available at no cost in public health services in South Africa since 1994, and now include the long-acting reversible contraceptives (LARCs) namely, the contraceptive implant and intrauterine device (IUD). The Department of Health's (DoH) policy on contraception and fertility planning, updated in 2014, expanding the method mix to give women greater choice for family planning [1]. According to the policy, "the methods of contraception were expanded to cover an increased access to LARC methods with with specific consideration of: increasing access to the copper intrauterine device (Cu IUD), with antibiotics at the time of insertion, and introduction of a single-rod progestogen implant..." [1]. The contraceptive implant, Implanon NXT, was the most common LARC on offer in South African public health services at no cost. It is a subdermal single-rod implant containing 68 mg of the progestin etonogestrel, which is highly effective in preventing pregnancy for a period of 3 years [2–4]. Despite the robust and supportive policies related to LARCs in the public sector, the use of the contraceptive implant among women is limited [5–7].

Among women, limited knowledge and awareness of the different contraceptive methods, including the implant, have been identified [7]. Additionally, concerns, myths and misconceptions about side effects and risks associated with the implant contribute to the limited uptake among women [8–10]. Research conducted among men on family planning use and support remains insufficient globally [11]. The few studies that have been conducted among men, show that male partner support for family planning influences women's behaviour towards the use of modern contraceptives [11–14]. One study has been undertaken among women showing that beliefs about and perceptions of the implant's side effects negatively influence men's support for its use by their female intimate partners [15]. Another South African study found that women report lack of male partner support for the use of the implant as one of the reasons for early removal and discontinuation of use [16].

This study aims to describe the specific factors affecting men's support for the future use of the contraceptive implant by their female intimate partners. Such an understanding can complement the women's perceptions of male partner support for family planning use and help design specific interventions to ameliorate the challenges affecting the implant use among women. Improving the implant uptake may significantly reduce unintended pregnancies which are highly prevalent among adolescents and adults in the country [7, 17]. Ultimately, this study hopes to contribute towards the intervention program development for the reduction of unplanned and or unintended pregnancies, as well as the unmet need for contraception in the country.

Methods

Research design and study setting

This quantitative, cross-sectional survey was conducted among adult men attending a public, primary health clinic in Cape Town, South Africa. The clinic was selected because it is a typical public clinic in a poor, peri-urban setting. It offered a range of public primary health services with a primary focus on STI, HIV and Tuberculosis (TB) services, including other sexual and reproductive health services. It is worth noting that historically, men poorly attend health care facilities and often delay seeking health care services when they are ill for various reasons, such as discomfort with female staff nurses, clinics being full of women, and fear of being labelled as "weak" according to gender norms [18–20]. Consequently in South Africa, "men only" clinics were initiated to help attract more men seeking health care service, particularly for STI testing and treatment including HIV services. This specific clinic, though not a "specialized" male clinic, it also had a "men only" section for STI treatment with dedicated male providers. Despite this effort, there were still few men attending the clinic.

Participant sampling

All men aged 18 years and above who were attending the clinic between February 2015 to February 2016 for sexual and reproductive health related services, including HIV and TB testing and treatment were invited to participate in this study. Although this study was conducted in a public health clinic which also included a "men only" section, very few men visited the clinic. Additionally, to be invited in the study, men had to be able to read and write in English or isiXhosa; not psychologically and or visually impaired. Hence, only 71 men were approached and recruited for this study over this period. Of the 71 sampled participants, 65 agreed to participate and completed the self-administered questionnaire. Those who declined to participate cited time constraints as the main reason.

Data collection tool

A paper-pencil questionnaire format, requiring approximately 10 min for completion, was used to collect data. Participants could complete it in their preferred language (either English or Xhosa). Because of the sensitive nature of the questions, we offered self-administered survey completion to give participants privacy to answer the questions as truthfully as possible.

Demographic questions included marital or relationship status, and whether they had main or casual sex partners, or both. A main sexual partner was defined as a sexual partner an individual has for six or more months and included wives while a casual partner was defined as a "secret" sexual partner an individual has sex with occasionally and included the "one-night-stands".

We included questions on partner's use of family planning methods, as well as knowledge and awareness of, and outcome expectancies related to the contraceptive implant. We also included questions about the number of pregnancies for the female intimate partner, and fertility intentions. We asked whether participants had heard of each of the different types of contraceptive methods, the sources of information about each method (health worker, friend, media, other), and whether the participant knew if his female intimate partner had ever used each method or was currently using it.

To assess knowledge of the contraceptive implant, participants were provided with a set of six statements regarding the safety (e.g., 'Most women can safely use the implant') and efficacy of the implant (e.g., 'The implant is very effective in preventing pregnancy). A three-point Likert scale was used (agree, disagree, and unsure). The internal consistency of the knowledge composite scale was adequate (Cronbach's Alpha: 0.64; 95% Confidence Interval (95% CI): 0.60–0.69).

To measure outcome expectancies of the contraceptive implant, participants were asked to imagine how it would be like for them if their female intimate partners were to use the implant. They were provided with eleven (11) statements each reflecting a positive or negative outcome expectancy (e.g., 'I think that if my partner were to use the implant it would be very good because it lasts for a long time' [positive] and 'I think that if my partner were to use the implant, the implant would move around her body [negative]). A three-point Likert scale was used (agree, disagree, or unsure). Finally, to measure men's support for their female intimate partners to use the implant in the future, participants were asked whether they would like their partners to use the implant in the future (response options: yes, no, or unsure). The implant was defined to the participants as a small plastic rod inserted under the skin of a woman's arm to prevent pregnancy. A copy of the questionnaire with the full statements is provided as an additional file [Additional file 1: Questionnaire]. Participants were offered a nominal reimbursement, a chocolate bar, for their time taken completing the survey.

Data analysis

Prior to analysis, items were rescored so that the valid knowledge statements and positive attitudes scored highest. Separate total scale scores were composed from the six items of knowledge composite and from the 11 items of the men's outcome expectancy composite for the implant use by their female intimate partners. However, the scale scores were not used in the analyses due to the low internal reliability as indicated by the Cronbach's Alpha statistic.

Data were analyzed using SPSS version 25. Descriptive statistics were performed to get an overview of the sample characteristics. A chi-square test was conducted to explore the associations between the demographic characteristics, knowledge scale, outcome expectancy items, and whether or not the men would like their female intimate partners to use the implant in the future. Significance level was set at p- value of equal to, or less than 0.05 ($p \leq 0.05$). Prior to conducting the chi-square test, some variables were collapsed to become dichotomous variables. This was done in order to ascertain non-violation of the minimum expected cell frequency for the chi-square test. Thus, a 2 by 2 table design was used in this study.

Results

A total of 65 men aged from 19 to 52 years with the mean (SD) of 31.2 (8.4) participated in this study. A small proportion, 23.1% ($n = 15$) were 24 years old or younger. Most had not completed secondary education (41.5%; $n = 30$) and 38.5% ($n = 25$) had completed secondary schooling. Only 15.4% ($n = 10$) had post-secondary school education. Most participants, 59.4%, ($n = 38$) reported they were unemployed. Most men, 87.2% ($n = 56$) were unmarried, but 81.3% ($n = 52$) reported to have a main sex partner and 43.8% ($n = 28$) reported to have a casual sex partner, while 18.8% ($n = 12$) did not have a main or casual partner. The reported reasons for being at the clinic on the day were for STI treatment by 61.5% ($n = 40$), 35.4% ($n = 23$) for an HIV test, and 4.6% ($n = 3$) for family planning.

Most participants, 76.6% ($n = 49$) endorsed the statement that both men and women should be responsible for family planning and 73.8% ($n = 48$) believed that men and women should decide together whether a woman should use contraception or not. Support for general contraception use by their female intimate partners was prevalent at 80.0% ($n = 54$). Awareness of the implant among men was relatively low, with 52.3% ($n = 34$) reporting they had never heard of the implant. Among those who had heard about the implant, 51.6% ($n = 15$) had heard about it from a friend, 32.3% ($n = 10$) from the healthcare worker and 32.3% ($n = 10$) from had heard about it from the media. Only 12.3% ($n = 8$) reported that their partners had used the implant before while the majority, 47.7% ($n = 31$) said their partners had never used the implant to their knowledge, and 38.5% ($n = 25$) said they did not know if their partners had ever used it. After having been informed by the data collector about the implant, 33.9% ($n = 20$) reported that they would like their partners to use the implant in the future, while 35.6% ($n = 21$) were unsure and 30.5% ($n = 18$) said they would not like their partners to use it.

Table 1 below compares men who reported they supported their partner using the implant in the future with those who did not support it or were unsure. Factors significantly associated with men's support included men's reports that their partner wished to have another child in future, knowledge that the implant is safe for use by women who have not had children, knowledge that the implant can effectively prevent pregnancy for 3 years, and the positive expectancy of the implant's long-lasting effectiveness.

Discussion

This study investigated factors associated with men's support for the future use of the implant by their female intimate partners. Among the men, there were relatively low levels of awareness about the implant and minimal support for its future use by their female intimate partners. However, support for general contraceptive use was high among the men in this study. Factors associated with men's support for the future use of the implant by their female intimate partners included: a) men knowing that the intimate partner wishes to have another child in future, b) knowing that the implant is safe for use by women who have not had children yet, c) knowing the timeframe within which the implant can effectively prevent pregnancy, and d) the perception that the implant last long. These findings are not unique, previous studies conducted elsewhere among men on women's contraceptive use also identified a strong association between men's awareness of contraceptive methods and their support for female intimate partner use [21–28]. Furthermore, men's awareness of and support for modern contraceptive use was strongly associated with women's desire to use contraception in Nigeria [21], and in Uganda [26]. Potentially, men may play an essential role in some women's decision to use or not use contraception. Therefore, to improve men's support for the use of the contraceptive implant by their female intimate partners, they need to be engaged with as well if efforts to improve the uptake of the implant among women in the country are to be realized. Thus, efforts to improve men's knowledge and awareness of the implant could potentially improve women's utilization of the contraceptive implant.

It is not clear why men who believe their partners want to have children in the future would be more likely to support the implant use. It is possible that the men's fertility intentions were not aligned to their partner's intentions, and they regarded the implant as an effective contraception. It is equally plausible that they supported their partner's use of the implant because of its reversable attribute, enabling their partner to become pregnant when the couple so desired.

It is well known that more women than men attend health facilities for reproductive healthcare services including family planning, but very little is being done to improve men's participation and involvement in reproductive health programmes in the country. Men do not come with their female intimate partners for family planning [5]. Therefore, most men, as well as some women generally have insufficient knowledge and understanding of female contraceptive methods, including the implant but men are hardly ever reached compared to women and continue to be distant in family planning programming. The findings of our study suggest the importance of actively engaging men in reproductive health and family planning programs, and the potential that men's support could have on improving contraceptive use among women.

There are, of course, some important limitations in interpreting the findings of this study. The cross-sectional nature of the study being the first important one, cannot infer causality, meaning that improving men's knowledge and awareness of the contraceptive implant will not necessarily result to improved uptake of the implant by the women. The other limitations are the small sample size of the men in this study, as well as the setting in which this study was undertaken and therefore, the findings cannot be generalizable. It is possible that most men were attending the "specialized" men only clinics where they will not be seen by female providers as well as not be amongst the many female patients who are filling up the waiting rooms in public health facilities [19]. Despite these limitations, the findings of this study highlight the need and importance of actively engaging men in reproductive health programming to improve contraceptive uptake and reduce the unmet need for contraception among women of reproductive age.

Conclusion

Men's perceptions about the implant's safety and long-lasting characteristics are associated with their support for the future use of the implant by their female intimate partners. Thus, improving knowledge and awareness of the contraceptive implant among men may be a step in the right direction towards improving the uptake of the implant by women in the country. Unless men are well-informed and involved in reproductive health or family planning programming, support for their female intimate partners to use contraception will remain a challenge for many women. Interventions and strategies to engage men in family planning programs and enhance their participation in these programs are needed.

Table 1 Associations between selected demographic characteristics, knowledge and outcome expectancy of the implant against whether the men would like their female intimate partners to use the implant in the future, Chi-Square results

Variables	Would you like your partner to use the implant in the future[a]		
	Yes n (%)	No or unsure n (%)	Chi-Square (*p*-value)
Demographics			
Age group			
< 25 years old	3 (21.4%)	11 (78.6%)	
> 25 years old	17 (37.8%)	28 (62.2%)	
			1.27 (.26)
Education			
Up to incomplete secondary school	11 (40.7%)	16 (59.3%)	
Secondary school and post-secondary	9 (28.1%)	23 (71.9%)	
			1.04 (.31)
Family planning responsibility and support			
Who is responsible for FP			
Woman or man	5 (35.7%)	9 (64.3%)	
Both man and woman	15 (33.3%)	30 (66.7%)	
			.03 (.87)
Who should decide a woman should use FP			
Woman or man	7 (46.7%)	8 (53.3%)	
Both man and woman	13 (29.5%)	31 (70.5%)	
			1.46 (.23)
How do you feel about your partner using FP			
Support partner	17 (34.7%)	32 (65.3%)	
I don't like it	2 (50.0%)	2 (50.0%)	
			.88 (.35)
Does your main partner/wife want a/another child			
Yes	14 (51.9%)	13 (48.1%)	
No or unsure	6 (18.8%)	26 (81.2%)	
			7.16 (.01)
Knowledge composite			
Most women can safely use the implant			
Agree	13 (50.0%)	13 (50.0%)	
Disagree or unsure	7 (21.2%)	26 (78.8%)	
			5.38 (.02)
Teenagers can safely use the implant			
Agree	13 (44.8%)	16 (55.2%)	
Disagree or unsure	7 (23.3%)	23 (76.7%)	
			3.04 (.08)
Women with no babies can safely use the implant			
Agree	11 (40.7%)	16 (59.3%)	
Disagree or unsure	9 (28.1%)	23 (71.9%)	
			1.04 (.31)
HIV positive women can safely use the implant			
Agree	11 (47.8%)	12 (52.2%)	
Disagree or unsure	9 (25.0%)	27 (75.0%)	

Table 1 Associations between selected demographic characteristics, knowledge and outcome expectancy of the implant against whether the men would like their female intimate partners to use the implant in the future, Chi-Square results *(Continued)*

Variables	Would you like your partner to use the implant in the future[a]		
	Yes n (%)	No or unsure n (%)	Chi-Square (*p*-value)
			3.26 (.07)
Implant is very effective in preventing pregnancy			
Agree	12 (40.0%)	18 (60.0%)	
Disagree or unsure	8 (27.6%)	21 (72.4%)	
			1.01 (.31)
Implant can prevent pregnancy for:			
About 3 years	9 (56.2%)	7 (43.8%))	
Don't know or other[b]	11 (25.6%)	32 (74.4%)	
			4.89 (.03)
Implant protects against STIs and HIV			
Agree	4 (28.6%)	10 (71.4%)	
Disagree or unsure	16 35.6%)	29 (64.4%)	
			.23 (.63)
Outcome expectancy composite			
Implant could be easily inserted			
Agree	10 (29.4%)	15 (70.6%)	
Disagree or unsure	10 (29.4%)	24 (70.6%)	
			7.2 (.39)
Implant could be easily removed			
Agree	8 (38.1%)	13 (61.9%)	
Disagree or unsure	12 (31.6%)	26 (68.4%)	
			.26 (.61)
Implant is convenient			
Agree	14 (42.4%)	19 (57.6%)	
Disagree or unsure	6 (23.1%)	20 (76.9%)	
			2.43 (.12)
Implant lasts for long			
Agree	14 (46.7%)	16 (53.3%)	
Disagree or unsure	6 (20.7%)	23 (79.3%)	
			4.44 (.04)
I'd worry about her gaining weight if she uses the implant			
Agree	10 (43.5%)	13 (56.5%)	
Disagree or unsure	10 (27.8%)	26 (72.2%)	
			1.54 (.21)
I'd worry about her monthly bleeding if she uses the implant			
Agree	5 (41.7%)	7 (58.3%)	
Disagree or unsure	15 (31.9%)	32 (68.1%)	
			.41 (.52)
Implant could stop her from falling pregnant even after she removes it			
Agree	8 (50.0%)	8 (50.0%)	
Disagree or unsure	12 (27.9%)	31 (72.1%)	
			2.27 (.13)

Table 1 Associations between selected demographic characteristics, knowledge and outcome expectancy of the implant against whether the men would like their female intimate partners to use the implant in the future, Chi-Square results *(Continued)*

Variables	Would you like your partner to use the implant in the future[a]		
	Yes n (%)	No or unsure n (%)	Chi-Square (*p*-value)
Implant could move around her body			
Agree	4 (50.0%)	4 (50.0%)	
Disagree or unsure	16 (31.4%)	35 (68.6%)	
			1.07 (.30)
Implant could be painful to her			
Agree	4 (44.4%)	5 (55.6%)	
Disagree or unsure	16 (32.0%)	34 (68.0%)	
			.53 (.47)
Implant could harm her future babies			
Agree	1 (16.7%)	5 (83.7%)	
Disagree or unsure	19 (35.8%)	34 (64.2%)	
			.88 (.35)

[a]Only those who reported to have a partner
[b]Other includes 6 months, about a year, about 5 years, more than 5 years, unsure
Bold is significant

Abbreviations

Cu IUD: Copper Intrauterine Device; HIV: Human Immunodeficiency Virus; IUD: Intrauterine device; LARC: Long-Acting and Reversible Contraceptives; STI: Sexually Transmitted Infections; SPSS: Statistical Package for the Social Sciences; TB: Tuberculosis

Acknowledgements

We thank Sekelwa Dumile, Amanda Mdlikiva, Brenda Skonje and Thembinkosi Mdlikiva for collecting the data; and the clinicians who referred their patients to participate in our study.

Authors' contributions

All authors participated in the conception and design of the study. KJ performed the data analysis and interpretation of the data and prepared the first draft of the manuscript. CM, MK, SK, and CM[d] contributed to analysis, interpretation of results and writing of the manuscript. All authors participated in the reviewing of the content for submission. All authors approved the final version of the manuscript.

Author details

[1]Health Systems Research Unit, South African Medical Research Council, Cape Town, South Africa. [2]Adolescent Health Research Unit, Department of Psychiatry and Mental Health, University of Cape Town, Cape Town, South Africa. [3]Department of Psychology, University of Connecticut, Storrs, Mansfield, CT, USA. [4]Liverpool School of Tropical Medicine, Liverpool, UK. [5]Women's Health Research Unit, School of Public Health and Family Medicine, University of Cape Town, Cape Town, South Africa. [6]Botswana-University of Pennsylvania Partnership, Gaborone, Botswana.

References

1. National Department of Health. National Contraception and Fertility Planning Policy and Services Delivery Guidelines: A Companion to the National Contraception Clinical Guidelines. Pretoria: Department of Health; 2014..
2. Patel M. Contraception: Everyone's responsibility. S Afr Med J. 2014;104(9): 644. https://doi.org/10.7196/SAMJ.8764.
3. Rowlands S, Searle S. Contraceptive implants. Curr Perspect. 2014;5:73–84. https://doi.org/10.2147/OAJC.S55968.
4. Dickerson LM, Diaz VA, Jordon J, et al. Satisfaction, early removal, and side effects associated with longacting reversible contraception. Fam Med. 2013; 45(10):701–7.
5. Adeagbo OA, Mullick S, Pillay D, et al. Uptake and early removals of Implanon NXT in South Africa: perceptions and attitudes of health workers. S Afr Med J. 2017;107(10):822–6. https://doi.org/10.7196/SAMJ.2017.v107i10.12821.
6. Mullick S, Chersich MF, Pillay Y, Rees H. Introduction of the contraceptive implant in South Africa: successes, challenges and the way forward. S Afr Med J. 2017 Oct;107(10):812–4.
7. Chersich MF, Wabiri N, Risher K, Shisana O, Celentano D, Rehle T, et al. Contraception coverage and methods used among women in South Africa: a national household survey. S Afr Med J. 2017;107(4):307–14. https://doi.org/10.7196/SAMJ.2017.v107i4.12141.
8. Foster DG, Barar R, Gould H, Gomez I, Nguyen D, Biggs MA. Projections and opinions from 100 experts in long-acting reversible contraception. Contraception. 2015;92(6):543–52.
9. Garrett CC, Keogh LA, Kavanagh A, Tomnay J, Hocking JS. Understanding the low uptake of long-acting reversible contraception by young women in Australia: a qualitative study. BMC Womens Health. 2015;15(1):72.
10. Spies EL, Askelson NM, Gelman E, Losch M. Young women's knowledge, attitudes, and behaviors related to long-acting reversible contraceptives. Womens Health Issues. 2010;20(6):394–9.
11. Marshall CJ, Gomez AM. Young men's awareness and knowledge of intrauterine devices in the United States. Contraception. 2015;92(5):494–500.
12. Oyediran KA, Ishola GP, Feyisetan BJ. Factors affecting ever-married men's contraceptive knowledge and use in Nigeria. J Biosoc Sci. 2002;34(4):497–510.
13. Duze MC, Mohammed IZ. Male knowledge, attitude, and family planning practices in northern Nigeria. Afr J Reprod Health. 2006;10(3):53–65.
14. Mesfin G. The role of men in fertility and family planning program in Tigray region. Ethiop J Health Dev. 2002;16(3):247–55.
15. Pillay D, Chersich MF, Morroni C, et al. User perspectives on Implanon NXT in South Africa: a survey of 12 public-sector facilities. S Afr Med J. 2017; 107(10):815–21. https://doi.org/10.7196/SAMJ.2017.v107i10.12833.
16. Pillay D, Morroni C, Pleaner M, Adeagbo OA, Chersich MF, Naidoo N, et al. Gaps in monitoring systems for Implanon NXT services in South Africa: an assessment of12 facilities in two districts. S Afr Med J. 2017;107(10):827–31.
17. National Department of Health (NDoH), Statistics South Africa (Stats SA), South African Medical Research Council (SAMRC), and ICF. South Africa demographic and health survey 2016. Pretoria: NDoH, Stats SA, SAMRC, and ICF; 2019.

18. Orner P, Cooper D, Myer L, Zweigenthal V, Bekker LG, Moodley J. Clients' perspectives on HIV/AIDS care and treatment and reproductive health services in South Africa. AIDS Care. 2008;20(10):1217–23.
19. Leichliter JS, Paz-Bailey G, Friedman AL, Habel MA, Vezi A, Sello M, Farirai T, Lewis DA. 'Clinics aren't meant for men': Sexual health care access and seeking behaviours among men in Gauteng province, South Africa. SAHARA J. 2011;8(2):81–8.
20. Braitstein P, Boulle A, Nash D, Brinkhof MW, Dabis F, Laurent C, Schechter M, Tuboi SH, Sprinz E, Miotti P, Hosseinipour M. Gender and the use of antiretroviral treatment in resource-constrained settings: findings from a multicenter collaboration. J Women's Health. 2008;17(1):47–55.
21. Ezeanolue EE, Iwelunmor J, Asaolu I, Obiefune MC, Ezeanolue CO, Osuji A, et al. Impact of male partner's awareness and support for contraceptives on female intent to use contraceptives in Southeast Nigeria. BMC Public Health. 2015;15(1):879.
22. Le Guen M, Ventola C, Bohet A, Moreau C, Bajos N. Men's contraceptive practices in France: evidence of male involvement in family planning. Contraception. 2015;92(1):46–54.
23. Nguyen BT, Shih G, Turok DK. Putting the man in contraceptive mandate. Contraception. 2014;89(1):3–5.
24. Mishra A, Nanda P, Speizer IS, Calhoun LM, Zimmerman A, Bhardwaj R. Men's attitudes on gender equality and their contraceptive use in Uttar Pradesh India. Reprod Health. 2014;11(1):41.
25. Shattuck D, Kerner B, Gilles K, Hartmann M, Ng'ombe T, Guest G. Encouraging contraceptive uptake by motivating men to communicate about family planning: the Malawi male motivator project. Am J Public Health. 2011;101(6):1089–95.
26. Anguzu R, Tweheyo R, Sekandi JN, Zalwango V, Muhumuza C, Tusiime S, Serwadda D. Knowledge and attitudes towards use of long acting reversible contraceptives among women of reproductive age in Lubaga division, Kampala district, Uganda. BMC Res Notes. 2014;7(1):153.
27. Ijadunola MY, Abiona TC, Ijadunola KT, Afolabi OT, Esimai OA, OlaOlorun FM. Male involvement in family planning decision making in Ile-Ife, Osun state, Nigeria. Afr J Reprod Health. 2010;14(4):45–52.
28. Vouking MZ, Evina CD, Tadenfok CN. Male involvement in family planning decision making in sub-Saharan Africa-what the evidence suggests. Pan Afr Medi J. 2014;19.

21

Contraceptive use and discontinuation among women in rural North-West Tanzania

Wende Safari[1], Mark Urassa[1], Baltazar Mtenga[1], John Changalucha[1], James Beard[1,2], Kathryn Church[2], Basia Zaba[2] and Jim Todd[1,2*]

Abstract

Introduction: Existing estimates of contraceptive use in Tanzania rely on cross-sectional or retrospective study designs. This study used a 2-year, retrospective, month-by-month calendar of contraceptive utilization among women aged 15–49 years.

Methods: We estimated the median duration of contraceptive use, factors associated with use, and contraceptive discontinuation rates in sexually active women, using life tables and Cox proportional hazard model.

Results: A total of 5416 women contributed to the analysis in the study. Of the 5416 women, 942 (17%) had never had sex, 410 (7.6%) had no sexual partner in the last year. Among the 5416 women, 4064 were sexually active during the period, 814 (21.1%) were pregnant or amenorrheic, 610 (15.0%) were using contraception, and 1203 (29.6%) did not want to get pregnant but were not using contraception. In the 1813 women who wanted to avoid pregnancy, contraceptive use was lower among women over 35 years compared to younger ones (OR = 0.28, 95%CI: 0.19, 0.41), and in HIV positive women (OR = 0.89, 95%CI: 0.60–1.32). On the other hand, use was higher among women who were married/living together compared to unmarried ones (OR = 2.23, 95% CI: 1.54, 3.23). Using a 2-year retrospective contraceptive calendar, 1054 women reported contraceptive use, 15.8% discontinued within 6 months and 30.5% discontinued within 12 months. Higher rates of contraceptive discontinuation were observed among women who used pills (OR = 1.86, 95%CI: 1.25, 2.77) or injections (OR = 2.04, 95%CI: 1.59, 2.61) compared to those who used implants.

Conclusion: Contraceptive use was significantly associated with age, education and parity, but not with HIV status. HIV status, number of living children and education are not statistically associated with discontinuation of contraceptive use Pills and injections had the highest rates of discontinuation. Wider choice and greater accessibility of long-acting contraceptive methods with better effectiveness and convenience may serve women better. Furthermore, special efforts may be needed to remove barriers to contraceptive use amongst younger women.

Keywords: Contraception use, HIV status, Life-tables, Retrospective contraceptive calendar

* Correspondence: jim.todd@lshtm.ac.uk
[1]National Institute for Medical Research (NIMR), Mwanza Centre, PO Box 1462, Mwanza, Tanzania
[2]London School of Hygiene and Tropical Medicine, London, UK

Introduction

The world population increases by 75 million people each year [1]. Tanzania has an annual fertility rate of 15.4 children per 100 women, with an estimated 1.6 million babies born in 2017 [2]. It is estimated that 20% of pregnancies in Tanzania are unintended or unplanned, with high unmet need for contraception, and limited access to safe abortion. There is a high maternal mortality ratio (MMR) in Tanzania with an estimated 398 [281–570] deaths per 100,000 live births [3, 4]. The challenge remains in Tanzania is to give women the ability to avoid unwanted pregnancy [5].

Despite the efforts that have been made in promoting contraceptive use and family planning in sub-Saharan Africa (SSA), contraceptive practice remains low. The Tanzania Demographic and Health Survey (TDHS) in 2016 showed a significant association between unintended pregnancy and low rates of contraceptive use [5, 6]. The contraceptive prevalence rate amongst women of reproductive age was reported to be 38.4% in 2016 [7]. Of the women who would like to avoid pregnancy, 20% reported they were not using any family planning methods [3, 6].

In some low and middle income countries (LMIC) rates of contraceptive discontinuation remain high and increasing, even among women who want to avoid pregnancy [8]. Results from a 2012 meta-analysis of 60 DHS surveys, which combined all contraceptive methods across 25 LMIC showed that, of women who started using a contraceptive method, on average 38% stopped within the first year, and two thirds (68%) stopped before 2 years [9]. More than half of the women who stopped contraceptive use, had experienced contraceptive failure or had method-related problems, and were still in need of an effective method to prevent unintended pregnancy [9, 10].

Wilcher and others noted that, countries with a high prevalence of HIV also have some of the highest levels of unmet need for family planning (2009) [11]. HIV-positive women have particular needs for contraception to avoid unwanted pregnancy in order to protect their own health, but also to reduce rates of mother-to-child (vertical) transmission of HIV [12]. There is a need to increase access to contraception among women with HIV who do not want to become pregnant, and it is important to integrate family planning with HIV services to meet this need [13]. Strengthening family planning programs will improve the reproductive health outcomes for among women in Tanzania.

The goals of this paper are: first, to provide a more comprehensive picture of contraceptive utilization among sexually active women of reproductive age in rural Tanzania; and second, to estimate contraceptive discontinuation rates from 2013 to 2016 stratifying by HIV status, contraceptive methods, socio-demographic characteristics such as age, marital status, education, and parity.

Materials and methods

Study design and population

We have analysed data from cross-sectional epidemiological serological survey (sero-survey) conducted during 2015/2016 nested within the Health and Demographic Surveillance System (HDSS) in Magu district, Tanzania. The Magu HDSS documents births, deaths and migration in a population of over 35,000 in an area of 115 km^2, as a component of the Kisesa observational HIV cohort study [14]. Every two to 3 years, all residents aged 15 years and above are invited to temporary clinics organized in each of the sero-survey working areas. The sero-survey participants are offered Voluntary Counselling and Testing (VCT), and if found to be HIV- positive are referred to the Care and Treatment Centre (CTC) at Kisesa health centre for treatment.

Data collection

A structured questionnaire was delivered, by same-sex interviewers using tablet computers, to all HDSS residents attending the sero-survey. All women of reproductive age (15–49 years of age) were asked about their sexual history, whether they had ever used contraceptives, whether they were currently using any contraceptive methods and their history of contraceptive use over the previous 2 years. The consort diagram in Fig. 1 presents the number of women in the study by their sexual history, and contraceptive use.

Data on the two-year history of contraceptive use was collected from all eligible women using a retrospective contraceptive calendar adapted from the 5-year calendar used in DHS surveys [15]. Use of one contraceptive method was recorded separately for each month per woman. From this monthly data, the number of method-specific episodes of contraceptive use were derived. An episode of contraceptive use was defined as the duration in months of continuous use of the same method, that may or may not have ended by the time of interview. For each episode of contraceptive use that ended in discontinuation, a reason for discontinuation was requested. A switch to a new method (or break between methods of at least 1 month) indicated the end of one episode, and the start of a new episode [9].

Case definition

Women were considered to be sexually active if they reported to have one or more sexual partners in the past year. Contraceptive use was defined as the proportion of all sexually active women who were currently using contraceptives. Women with met needs for contraception were defined as sexually active, non-pregnant women,

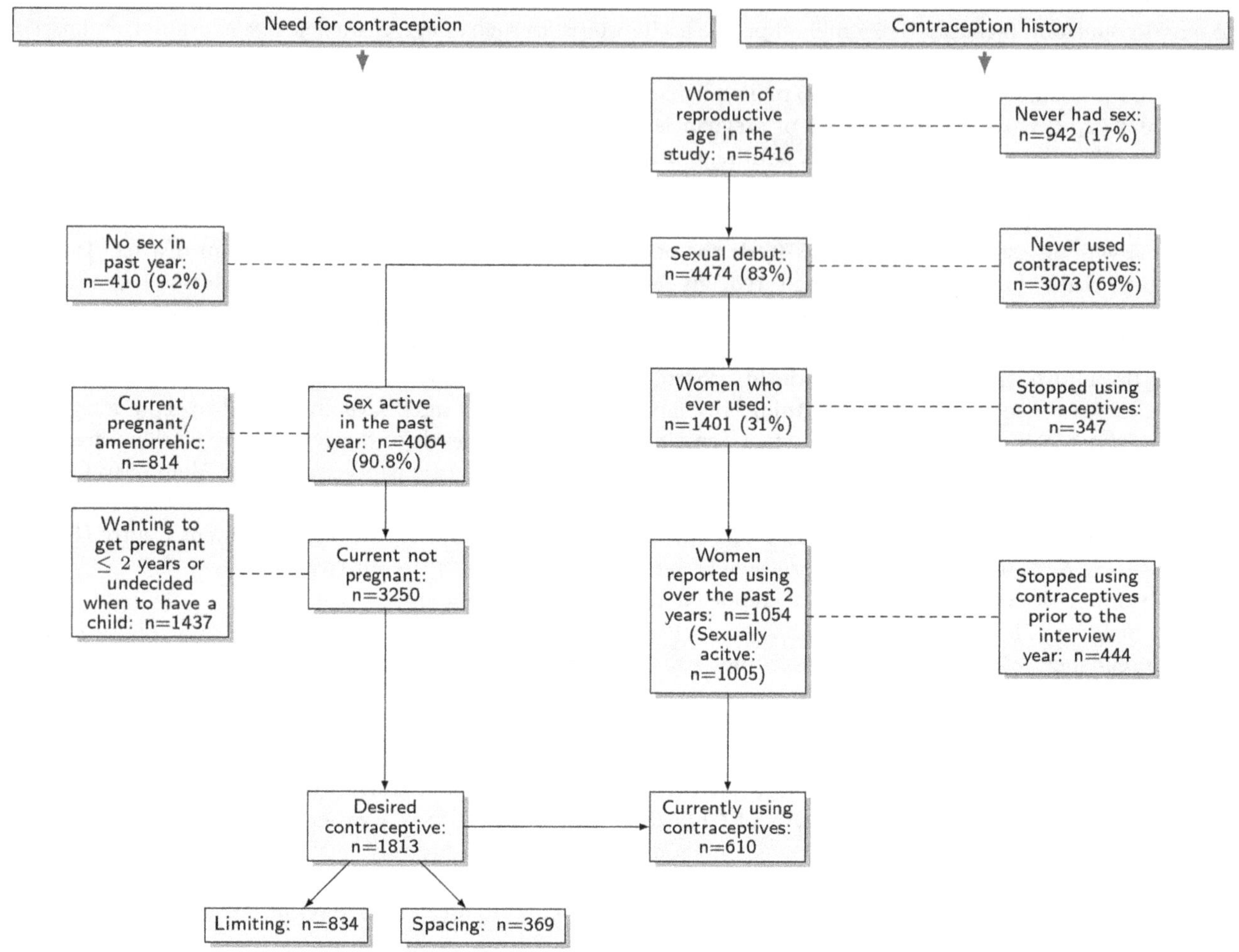

Fig. 1 Flowchart of the need for contraception and history of contraceptive use among 5416 women of reproductive age in Kisesa cohort

who were currently using contraception to avoid pregnancy. Women with unmet need for contraception are those who didn't want to have a child (limiting) or who did not want to have a child in the next 2 years (spacing) but were not currently using contraception (see Fig. 1) [16]. Women were considered HIV negative or HIV positive based on the HIV test at the same sero-survey.

Statistical analysis

The analysis was restricted to sexually active women, and findings are presented in three sets. Firstly, among all sexually active women a description of the background variables and types of contraceptive use, for both traditional and modern contraceptives.

Secondly, to examine factors associated with current contraceptive use, unadjusted and multivariable logistic regression models were fitted to obtain Odds ratio (OR) with 95% confidence interval (95% CI). This analysis was based on sexually active, non-pregnant women who reported wanting to avoid pregnancy, comparing those using contraceptives and those with unmet need for contraceptives, to assess the effect of each independent variable on the current use of contraceptive methods, and the adjusted effect after controlling for possible confounders.

Finally, from the women who reported contraceptive use during the past 2 years, we constructed a life table of the contraceptive discontinuation rates for the first six and 12 months from the initial use of the contraception. The information was collected in a month-by-month calendar of contraceptive use, from the women who reported use of contraceptives in the past 2 years. The discontinuation rates were calculated overall and for the different contraceptive methods. Cox proportional hazard model was used to obtain adjusted hazard ratios (aHR) and 95% confidence intervals for the association between discontinuation and individual characteristics, the number of living children and the different method types, with discontinuation rates. The unit analysis for this is month of contraceptive use, and the outcome is the discontinuation of contraceptive use [9]. For the analyses of discontinuation rates, the calendar data were truncated at a point 3 months before the interview date to avoid potential bias due to under reporting of first trimester pregnancies [9, 17].

Analyses were done using STATA software, and statistical significance was considered at p-value less than 0.05. With 4000 women taking part in the sero-survey, the analysis would have 80% power to detect an 8% difference in contraceptive use between HIV positive and HIV negative women with 5% significance.

Ethical approval

The eighth round sero-survey had ethical approval from the Lake Zone Institutional Review Board (LZIRB), and the London School of Hygiene & Tropical Medicine (LSHTM). All participants of the eighth sero-survey (including women contributing data for this work) were asked for written informed consent.

Results

Background characteristics of the study population

Figure 1 shows the characteristics of 5416 women of reproductive age (15–49 years) in the study population. Among the study respondents, 942 (17%) had never had sex, whereas 4474 (83%) reported sexual debut, and 4064 were sexually active (one or more sexual partner in the last year) and 856 were currently pregnant. Of the 1813 sexually-active, non-pregnant women who did not want another pregnancy at this time, 610 (33.6%) of the women had met need for contraception, and 1203 (66.4%) were not using contraceptives. Of the 1203 women with unmet need in this study, 331 (18.2%) had unmet need for spacing, and 834 (46.0%) had unmet need for limiting.

Excluding 410 (9%) women who were not sexually active, (with no sexual partners in the past year), Table 1 shows the characteristics of the 4064 sexually active women. Eight percent of the sexually active women were HIV-positive and included women aged 15–24 years (34%), 25–34 years (36%), and 35 years and above (30%). Half of women had completed primary school, and only 15% had attended or completed secondary education. More than half of the women (54%) had three or more children.

Table 1 Demographic characteristics of 4064 sexually active women in Kisesa from 2015/16

Characteristic	Value (%)
HIV status	
Positive	328 (8.1)
Negative	3724 (91.9)
Age	
15–24	1401 (34.5)
25–34	1474 (36.3)
35+	1189 (29.2)
Education	
None/some primary	1394 (34.3)
Completed primary	2086 (51.4)
Secondary+	580 (14.3)
Number of living children	
< 3	1858 (45.7)
3+	2206 (54.3)

Characteristics of women using contraceptive methods

The contraceptive choices of the 4064 sexually active women (of reproductive age) who had ever had sex is shown in Table 2. In total, 1054 women reported one or more episodes of contraceptive use over the 2 years period prior to the survey, although 49 women were not sexually active in the last year. The most popular contraceptive method was injections with 529 women using this for 535 distinct episodes during the 2 year period (Table 2).

As shown in Table 2, injections and implants were chosen more often by HIV positive women. Injectables were chosen more often by women who have completed primary school, users who are 25–34 years old and users with three or more children. Implants were chosen more often by women with post primary education.

Factors associated with current contraceptive use

Table 3 presents unadjusted and adjusted effects of the predictors for currently using contraceptives among the 1813 sexually active, non-pregnant women wanting to avoid pregnancy. There was an independent effect of age, education and marital status on the current use of contraceptives by these women (Table 3). Compared to the youngest age group (15–24 years), the odds of currently using contraceptive are 0.28 times for women who are 35 years and above (OR = 0.28, 95% CI: 0.19, 0.41). Contraceptive use was lower among HIV positive women compared to HIV negative women although this effect was not significant (OR = 0.89, 95%CI: 0.60–1.32). On the other hand, the odds of current use of contraceptives are higher among women who completed primary education or those with post primary school (OR = 1.67, 95% CI: 1.32, 2.13; OR = 1.95, 95% CI: 1.36, 2.80, respectively) compared to women with no formal education. Notably, contraceptives use varied by marital status and was significantly higher among women who were married/ cohabiting (OR; 2.23, 95% CI 1.54, 3.23) and those who were divorced/separated/widowed (OR; 2.14, 95% CI 1.33, 3.44) as compared to unmarried ones.

Reasons for discontinuing using contraceptives over the past two years

A total of 1054 women reported some use of contraceptives over the past 2 years, and reported their history of contraceptive use over the previous 2 years. Of these

Table 2 The background characteristics of 4064 sexually active women in Kisesa in 2015/16 and use of contraceptives over the past two years

Contraceptive history	Pill	Injection	Condom	Implants	IUD	Sterilization	Traditional methods	No. methods	Total no. of women
Ever used	215 (5.3)	812 (20)	22 (0.5)	385 (9.5)	85 (2.1)	17 (0.4)	22 (0.5)	2741 (67.4)	4064
Past 2 years	102 (2.5)	529 (13.1)	14 (0.3)	328 (8.1)	56 (1.4)	15 (0.4)	21 (0.5)	3059 (75.3)	4064
Past 2 years segment used	103	535	17	330	56	15	21		
Background characteristics on contraceptive use in the past 2 years									
HIV status									
Positive	5 (1.5)	39 (11.9)	0 (0)	25 (7.6)	5 (1.5)	4 (1.2)	3 (0.9)	244 (74.4)	328
Negative	97 (2.6)	488 (13.1)	14 (0.4)	302 (8.1)	51 (1.4)	11 (0.3)	18 (0.5)	2811 (75.5)	3724
Age									
15–24	16 (1.1)	127 (9.1)	8 (0.6)	101 (7.2)	9 (0.6)	0 (0)	3 (0.2)	1163 (83.0)	1401
25–34	53 (3.4)	278 (18.9)	3 (0.2)	173 (11.7)	23 (15.6)	2 (0.1)	7 (0.5)	969 (65.7)	1474
35+	33 (2.8)	124 (10.4)	3 (0.3)	54 (4.5)	24 (2.0)	13 (1.1)	11 (0.9)	931 (78.3)	1189
Education									
None/some primary	25 (1.8)	113 (8.1)	3 (0.2)	90 (6.5)	16 (1.1)	7 (0.5)	4 (0.3)	1141 (81.9)	1394
Completed primary	62 (3.0)	308 (14.8)	4 (0.2)	176 (8.4)	31 (1.5)	8 (0.5)	10 (0.5)	1490 (71.4)	2086
Secondary+	15 (2.6)	62 (10.7)	7 (1.2)	62 (10.7)	9 (1.6)	0 (0)	7 (1.2)	429 (74.0)	580
Number of living children									
< 3	38 (2.0)	159 (8.6)	10 (0.5)	121 (6.5)	14 (0.8)	0 (0.0)	4 (0.2)	1531 (82.4)	1858
3+	64 (2.9)	319 (14.5)	4 (0.2)	207 (9.4)	42 (1.9)	15 (0.7)	17 (0.8)	1546 (70.1)	2206

1054 women, 383 (36%) reported 394 discontinuation events for contraceptive methods, and 66 switching events over the past 2 years (Table 5). There were 98 women who stopped because they desired to have a child, and among them 49 (50%) reported being pregnant prior to the interview date. The remaining 343 women who discontinued contraceptives, did not report wanting to get pregnant, although 129 (38%) of them reported a pregnancy following discontinuation (Table 5). The reasons for discontinuation included infrequent sex $n = 45$ (13.1%), inconvenient to use $n = 19$ (1.4%), health concerns $n = 89$ (20.2%) and other reasons $n = 49$ (11.1%). There were 122 women who reported no reason for discontinuing contraceptive use, of which 83 (68%) became pregnant within 3 months of discontinuation, and an additional six women reported contraceptive failure as the reason for the pregnancy. Over the 2-year period, there were a total of 89 pregnancies in the 1054 women who reported taking contraceptives prior to the pregnancy.

Contraceptive discontinuation rates

There were 15 women who reported sterilisation as their contraceptive method, and who were excluded from the calculation of discontinuation rates for contraceptive use. A further 102 women only reported contraceptive use in the last 3 months prior to the survey and were also excluded from the discontinuation rates estimation, as women may be unaware of contraception failure if it happened in the 3 months prior to the survey. Table 4 shows the percentage of the 952 women who discontinued contraception, for all methods, and for each specific method, at 6 and 12 months. The overall discontinuation rates for the 952 women who reported using a contraceptive method during the 21 months were 15.8% at 6 months and 30.5% at 12 months. However, some of these women switched to another method during the study period, with 58 (6.1%) women using more than one method of contraception during the study period, sometimes immediately following the discontinuation and other times after a period of non-use (Table 5).

The median duration of use for all modern methods (except for sterilization) was 21 months. Pills and injections show a similar pattern of discontinuation with around 40% of women discontinuing within 12 months, and median use of 15.5 months. A lower discontinuation rate was estimated for women using intrauterine devices (IUD) or implants methods with only 9.6% of IUD users, and 12.8% of women who used implants stopping within 6 months. The median time for discontinuation of these methods was longer than the observation period of the study.

Results of the Cox regression on the factors associated with discontinuation in 952 women who used contraception during the past 2 years are shown on Table 6. All coefficients in the table, pass the assumption of proportional hazards. As expected, discontinuation varied by method and was significantly higher among users of the pills (aHR;

Table 3 The odds ratio for the determinants of current use of contraception among 1813 non-pregnant, sexually active women of reproductive age, who say they do not want to get pregnant

Categories	Total	Current use	Unadjusted model		Adjusted model	
			Odds Ratio		Odds Ratio	
	N = 1813	N = 610	(95% C.I.)	p-value	(95% C.I.)	p-value
Intercept					1.00	
HIV status[a]						
Negative	1651	566	1.00			
Positive	155	42	0.71 (0.49,1.03)	0.0714	0.89 (0.60,1.32)	0.5598
Age						
15–24	373	144	1.00			
25–34	643	312	1.50 (1.16,1.94)	0.0022	1.17 (0.84,1.64)	0.3578
35 and above	797	154	0.38 (0.29,0.50)	<.0001	0.28 (0.19,0.41)	< 0.0001
Martial status						
Unmarried	207	55	1.00			
Married/Living together	1418	494	1.48 (1.07,2.05)	0.0194	2.23 (1.54,3.23)	< 0.0001
Divorced/Separated/Widowed	188	61	1.33 (0.86,2.05)	0.2008	2.14 (1.33,3.44)	0.0017
Education						
None/some primary	593	150	1.00			
Completed primary	977	360	1.72 (1.46,2.18)	< .0001	1.67 (1.32,2.13)	< .0001
Secondary+	270	100	2.11 (1.54,2.89)	< .0001	1.95 (1.36,2.80)	0.0003
Number of living children						
< 3	539	203	1.00			
3+	1274	407	0.78 (0.63,0.96)	0.0187	1.25 (0.91,1.71)	0.1665

Note: Both unadjusted and adjusted odds ratios shown in this table are estimated using logistic regression. Unadjusted odds ratio are based on separate logistic regressions for each predictor variable with that variable as the only predictor variable. Adjusted odds ratios are based on a single logistic regression consisting of all the predictor variables in the table. For any given predictor variable in the adjusted column, the set of control variables consists of all the other predictor variables in the table
42 women reported to currently using contraceptives whereas they were pregnant/breastfeeding
[a]Contains 8 missing observations (but less than 10%)

1.86, 95% CI 1.25,2.77) and injection (aHR; 2.04, 95% CI 1.59,2.77) as compared to users of implants. Further, results show that being over 25 years old, is significantly associated with a decreased rate of method discontinuation. Notwithstanding, HIV status, number of living children and education are not statistically associated with discontinuation of contraceptive use.

Discussion

Access to contraception is a crucial goal for sustainable development in many LMIC including Tanzania [18]. The policies on access to contraception are important for family planning, and also for prevention of mother to child transmission of HIV (PMTCT). Our results show that 16% of sexually active women in this rural area of Tanzania were

Table 4 Life table discontinuation rates for 1056 women in Kisesa in 2015/16, and median duration of use by method

Method	6-month discontinuation rate	12-month discontinuation rate	Median duration of use (in months)
Pills	27.8	43.6	15.5
Injections	21	41.9	15.5
Implants	12.8	24.9	–
IUD	9.6	13.7	–
All methods (Including traditional methods)	15.8	30.5	–
All modern methods (excluding sterilization)	16.9	32	21

Table 5 Reasons for discontinuation among women who used contraceptives in the past two years

	Number of women	Discontinuation events	Women who became pregnant (%)
Did not discontinue	613	0	0
Switched	58	66	0
Discontinued	383	394	178 (45.2)
Desired for pregnancy	98 (22.2)	100	49 (50)
Not reported desired for pregnancy	343 (77.8)		129 (38)
Reasons for discontinuation			
Infrequent sex	58 (13.1)		6 (10.3)
Health concerns	89 (20.2)		13 (14.6)
Inconvenient to use	19 (4.3)		4 (21.1)
Contraceptive failure	6 (1.4)		6 (100)
Other reasons	49 (11.1)		17 (34.7)
No reason reported	122 (27.7)		83 (68.0)

currently using contraceptives, while 20% were currently pregnant or amenorrheic. Among all sexually experienced women of reproductive age (15–49 years), only 31% had ever used contraception, although 86% women in this population knew about family planning and contraceptive methods. The low use of contraception in this study concurs with previous studies showing low usage of modern contraceptives in other countries in sub-Saharan Africa [19, 20]. Injections, implants and pills were found to be the most common contraceptive methods used by women in this study. There were few women who used condoms (either male or female) for contraception, female sterilization, or who reported using traditional methods of contraception.

Table 6 Cox proportional hazards model on time until discontinuation of baseline method, by demographic. characteristics, number of living children, HIV status, and method type, $N = 952$.

Factors	Number of discontinuations	Rates (95% CI) per 100 women	Unadj HRs (95% CI)	*p*-value	Adjusted HRs (95% CI)	*p*-value
HIV status						
Negative	341	3.17 (2.85,3.52)	1			
Positive	32	2.94 (2.08,4.16)	0.83 (0.59,1.17)	0.2800	0.89 (0.63,1.29)	0.5200
Methods						
Implants	90	2.17 (1.76,2.66)	1			
Pills	35	3.70 (2.66,5.16)	1.73 (1.17,2.56)	0.0060	1.86 (1.25,2.77)	0.0020
Injection	225	4.19 (3.68,4.78)	1.97 (1.54,2.52)	0.0001	2.04 (1.59,2.61)	0.0001
IUD	11	1.24 (0.69,2.25)	0.56 (0.30,1.05)	0.0710	0.60 (0.32,1.13)	0.1160
Other methods	12	2.08 (1.18,3.66)	0.96 (0.52,1.75)	0.8850	1.07 (0.58,1.99)	0.8190
Age						
15–24	92	3.90 (3.18,4.78)	1			
25–34	184	3.05 (2.64,3.53)	0.77 (0.60,0.99)	0.0390	0.72 (0.56,0.93)	0.0110
35+	97	2.74 (2.25,3.35)	0.68 (0.51,0.90)	0.0080	0.67 (0.50,0.90)	0.0070
Education						
None/some primary	98	3.32 (2.72,4.05)	1			
Completed primary	222	3.06 (2.68,3.48)	0.92 (0.72,1.16)	0.4700		
Secondary+	52	3.05 (2.33,4.01)	0.92 (0.66,1.29)	0.6180	–	–
Number of living children						
< 3	127	3.44 (2.89,4.09)	1			
3+	246	2.99 (2.64,3.39)	0.86 (0.69,1.06)	0.160	–	–

In this study 66% of all sexually-active, non-pregnant women who wanted to avoid pregnancy had an unmet need for contraception. We did not ask pregnant women about whether their pregnancy was wanted or not, and are therefore unable to ascertain the overall unmet need for contraception in this study. The unmet need for contraception in this study is higher than the unmet need for contraception reported in Uganda (34%) or Ghana (36%) [21].

Our results agree with the paper by MacQuarrie et al. [22] as we find no significant difference in the use of contraception by HIV status. However, women who were older, had attained higher educational levels and were married, had significantly higher levels of current contraceptive use. The positive association between education and contraceptive use is in line with findings from other studies [14, 23]. Women who have more years of education are more likely to understand the uses of contraception in reducing fertility, maternal and child morbidity and mortality. Educated women can also avoid the negative effects of family planning methods because they might have an awareness of the side effects of contraceptive methods, and be able to choose the most convenient method to use, and thereby increasing their consistent use [23]. In this study only 14% of the women had any secondary education, and the contraceptive discontinuation rate was lower in women with primary and secondary education compared to those with no education.

This study also showed around one third of women discontinue contraceptive use within a year, although this varies according to the type of contraceptives. The discontinuation rates were lowest among women using IUD (13.7% per year) or implants (24.9% per year), and higher for women using pills (43.6% per year) or injections (41.9% per year). The discontinuation rate for IUD is similar to that reported in Pakistan (19.1% in 10 months) and Senegal (18.4% in 12 months) [24, 25]. The discontinuation rates were lower among users of IUD and implants methods because these methods are long-lasting, and also removal of the devices requires help from a health professional [26]. Age, education and parity had a significant effect on contraceptive discontinuations, and discontinuation rates were higher among women who used pills and injections than those who used implants.

To understand the low contraceptive usage and high rates of discontinuation in this study, women were asked their reasons for stopping contraceptive use over the past 2 years. Around a quarter of the women who discontinued contraceptive use said they discontinued because they wanted to get pregnant. A further 28% become pregnant without giving a reason, perhaps reflecting an unplanned pregnancy, although only 6 women gave contraceptive failure as the reason for the pregnancy. Other than pregnancy, the most cited reasons for discontinuation of the use of contraceptive methods were fear of side effects, health concerns, inconvenience to use and infrequent sex. There was a very low discontinuation due to cost, problems in accessing contraception or marital dissolution. No one reported stopping due to religious or family opposition to contraceptive use.

This study shows that Tanzania is a long way from reaching its national family planning target of 60% contraceptive prevalence rate [27]. Results from this analysis emphasize the low uptake of contraception, and the high rates of contraceptive discontinuation, even among women who want to avoid pregnancy. Providing education on contraception, and universal access to contraceptives and family planning would empower women to overcome cultural barriers to the use of contraception. This would enable them to choose the number and spacing of children, to prevent unintended pregnancies, to reduce vertical transmission of HIV, and ultimately to improve maternal and child health. The high unmet need in this population underscores the importance of improving and expanding the provision of contraceptive use for women through different programmes, and making those programmes more accessible to younger women. Despite the benefits of contraception in preventing vertical transmission of HIV, the use of contraception was no higher among HIV positive women than HIV negative women. The PMTCT programme could be used to encourage HIV positive women to increase their use contraception for family planning and HIV prevention purposes.

Strengths and limitations

This study reports on the behaviour of a large sample of sexually-active women of reproductive age, living in a defined area covered by the Kisesa HDSS. It reports the current use of contraception of both married and unmarried women. One limitation is that, it relies on the woman's report of contraception use, and women may not accurately recall this over the 2 years. Secondly, young, unmarried women might not be honest regarding sexual debut, and they are the least likely to access contraception, or report contraception use, and this may underestimate the unmet need for contraception in this population. Thirdly, the study did not ask pregnant women or those with postpartum amenorrhea whether the pregnancy was intended or not, which may also lead to an underestimate of the unmet need for contraception. There are methodological limitations around censoring of episodes at the beginning and end of the 24-month calendar of contraceptive use, which may underestimate changes in contraceptive use, and hence the discontinuation rate. Finally, the study failed to take into consideration the competing risk events (such as switching between methods), and considered all switches to be discontinuation events, which would over-estimate the discontinuation rate in this population.

Conclusions and implications

In conclusion, findings showed that a large proportion of sexually active women were not using any modern contraceptive, despite their high knowledge of contraceptives. Almost one fifth of sexually-active women had an unmet need for contraception in this population, which if translated across Tanzania would mean 2 million women needing contraceptive services. Using the Kisesa HDSS, we found non-significant association between women's HIV status and both contraceptive use and discontinuation. Although there was no significant association, none of the HIV positive woman reported using condoms. There were significant relationships between contraceptive use and contraceptive discontinuation with age, education and parity. The predictors of contraceptive discontinuations indicated that, better interventions should be developed to target the needs of younger women. Women who used pills or injections had the highest rates of discontinuation, and a wider choice of long-acting contraceptive methods with better effectiveness and convenience may be better suited to their needs.

Abbreviations

95% CI: 95% confidence interval; aHR: adjusted hazard ratios; CPR: Contraceptive prevalence rate; CTC: Care and Treatment Centre; HDSS: Health and Demographic Surveillance System; IUD: Intrauterine devices; LMIC: Low and middle income countries; LSHTM: London School of Hygiene & Tropical Medicine; LZIRB: Lake Zone Institutional Review Board; MMR : Maternal mortality ratio; OR: Odds Ratio; PMTCT: Prevention of mother-to-child transmission; SSA: Sub-Saharan Africa; TDHS: Tanzania Demographic and Health Survey; VCT: Voluntary Counselling and Testing

Acknowledgements

We thank the regional and district health authorities for permission to carry out the study. We acknowledge the hard work of the study teams in collecting and managing the data for the study. We acknowledge the inputs from the TAZAMA project, and the National Institute for Medical Research in Mwanza to organize the study. We thank the study participants for their time and patience in attending the survey and providing the responses for these data.

Authors' contributions

The study and questions for data collection were conceived by MU, JC, KC, BZ and JT. The initial data were managed and cleaned by BM and JB. The data were analysed by WS, MU, JB and JT. The paper was initially drafted by WS. All authors contributed to the preparation and finalisation of the manuscript. All authors, except BZ who died in 2018, read and approved the final manuscript.

References

1. Wikipedia: Population growth. https://en.wikipedia.org/wiki/Populationgrowth. Accessed 16 Apr 2018.
2. THE WORLD FACTBOOK. https://www.cia.gov/library/publications/the-world-factbook/geos/tz.html. Accessed 16 Apr 2018.
3. The Guttmacher Institute: Contraception 2017. https://www.guttmacher.org/infographic/2016/1-5-women-tanzania-have-unmet-need-contraception. Accessed 31 Mar 2018.
4. Shoo RS, Mboera LE, Ndeki S, Munishi G. Stagnating maternal mortality in Tanzania: what went wrong and what can be done. Tanzan J Health Res. 2017;19(2):1–12.
5. Cleland J, Bernstein S, Ezeh A, Faundes A, Glasier A, Innis J. Family planning: the unfinished agenda. Lancet. 2006;368(9549):1810–27 PMID:17113431.
6. Tanzania Demographic and Health Survey and Malaria Indicator Survey, 2015/16. https://dhsprogram.com/pubs/pdf/fr321/fr321.pdf. Accessed 16 Apr 2018.
7. The World Bank Data. Contraceptive prevalence, any methods, 2016. https://data.worldbank.org/indicator/SP.DYN.CONU.ZS?locations=TZ&view=chart Accessed: 4 Feb 2019.
8. Rizvi F, Irfan G. Reasons for discontinuation of contraceptive methods among couples with different family size and educational status. J Ayub Med Coll Abbottabad. 2012;24(1):101–4 PMID:23855108.
9. Ali, M.M., Cleland, J.G., Shah I.H.: Causes and consequences of contraceptive discontinuation: evidence from 60 demographic and health surveys (2012). World Health Organisation ISBN: 978 92 4 150405 8. At https://www.who.int/reproductivehealth/publications/family_planning/9789241504058/en/.
10. Castle S, Askew I. Contraceptive Discontinuation: Reasons, Challenges, And Solutions. Family Planning 2020. New York: The Population Council; 2015. At: http://www.familyplanning2020.org/resources/contraceptive-discontinuation-reasons-challenges-and-solutions
11. Wilcher R, Cates W Jr, Gregson S. Family planning and HIV: strange bedfellows no longer. AIDS (London, England). 2009;23(Suppl 1):1 PMID:20081381.
12. Haddad LB, Philpott-Jones S, Schonfeld T. Contraception and prevention of hiv transmission: a potential conflict of public health principles. J Fam Plann Reprod Health Care. 2014;41(1):20–3 PMID:25323410.
13. MeasureEvaluation: Family Planning and HIV. https://www.measureevaluation.org/prh/rhindicators/family-planning/family-planning-and-HIV. Accessed April 2018.
14. Kishamawe C, Isingo R, Mtenga B, Zaba B, Todd J, Clark B, Changalucha J, Urassa M. Health & demographic surveillance system profile: the Magu health and demographic surveillance system (Magu HDSS). Int J Epidemiol. 2015;44(6):1851–61 PMID:4911678.
15. MeasureEvaluation: Womens questionnaire. At: https://www.dhsprogram.com/pubs/pdf/DHSQ7/DHS7-Womans-QRE-EN-17Dec2018-DHSQ7.pdf. Accessed July 2019.
16. Bradley SE, Croft TN, Fishel JD, Westoff CF. Revising unmet need for family planning, DHS analytical studies no. 25. Calverton, Maryland: ICF International; 2012. At: https://www.dhsprogram.com/pubs/pdf/AS25/AS25[12June2012].pdf
17. Curtis SL, Hammerslough CR. Model further analysis plan: contraceptive use dynamics, DHS analytical studies no. 59. Calverton, Maryland: ICF International; 1995. At: https://www.dhsprogram.com/pubs/pdf/FA59/FA59.pdf
18. Sustainable Development Goals. 2015. http://www.un.org/sustainabledevelopment/sustainable-development-goals/. Accessed 16 June 2017.
19. Mosha I, Ruben R, Kakoko D. Family planning decisions, perceptions and gender dynamics among couples in Mwanza, Tanzania: a qualitative study. BMC Public Health. 2013;13(1):523 PMID:23721196.
20. Bongaarts J, Bruce J. The causes of unmet need for contraception and the social content of services. Stud Fam Plan. 1995;26(2):57–75 PMID:7618196.
21. Sedgh G, Ashoford LS, Hussain R. Unmet need for contraception in developing countries: examine women's reasons for not using a method. New York: Technical report, the Guttmacher institute; 2016. At https://www.guttmacher.org/report/unmet-need-for-contraception-in-developing-countries
22. MacQuarrie K, Bradley S, Gemmill A, Staveteig S. Contraceptive dynamics following HIV testing, DHS analytical studies 47. Calverton, Maryland: ICF International; 2014. At: https://www.researchgate.net/publication/266202360_Contraceptive_Dynamics_following_HIV_Testing
23. Asiimwe JB, Ndugga P, Mushomi J, Ntozi JPM. Factors associated with modern contraceptive use among young and older women in Uganda; a comparative analysis. BMC Public Health. 2014;14(1):926 PMID:4169837.
24. Azmat SK, Hameed W, Mustafa G, Hussain W, Ahmed A, Bilgrami M. IUD discontinuation rates, switching behavior, and user satisfaction: findings from a retrospective analysis of a mobile outreach service program in Pakistan. Int J Women's Health. 2013;5:19 PMID:23359788.
25. Barden-O'Fallon J, Speizer IS, Calhoun LM, Corroon M. Women's contraceptive discontinuation and switching behavior in urban Senegal, 2010–2015. BMC Womens Health. 2018;18(1):35 PMID:5800088.

26. Bradley, S.E., Schwandt, H., Khan, S.: Levels, trends, and reasons for contraceptive discontinuation. DHS analytical studies 20 (2009) At: https://www.researchgate.net/publication/242569444_Levels_Trends_and_Reasons_for_Contraceptive_Discontinuation
27. Ministry of Health and Social Welfare, Tanzania: The National Family Planning Costed Implementation Program 2010–2015. http://www.rchs.go.tz/index.php/en/resources/family-planning/strategy-policy-8/131-national-family-planning-costed-implementation-program-2010-2015-updated-2013/file.html. Accessed 16 Apr 2018.

22

Long acting reversible contraceptives utilization and associated factors among women of reproductive age in Arsi Negele town, Southeastern Ethiopia

Desalegn Tsegaw Hibstu[1*] and Akalewold Alemayehu[2]

Abstract

Background: Ethiopia is the second populous country in Africa with a total fertility rate of 4.6 and contraceptive prevalence of 35%, where implant and intrauterine contraceptive devices account for 8 and 2% respectively. The aim of this study was to determine the magnitude of long acting reversible contraceptives utilization and its associated factors among women of reproductive age in Arsi Negele town, Southeastern Ethiopia.

Methods: Facility-based cross-sectional study was conducted from April 01–May 30, 2017. A total of 361 women using modern contraceptives were selected by a systematic random sampling technique. Pre-tested and interviewer administered structured questionnaire was used to collect quantitative data. Bivariate and multivariate logistic regressions were performed using SPSS version 20.0 software.

Result: The magnitude of long acting reversible contraceptives (LARCs) utilization was 33.5% [95% CI, 28.5–38.8]. Husband with no formal education [AOR = 0.41, CI: 0.16, 0.78] and unemployed women [AOR = 0.35, CI: 0.42, 0.65] were negative predictors while having media exposure [AOR = 7.14, CI: 3.85, 13.25], women who desired only one child [AOR = 3.28, CI; 1.28, 8.39] and husband support [AOR = 7.33, CI: 3.48, 15.43] were positive predictors of LARCs utilization.

Conclusion: The overall utilization of LARCs is 33.5%. Creating employment opportunities, male involvement, advertisement and advocacy activities through mass media need to be considered to improve utilization of LARCs.

Keywords: Arsi Negele town, Long acting and reversible contraceptive, Magnitude, Factors

Background

Long acting reversible contraceptives (LARCs) are birth controls providing effective pregnancy protection for an extended duration without user action. These methods include implants and intrauterine contraceptive devices (IUCDs) [1].

* Correspondence: desuethiopia@yahoo.com
[1]Department of Reproductive Health, School of Public Health, College of Medicine and Health Sciences, Hawassa University, Hawassa, Ethiopia

Globally in 2017, 12% of married women were estimated to have an unmet need for family planning. The severity was higher in Africa (22%) compared to other regions, where the unmet need for family planning is estimated to be as low as 10 % in developed countries [2].

In the developing world, two to three among ten women using oral contraceptives or injectable discontinued within 2 years of use due to side effects, use inconsistency, user run out of the method or other related concerns and as a result majority of women can be benefited if they use LARCs [3].

According to the 2007 population census, Ethiopia is the second populous country in Africa next to Nigeria [4] with a total fertility rate of 4.6 and contraceptive prevalence of 35%. Of the total contraceptive utilization, long acting and permanent contraceptive methods account for 10%, IUCD and implant account for 2 and 8% respectively [5].

Depending on setting, a number of factors have been described in literature to affect adoption of LARCs among contraceptive users. Evidence suggest from other countries and in Ethiopia indicated that desire to more children, opposition to use, lack of knowledge, side effects of contraceptives, age of women, educational status of women and men, and family income are the potential factors affecting utilization of LARCs [4, 6].

The Federal Ministry of Health, Ethiopia considered the role of LARCs for birth spacing and limiting, and planned to increase implant and IUD to 33 and 15% respectively in the method mix by the end of 2020 [7]. In Ethiopia, all contraceptives including long acing and permanent contraceptive methods are rendered free [8]. In the country, many governmental and nongovernmental organizations are delivering LARCs through static and outreach outlets at all levels of health facilities (hospitals, health centers and health posts) [9].

Increasing contraceptive method mix played a big role in reducing discontinuation rates due to short-acting hormonal methods that are primarily chosen by contraceptive users in SSA [7, 10] where about 1.8 million unplanned pregnancies would been avoided within 5 years if one-fifth of women utilizing oral contraceptives and injectable shift to LARCs [11]. Therefore, the aim of this study was to determine the magnitude of long acting and permanent contraceptive utilization among women of reproductive age using modern contraceptives in Arsi Negele town, southeastern Ethiopia.

Methods

Study design and setting

Facility-based quantitative cross-sectional study was employed from April 01–May 30, 2017. The study was conducted in Aresi Negelle town. The town is located in West Arsi Zone of Oromia regional state in southeastern Ethiopia at a distance of 225 Kilometer) KM from Addis Ababa, capital city of Ethiopia. According to the 2007 Ethiopian population and housing census, the total population of the town was 36,699 (17,618 female) [Arsi Negele town Health Office, Annual report, 2017, Unpublished].

The town has one health center providing preventive, promotive, curative and rehabilitation services for the community and other surrounding communities. The source populations were all women of reproductive age group living in Aresi Negelle town and the study populations were all women of reproductive age group (15–49 years old) using modern contraceptives in Arsi Negele town. However, women who were diagnosed by a physician as seriously ill and unable to hear were excluded.

Sample size determination and sampling procedure

Sample size was determined using single population proportion formula considering the following assumption: 95% confidence level ($z_{\alpha/2}{}^2$), 4% margin of error (d) and expected proportion (p) of long acting reversible contraceptive users was 19.5% [12].

$$\frac{n = z_{\alpha/2}{}^2 p\,(1-p)}{d^2} = \frac{(1.96)^2 x\ 0.195(0.805)}{(0.04)^2} = 376$$

Study participants were selected using a systematic random sampling technique with an interval of two where the interval constant was obtained by dividing the total modern contraceptive users in the health center to the sample size from their family planning registration book.

Data collection tool and procedure

Pre-tested and interviewer-administered structured questionnaire, first prepared in English and translated to Amharic language was employed to collect quantitative data. Six registered female nurses were participated to collect the data. Training was given to data collectors for 2 days. The training focused on the study objectives, questionnaire and process of data collection. One bachelor degree holder with principal investigator supervised the data collection process and checked filled questionnaire for consistency and completeness.

Statistical analysis

After data collection, data were edited and cleaned before analysis, each questionnaire was checked for completeness and code was provided. Data were entered into computer using EPI Info version 3.5.4 and the analysis was done using SPSS version 20.0. Frequency, percentage and descriptive summaries were used to describe the study variables. Logistic regression was carried out to identify factors associated with utilization of LARCs. Variables with p-value ≤0.2 in the bivariate analysis were transferred for multivariable logistic regression analysis to control the effect of confounders. Adjusted odds ratios (AOR) with 95% confidence interval (CI) and p-value of less than 0.05 were considered to have significant association between the outcome and the explanatory variables.

Results

Socio demographic and economic characteristics

A total of 361 of reproductive aged women were included in the study. The mean age of the study subjects was 27.4 years (+ 4.9, standard deviation (SD)). Two hundred and twenty seven (62.9%) study subjects were found in the age group 25–34 years. One hundred and eighty eight (52.1%) of the respondents were followers of orthodox religion and 191 (52.9%) were Oromo by ethnicity. Among the total study participants, 342 (94.7%) were currently married and about nine in ten, 338 (93.6%) living in urban area.

One hundred and sixty seven (46.3%) women had acquired only primary education and 159 (44%) of all partners had acquired at least a secondary education. As shown in Table 1, about six in ten, (62.3%) were unemployed and 340 (94.2%) of their husbands were employed. Almost one among four, 94 (26%) mothers had monthly income between 1001 and 2000 Ethiopian birr (≈ 46 USD – 93 USD) (Table 1).

Reproductive history of women

As indicated in table two below, of the total women, about nine in ten women 322(89.2%) had history of giving birth and 152 (42.1%) gave more than three live births with 151(41.8%) alive currently during the study period. One hundred fifty four (42.7%) women desired to have two and above children in their reproductive life and 109 (30.2%) wish to have more children within the next 2 years. About three fourth 275 (76.2%) of the desired number of children was decided jointly (by the husband and wife). The average number of parity,

Table 1 Socio demographic and economic characteristics of the study participants in Arsi Negele town, Southeastern Ethiopia, 2017

Variables	Category	Frequency(n)	Percentage (%)
Age in years	15–24	100	27.7.9
	25–34	227	62.9
	> 35	34	9.4
Ethnicity	Oromo	191	52.9
	Amhara	91	25.2
	Guraghe	35	9.7
	Tigre	25	6.9
	Wolayita	19	5.3
Religion	Orthodox	188	52.1
	Protestant	94	26.0
	Muslim	79	21.9
	Catholic	11	3.0
Marital status	Currently married	342	94.7
	Currently unmarried	19	5.3
Residence	Urban	338	93.6
	Rural	23	6.4
Women education	No formal education	84	23.3
	Primary education	167	46.3
	Secondary & above	110	30.5
Husband /partner education	No formal education	59	16.3
	Primary education	143	39.6
	Secondary & above	159	44.0
Women occupation	Unemployed	225	62.3
	Employed	136	37.7
Husband occupation	Unemployed	21	5.8
	Employed	340	94.2
Monthly income (Ethiopian Birr)	≤ 1000	64	17.7
	1001–2000	94	26.0
	2001–3000	78	21.6
	> 3000	125	34.6

currently living children, desired number of children in the reproductive life were 2.4 (+ 1.6 standard deviation (SD)), 2.3 (+ 1.5 SD) and 2.4 (+ 1.3 SD), respectively (Table 2).

Contraceptive related characteristics

As shown in Table 3, of the total modern contraceptives users, nearly four in five women heard about LARCs. Among the total women, 193 (53.5%) had media exposure about LARCs where 170(88.1%) were exposed to Television (TV). Injectable contraceptive method was the most known type by women, 338 (93.6%) and vasectomy was the least known method, 13 (3.6%). More than two in five, 229 (63.4) women mentioned limiting family size, prevents maternal and child health and child spacing as a benefit of LARCs.

The overall utilization of LARCs among women using modern contraceptive was 121 (33.5%) [95% CI, 28.5–38.8]. Ninety four (26%) and 27 (7.5%) women practiced implant and intrauterine contraceptive device (IUCD). Almost four among five, 287 (79.5%) women had discussion with their husbands on contraceptive utilization and 229 (63.4%) respondents' utilization of contraceptive was approved by their husbands (Table 3).

Factors associated with LARC utilization

As indicated in Table 4, in the multivariate logistic regression analysis; husband education, women occupation, media exposure, desired number of children and approval of partner to use contraceptive were examined to be independent predictors of long acting reversible contraceptive methods.

The study demonstrated that the probability LARCs utilization among women whose husbands with no formal education was 59% [AOR = 0.41, 95%CI; 0.16, 0.78] less likely to adapt LARCs compared with husbands attended secondary and above education. The study identified that practicing LARCs decreased by 65% among unemployed women compared with employed women [AOR = 0.35, CI: 0.42, 0.65].

Another important factor was media exposure to LARCs. Women having media exposure to LARCs were seven times more likely to use LARCs liken with women with no media exposure [AOR = 7.14, CI: 3.85, 13.25].

On the other hand, desired number of children and husband approval/support were identified as determinants of LARCs utilization. The odds of using LARCs was nearly three times more likely to be increased among women whose desired number of children was one compared to three and above [AOR = 3.28, CI: 1.28, 8.39]. Women who got support/approval from their husband about contraceptive methods were seven times more likely to practice LARCs [AOR = 7.33, CI: 3.48, 15.43].

Discussion

In the present study, it was indicated that long acting reversible contraceptives (LARCs) utilization was 33.5%.

Table 2 Reproductive history of study participants in Arsi Negele town, Southeastern Ethiopia, 2017

Variables	Category	Frequency (n)	Percentage (%)
History of giving birth	Yes	322	89.2
	No	39	10.8
Number of ever born births	None	39	10.8
	One	74	20.5
	Two	96	26.6
	Three and above	152	42.1
Number of alive children	None	42	11.6
	One	72	19.9
	Two	96	26.6
	Three and above	151	41.8
Desired number of children	One	86	23.8
	Two	154	42.7
	Three and above	121	33.5
Desire to have more children	Yes	109	30.2
	No	252	69.8
Decision maker on number of children.	Woman	23	6.4
	Husband	34	9.4
	Jointly[a]	275	76.2
	God	29	8.0

[a]both woman and husband

Table 3 Contraceptive related characteristics of women of reproductive age groups in Arsi Negele town, Southeastern Ethiopia, 2017

Variables	Category	Frequency (n)	Percentage (%)
Heard of LARCs	Yes	295	81.7
	No	66	18.3
Media exposure to LARCs	Yes	193	53.5
	No	168	46.5
Type of media exposed	Television	170	88.1
	Radio	23	11.9
Known contraceptive	Pills	301	83.4
	Injectable	338	93.6
	Implant	282	78.1
	IUCD	243	67.3
	Condom	29	8
	Tuba ligation	46	18
	Vasectomy	13	3.6
Benefits of LARC[a]	Limiting family size	27	7.5
	Improves maternal and child health	13	3.6
	Child spacing	23	6.4
	Used for all[a]	229	63.4
	Don't' know uses	69	19.1
Utilization of LARC	Yes	121	33.5
	No	240	66.5
Type of LARC used (n = 121)	Implant	94	26.0
	IUCD	27	7.5
Contraceptive discussion among couples	Yes	287	79.5
	No	69	20.5
Approval of husband to use contraceptive	Yes	229	63.4
	No	132	36.6

Used for all[a]: indicate benefits of LARC for limiting family size, improves maternal and child health and child spacing

This finding was nearly in line with a study conducted in Ethiopia: Areka town (29.7%) and Adigrat town (37.3%) [13, 14] and higher than studies done in Ethiopia: Debremarkos (19.5%) and Mekelle (12%) [12, 15]. The increased prevalence noticed in this research might be due to the difference in time and study setting (institutional versus community based) and, improved awareness of women and advocacy of long acting and permanent contraceptives by governmental and non-governmental organization through mass media and health professionals.

The most widely used long acting reversible contraceptive method in this study was implant (26%). This result was similar with other findings in Ethiopia: Arbaminch and west Ethiopia, [16, 17]. Only 7.5% of the study participants practiced intrauterine contraceptive (IUCD) device which is nearly similar with a study conducted in Nigeria (7%) [18], and lower than the findings in Indonesia (52%) [19]. The possible explanation in this study could be women might have misconception about IUCD and its side effects such as interference with sexual intercourse, cancer, delays pregnancy, restriction from working normal activity and invasion of privacy during its insertion and removal [15].

In the current study, it was figured out that utilization of LARCs was higher among women whose husbands completed secondary and above education compared with women who did not attend formal education. This finding is agreed with studies in Ethiopia: Adigrat town and west Ethiopia [14, 17]. This might be explained by the fact that there is no question that better educated family members would have access for information on LARC methods and their increased knowledge on modern contraceptives. It is also thought that increased educational status in particular secondary education and above could have a positive outcome service use and female decision-making power on reproductive health services including family planning.

Table 4 Multivariate logistic regression model predicting utilization of LARCs among women in Arsi Negele town, Southeastern Ethiopia, 2017

Variables	Category	Use of LARC		*COR* (95% CI)	AOR* (95% CI)	*P*-value
		No	***Yes***			
Age of women (years)	15–24	79	21	0.30(0.13, 0.68)	0.44(0.14,1.36)	0.154
	25–34	*143*	84	0.66 (0.32, 1.37)	0.50 (0.19,1.35)	0.171
	≥ 35	*18*	16	1.00	1.00	
Husband education	No formal education	47	12	0.48 (0.24, 0.99)	0.41 (0.16,0.78)	0.006
	Primary education	89	54	1.15 (0.72, 1.84)	0.75 (0.65,0.98)	0.005
	Secondary and above	104	55	1.00	1.00	
Women occupation	Unemployed	162	63	0.52 (0.33, 0.82)	0.35 (0.42,0.65)	0.001
	Employed	*78*	*58*	1.00	1.00	
Heard of LARCs	Yes	180	115	6.39 (2.67, 15.27)	1.50 (0.53,4.29)	0.450
	No	*60*	*6*	1.00		
Media exposure to LARCs	Yes	89	104	10.38 (5.84,18.46)	7.14 (3.85,13.25)	0.002
	No	151	17	1.00	1.00	
Desire for more children	Yes	81	28	0.59 (0.36, 0.97)	0.73 (0.38,1.38)	0.329
	No	159	93	1.00	1.00	1.00
Desired number of children	One	46	40	4.14 (2.20, 7.80)	3.28 (1.28,8.39)	0.023
	Two	94	60	3.04 (1.72, 5.38)	2.58 (1.16,5.71)	0.020
	Three and above	100	21	1.00	1.00	
Discussion among couples	Yes	*81*	*28*	2.55 (1.36, 4.78)	0.493 (0.14,1.69)	0.261
	No	159	93	1.00	1.00	
Husband Support to use contraceptive	Yes	118	111	2.55 (1.36,4.78)	7.33 (3.48,15.43)	0.000
	No	122	121	1.00	1.00	

The study also revealed that utilization of LARC was increased among employed women than unemployed women. This finding was consistent with studies in Ethiopia: Adigrat town and west Ethiopia [14, 17]. This could happen because employed women would have a positive outcome in utilization of LARC by having frequent health institution contact to access the service with payment though it is provided free of charge in Ethiopia.

Significant association was observed concerning media exposure. It was figured out that utilization of LARC was more likely to increase among women had exposure of media. This finding is in line with study conducted in Ethiopia [17]. This could be explained as media has a power in explaining the different methods available, their benefits and where the methods are available and enhances women to utilize the methods.

On the other hand, desired number of children and approval of husband/partner plays significant role on utilization of long acting and permanent contraceptive. Women whose desired number of children only one were more likely to use LARC. Women who had approval from their husband/partner were more likely to use LARC. This finding was congruent with the studies done in Ethiopia: Debremarkos, Arbaminch and Butajira [12, 16, 20].

Limitations

When interpreting the findings of this study, researchers need to consider the following limitations. First, the cross sectional nature of the data had made impossible to arrive at the causal relation between the different explanatory variables and knowledge of long acting and permanent contraceptives. Second, as the study is based on a sample of all reproductive age group women who are using modern contraceptives, possible selection bias needs to be seen since it did not address the main characteristic of the general population in the study.

Conclusions

In general, in this study, the magnitude of long acting reversible contraceptive was 33.5%. Husband education, women occupational status, media exposure, desired number of children and approval of husband/partner to use contraceptives were predictors of

LARCs among women in Arsi Negele town, Southeastern Ethiopia.

Creating employment opportunities, male involvement, advertisement and advocacy activities through mass media need to be considered to improve utilization of LARCs.

Abbreviations

AOR: Adjusted odd ratio; CI: Confidence Interval; EDHS: Ethiopian Demographic and Health Survey; IUCD: Intra-uterine device; KM: Kilometer; SD: Standard deviation; LARC: Long acting reversible contraceptive; SSA: Sub Saharan Africa; SPSS: Statistical Package Software for Social Sciences

Acknowledgements

Arsi Negele town health office should be acknowledged for facilitating the data collection process. The study subjects need to be given respect, without their consent and the provision of the demanded information, this research work would not have been come into existence.

Authors' contributions

DTH took part in planning and designing the study, monitoring data collection process and analyzes the data. **AA** participated in planning the study, supervising data collection process and writing the manuscript. Both authors read and approved the final manuscript.

Author details

[1]Department of Reproductive Health, School of Public Health, College of Medicine and Health Sciences, Hawassa University, Hawassa, Ethiopia. [2]Department of Epidemiology, School of Public Health, College of Medicine and Health Sciences, Hawassa University, Hawassa, Ethiopia.

References

1. Stoddard A, McNicholas C, Peipert JF. Efficacy and safety of long-acting reversible contraception. Drugs. 2011 May 1;71(8):969–80.
2. United Nations, Department of Economic and Social Affairs, Population Division. Model-based estimates and projections of family planning indicators 2017. New York: United Nations; 2017b.
3. Ali M, Cleland J. Determinants of contraceptive discontinuation in six developing countries. J Biosoc Sci. 1999 Jul;31(3):343–60.
4. Federal Democratic Republic of Ethiopia, Planning and Programming Department, Ministry of Health Of Ethiopia. Health and health related indicators. Addis Ababa; 2007.
5. Demographic E. Health survey: Addis Ababa. Ethiopia and Calverton, Maryland, USA: central statistics agency and ORC macro; 2016. p. 2016.
6. Lauro D. Abortion and contraceptive use in sub-Saharan Africa: how women plan their families. Afr J Reprod Health. 2011;15(1).
7. Federal Democratic Republic of Ethiopia Ministry of Health. HSTP Health Sector Transformation Plan 2015/16–2019/20 (2008–2012 EFY). 2015.
8. Ministry of Health Ethiopia, PMNCH, WHO, World Bank, AHPSR, Participants in the Ethiopia multi-stakeholder policy review (2015). Success Factors for Women's and Children's Health: Ethiopia. 2015.
9. Federal Democratic Republic of Ethiopia Ministry of Health. National Guideline for family planning Services in Ethiopia. 2011.
10. Scott A, Glasier A. Evidence based contraceptive choices. Best Pract Res Clin Obstet Gynaecol. 2006 Oct 1;20(5):665–80.
11. Hubacher D, Mavranezouli I, Mc GE. Unintended pregnancy in subSaharan Africa: magnitude of the problem and potential role of contraceptive implants to alleviate it. Contraception. 2008;78(1):73–8.
12. Bulto GA, Zewdie TA, Beyen TK. Demand for long acting and permanent contraceptive methods and associated factors among married women of reproductive age group in Debre Markos town, north West Ethiopia. BMC Womens Health. 2014 Dec 1;14(1):46.
13. Kabalo MY. Utilization of reversible long acting family planning methods among married 15–49 years women in Areka town, Southern Ethiopia. Int J Sci Rep. 2016;2(1):1–6.
14. Gebreyesus B, Berhe S, Bayray A. Assessment of long acting and permanent contraceptive method utilization and associated factors among married women of reproductive age group in Adigrat town. Tigray Reg Ethiop. 2015;2:36–45.
15. Alemayehu M, Belachew T, Tilahun T. Factors associated with utilization of long acting and permanent contraceptive methods among married women of reproductive age in Mekelle town, Tigray region, North Ethiopia. BMC Pregnancy Childbirth. 2012 Dec;12(1):6.
16. Gultie T, Hailu D, Workineh Y. Predictors of long acting contraceptives utilization among reproductive age women in Arba Minch Zuria district, Ethiopia. Qual Prim Car. 2016;24(1):17–22.
17. Melka AS, Tekelab T, Wirtu D. Determinants of long acting and permanent contraceptive methods utilization among married women of reproductive age groups in western Ethiopia: a cross-sectional study. Pan Afr Med J. 2015;22(1).
18. Chigbu B, Onwere S, Aluka C, Kamanu C, Okoro O, Feyi-Waboso PJ. Contraceptive choices of women in rural Southeastern Nigeria. Niger J Clin Pract. 2010;13(2).
19. Schoemaker J. Contraceptive use among the poor in Indonesia. Int Fam Plan Perspect. 2005;1:106–14.
20. Mekonnen W, Worku A. Determinants of low family planning use and high unmet need in Butajira District, South Central Ethiopia. Reproductive Health. 2011;8(1):37.

Patterns of triggers, ideation and motivational factors of contraceptive utilization among women and gate-keepers in Nigeria: A scoping study on the resilient and accelerated scale up of DMPA-SC in Nigeria (RASUDIN)

Kehinde Osinowo[1*], Michael Ekholuenetale[1,2], Oluwaseun Ojomo[1], Abiodun Hassan[1,3] and Oladapo Alabi Ladipo[1]

Abstract

Background: Women have unfair share in the burden of unintended pregnancy outcome and unhealthy interpregnancy intervals. An understanding of the triggers, ideation and motivational factors influencing utilization of modern contraceptives is relevant for efforts aimed at increasing utilization among the general public, specifically sexually active women. The objective of this study is to explore the triggers, ideation and motivational factors influencing the use of modern family planning methods including depot-medroxyprogesterone acetate subcutaneous (DMPA-SC).

Methods: Qualitative methods which include; Focus Group Discussions (FGDs) and In-depth Interviews (IDIs) were used to elicit information from women of reproductive age and gate-keepers in selected Nigerian states; Rivers, Ogun, Kwara, Niger, Anambra, Delta, Lagos, Enugu and Oyo. The categories of respondents include; unmarried women aged 18-25 years, women in union aged 18-24 years using modern family planning (FP), women in union aged 25-49 years using modern FP, women in union aged 26-49 years non-users of modern FP, community leaders, health facility focal person, husbands of current users of modern FP, husbands of non-users of modern FP, religious leaders, state FP coordinators and women aged 18-49 years who currently use DMPA-SC. Maximum variation sampling techniques was used to enlist participants to participate in both FGDs and IDIs.

(Continued on next page)

* Correspondence: osinowo.k@arfh-ng.org
[1]Association for Reproductive and Family Health, 1st Floor, Block C, Millennium Builders Plaza, Abuja, Nigeria

(Continued from previous page)

Results: Respondents reported being motivated to use FP for reasons such as benefits of the method, economic situation, suitability of the methods, fear of unwanted pregnancy and its convenience. Further analysis showed that the unmarried respondents discussed more about fear of unwanted pregnancy and accessibility and affordability as a key motivator; while women in union discussed more on economic situations, encouragement from partners and benefits of FP when compared with the unmarried. In addition, respondents reported that their partners, health workers and friends influenced their decisions to use FP. Partners' encouragement, personal experience, accessibility and availability, awareness of FP and its benefits; willingness to space children and costs were notable enablers of FP use. The triggers for FP use were; appointment cards, phone calls from health workers, reminders (text messages, phone alarms and partners' support).

Conclusion: Increasing utilization therefore requires a well-planned horizontal approach that considers all enabling factors influencing utilization including women's empowerment. Family planning programmes that are client centered, address socio-cultural and gender norms and ensure access to contraceptive mix methods are recommended to improve utilization rate. This study recommends improved care-seeking behaviour through community-based awareness creation to address myths and misconceptions of family planning use, establishment of contraceptive delivery teams to prevent challenges of availability and accessibility, value clarification and tasks shifting among others to deal with the issue of inadequate family planning utilization.

Keywords: Family planning, women's autonomy, Enabling factors, Parity, Pregnancy

Background

In the past decades, Nigeria has become one of the fastest growing population in the world due to low contraceptive use [1]. The estimated population is over 170 million while more than 40,000 women in Nigeria die annually from childbirth and related complications from unplanned pregnancies [2, 3]. Globally, family planning is the major approach to population growth control and enhance the economic dividends of the country. A recent report confirmed majority of people living below poverty line in Nigeria [4]; and this brings to limelight the benefits of family planning and the need to provide the opportunity to decide freely the number, timing and spacing of childbirth. Notably, more children survive and thrive when their parents can efficiently plan for their future and cater for them. Family planning is the nexus to the development of any nation and has been observed to be the gateway intervention to achieving the third Sustainable Development Goal (SDG-3) [5, 6].

Contraceptive use remains a prominent strategy to reduce the country's maternal and infant mortality rates and prevent the spread of communicable diseases such as Human Immunodeficiency Virus (HIV)/Acquired Immunodeficiency Syndrome (AIDS) [7, 8]. Only healthy mothers can produce healthy children as family planning makes it easier for the mother to regain her strength and health after any delivery, she is able to focus on her own personal advancement and actively participate in paid employment, which invariably positively contributes to the country's economy. Moreover, evidence have shown that many families are doing better because of their decision to uptake family planning [9], they can easily invest on their children and improve their overall wellbeing. Family planning has been proven to be a major contributing factor to gender equality and women empowerment which stands as a key factor in reducing poverty, sustaining economic growth and national development [9].

Regrettably, many women, especially those living in rural communities face many hardships while trying to access family planning, which are fueled by economic, social and cultural barriers. Some women live in communities where there are widespread socio-cultural beliefs that discourage them from using family planning, while some are misinformed, others do not have the resources or means to services [10, 11]. There are many cases of women who may want to uptake family planning, but are unable to do so because of key influencer decision makers in her life such as her husband, mother or mother-in-law. Some of these people may have strong negative influence on the woman, which may make it difficult for her to access such services, especially in Northern Nigeria. According to the Nigeria Demographic and Health Survey (NDHS), in spite of the gloomy situation, about one-fifth of women who desired to use one form of contraceptive method, were not using any method. This unmet need has not reduced, in spite of the huge investment in family planning interventions [12]. The implication of this is that a lot of sexually active individuals, are not using any contraceptives to prevent unintended pregnancies.

In this study, we explore the patterns of triggers, ideation and motivational factors affecting uptake of family planning in selected states of Nigeria. One of the flagship projects of the Association for Reproductive and Family Health (ARFH), Nigeria. This study sought to review factors and triggers and the determinants of contraceptive use, with interest and focus on ideational variables through the views and perceptions that women and gate-keepers. These views and ideas reflect individuals' knowledge, opinions, ideas and views. Notably, mass media and social interaction channels contribute to shaping people's views and ideas about family planning [2, 11, 13, 14]. There has been different assertion suggesting that ideational changes in the way people think as a key factor in fertility decline, changing moral values and decision making.

In the context of Social and Behaviour Change (SBC), there has been a lot of contextual association between different factors influencing the uptake of family planning services. It is important to determine the variables to close up the gaps and barriers to inform the appropriate SBC strategies for family planning intervention design. Giving the low contraceptive prevalence rate in Nigeria [15, 16], it is important to determine factors associated with modern contraceptive use staggering at approximately 10% among currently married women [12], which is significantly lower than the regional prevalence.

Furthermore, we set out to identify or do a deeper dive of major factors of modern contraceptive method uptake; some of which include poor spousal communication and support, sociocultural and religious norms, desire for a large family, fear of side-effects, lack of knowledge of different contraceptive methods as well as distance barrier to health facility amongst others [17–19]. The exploration of the triggers, ideation and motivational factors associated with family planning becomes very important prior to SBC which the "Resilient and Accelerated Scale Up of Depot-medroxyprogesterone acetate subcutaneous in Nigeria (RASUDIN)" project is set to adopt. Contraceptive use is influenced by people's beliefs, ideas and changing the motivational factors can change people's behaviour using multiple communication channels to foster understanding about family planning, increase social approval, and improve accurate knowledge about contraceptive methods. This study explored the use of the baseline findings from community audit in a project titled "Resilient and accelerated scale up of DMPA-SC/self-injection in Nigeria (RASUDIN)". The project is being conducted in Ten Nigerian states to expand the acceptance, utilization, availability and accessibility of DMPA-SC within a broader contraceptive method mix, and kick start the roll out of Self-injection among women of reproductive age.

Methods

Study design

In this study, we utilized qualitative methods such as Focus Group Discussion (FGDs) and In-depth Interviews (IDIs) to elicit information from respondents. The qualitative study component utilized a phenomenological approach to explore the triggers, ideation and motivational factors influencing the use of modern family planning including DMPA-SC methods. This design was useful in understanding and describing the experiences of users and non-users of modern family planning methods including DMPA-SC methods. The qualitative study was conducted in nine [9] project states. See Table 1 for the details.

Data collection

Study guides were developed for data collection to address knowledge, attitude, perception and barriers to modern family planning. In addition, the guide covered motivations, enablers and promoters of modern family planning including DMPA-SC. The FGD guide was used to facilitate group discussion and elicit response from participants; the paper-based note taking template was also used to document all responses in addition to audio recording of every session. Furthermore, IDI guide and note taking tool were also used. One-on-one interviews were conducted with identified stakeholders and persons with experiences, relevant to the focus of the research. Digital recording devices were used during the FGD and IDI sessions to record all discussions and interviews. Audio recordings were complementary to the notes taken in other to ensure comprehensiveness of notes.

Table 1 Study carried out in nine out of 10 RASUDIN project states

State	Local government areas
Rivers	Phalga; Eleme; Obio-Akpor
Ogun	Ifo, Ado-Odo; and Abeokuta South
Kwara	Offa; Moro; Ilorin West; and Ilorin North.
Niger	Chanchaga; Busso; and Wushishi
Anambra	Aguata; Anaocha; and Idenmili
Delta	Isoko North; Oshimili South; Aniocha North; Ethiope East; Patani; and Sapele
Lagos	Lagos Mainland; and Ikorodu
Enugu	Enugu South; Enugu East; Enugu North; Udi-Agwu; and Nkanu West
Oyo	Akinyele; Ibadan South; Ogbomosho North; and Oyo West.

Both FGDs and IDIs interview sessions were facilitated by trained research assistants and note takers. A total of 56 FGDs and 71 IDIs were conducted across the 9 states. Total number of study participants for both FGD and IDI was 590. Table 2 shows a matrix of specific audience groups for FGDs and IDIs. The duration for FGDs and IDIs were approximately 60 min.

Sampling approach

Stratified purposeful and maximum variation sampling techniques was used to enlist participants to participate in both FGDs and IDIs. Stratification allowed the team to study subgroups of interest which included women of reproductive age disaggregated into two groups: age 18–24; and 25-49 years; users of modern contraceptives and non-users; husbands of users and non-users; women who use DMPA-SC; community and religious leaders; and family planning focal persons at the state and facility levels. Maximum variations sampling allowed us to explore how norms and perceptions varies across different groups and locations and socio-demographic variables such as age groups and marital status. Recruitment of target group was supported by staff of State Ministry of Health and ARFH state-based staff who served as mobilizers. These mobilizers ensured the right participants were selected and ready to participate in the interviews/FGD. Communication with the respondents was both in English and local dialects. The local dialects were later transcribed by experts of local dialects.

Ethical approval

Ethical approval was obtained from National Health Research Ethics Committee (NHREC) of Nigeria – Protocol approval number: NHREC/01/01/2007–17/10/2018. In addition, permission to conduct the survey was also obtained from individual State Ministry of Health. All women and gate-keepers were informed of the purpose of the study, and they were assured of the confidentiality of information obtained. No names or specific contact information were obtained from study participants. Written informed consents for both the discussions and the audiotaping were obtained from the participants. Where the consent cannot be obtained in writing, the non-written consent was formally documented and witnessed. They were informed that evidence generated from the study could inform policies made and change practices leading to the reduction of maternal mortality. They were also informed that they would incur no risk if they opt out of the interview at any time. Only those who agreed to participate in the fully explained study and gave consent were recruited for the study.

Data management

Recordings from interviews and focus group discussions were transcribed verbatim by a team of research assistants. Recordings in Hausa, Igbo and Yoruba languages were translated by experienced research assistants who also conducted the interviews in local dialects. All transcripts were exported into Dedoose 8.0, a qualitative software and analyzed based on thematic approach to

Table 2 Matrix of specific audience groups for FGDs and IDIs

Interviews	RASUDIN project states								
	Anambra	**Delta**	**Enugu**	**Kwara**	**Lagos**	**Niger**	**Ogun**	**Oyo**	**Rivers**
Unmarried women aged 18-25 years	FGD = 3	NA	NA	NA	NA	FGD = 3	NA	NA	FGD = 3
Women in union aged 18-24 years using modern FP	FGD = 2	FGD = 3	FGD = 3	FGD = 3	NA	FGD = 2	FGD = 4	FGD = 3	FGD = 3
Women in union aged 25-49 years using modern FP	FGD = 3	FGD = 3	FGD = 3	FGD = 3	FGD = 1	FGD = 3	FGD = 2	FGD = 3	FGD = 3
Women in union aged 26-49 years non-user of modern FP	IDI = 2	IDI = 2	IDI = 2	IDI = 2	IDI = 1	IDI = 3	IDI = 1	IDI = 1	IDI = 2
Community leader	IDI = 1	IDI = 1	NA	IDI = 1	NA	IDI = 1	IDI = 2	IDI = 1	IDI = 1
Health facility focal person	IDI = 1	IDI = 1	IDI = 1	IDI = 1	IDI = 1	IDI = 1	IDI = 1	IDI = 1	IDI = 1
Husbands of current users of modern FP	IDI = 1	IDI = 1	IDI = 1	IDI = 1	IDI = 1	IDI = 1	IDI = 1	IDI = 1	IDI = 1
Husbands of non-users of modern FP	IDI = 1	IDI = 1	IDI = 1	IDI = 1	NA	IDI = 1	IDI = 2	NA	IDI = 1
Religious leader	IDI = 1	IDI = 1	IDI = 1	IDI = 1	NA	IDI = 1	NA	NA	IDI = 1
State FP coordinator	IDI = 1	IDI = 1	IDI = 1	IDI = 1	NA	IDI = 1	IDI = 1	IDI = 1	IDI = 1
DKT State team	NA	NA	NA	NA	IDI = 1	NA	NA	NA	NA
Women aged 18-49 years who use DMPA-SC	NA	IDI = 1	IDI = 1	IDI = 1	IDI = 1	IDI = 1	IDI = 1	NA	NA
Total	**FGD = 8 IDI = 8**	**FGD = 6 IDI = 9**	**FGD = 6 IDI = 8**	**FGD = 6 IDI = 9**	**FGD = 1 IDI = 5**	**FGD = 8 IDI = 10**	**FGD = 6 IDI = 9**	**FGD = 6 IDI = 5**	**FGD = 9 IDI = 8**

NA Not Applicable, *FGD* Focus Group Discussion, *IDI* In-depth Interview

identify themes and patterns across research objective areas. Coding of transcripts was carried out by a team of researchers from ARFH and Centre for Communication and Social Impact (CCSI). The initial phase involved deductive coding where a set of predetermined codes reflecting main topical areas of the discussion guide applied. A harmonized coding structure was finalized by the research team who worked together to ensure consistent coding pattern, relevant themes were captured, and codes reflected the research objectives. Thereafter, inductive coding of transcripts was carried using themes and categorizing responses aimed at addressing the study objectives. Comparative assessments of patterns and themes were examined within themes and across sub-groups, and socio demographic variables used in the study; and emerging themes were identified and documented during the iterative coding process. Themes were identified with associated sub codes.

Results

Ideation and motivational factors

Motivations to use modern family planning (FP)

Concerning what motivates women to use family planning, it was observed that respondents were motivated to use FP for reasons such as benefits of the method, economic situation, and suitability of the methods, fear of unwanted pregnancy and its convenience. Further analysis showed that the unmarried respondents discussed more around fear of unwanted pregnancy and accessibility and affordability as a key motivator; while women in union discussed more around economic situations, encouragement from partners and benefits of FP when compared with the unmarried (See Table 3) below.

> *"The condition of Nigeria influenced my decision to take up family planning"* **[FGD, women aged 18–24 years, Anambra].**

Table 3 Motivating factors for women to use modern family planning

Motivations	Number of coded segments
Fear of unwanted pregnancy	44
Benefits of FP	107
Economic situation	62
Affordability and accessibility	22
Personal conviction	33
Suitability and convenience	40
Referrals	8
Encouragement from partners	6
Others	31

> *"Because if you born pass your level, who will feed them and take care of them, and the present state of the country ..."* **[FGD, women in union 18-24 years, Enugu]**

> *"The biting economy has made me use family planning"* **[FGD, women in union aged 18-24 years using modern FP]**

Further analysis to explore what respondents described as benefits of FP which motivates them include rest, good spacing leading to healthy mothers and children (Fig. 1, Table 4).

Influencers of modern FP

More respondents reported that their partners influenced their decisions to use FP. Other influencers identified during the FGD/interview sessions include: health workers, self and friends.

This study revealed that the decision-making process regarding utilization of family planning services, is influenced by the decision maker in the family. Men are dominant in this process, but some women are also involved in making the decision as well. Excerpts from some respondents are stated as below (Table 5):

> *"It is the couple but sometime the wife would sneak out and do it (family planning) if the man doesn't care about her well-being"* **[FGD, women in union, 25–29 years, Enugu]**

> *"Persistent request for sexual intercourse"* **[FGD, women aged 25-49 years, Oyo]**

Another respondent from Anambra has this to say:

> *"What made me to start using a family planning method was when I gave birth to my second daughter, she was like 7 months and I now took in again. It was too stressful with the pregnancy and I am going to work, taking care of the other child, school runs and the rest so it was not that easy, when I give birth to the third child, I and my doctor, we now discuss on the family planning because I asked the doctor if there is any way to avoid taking in so soon, so he now introduce the family planning to me. Initially I don't like the idea but when he now explains the benefits and the rest and no side effects, I now admitted it, that was my experience"* **[FGD, women in union 18-24 years using modern FP, Anambra]**

Interestingly, most of the women were motivated to take up modern family planning method following

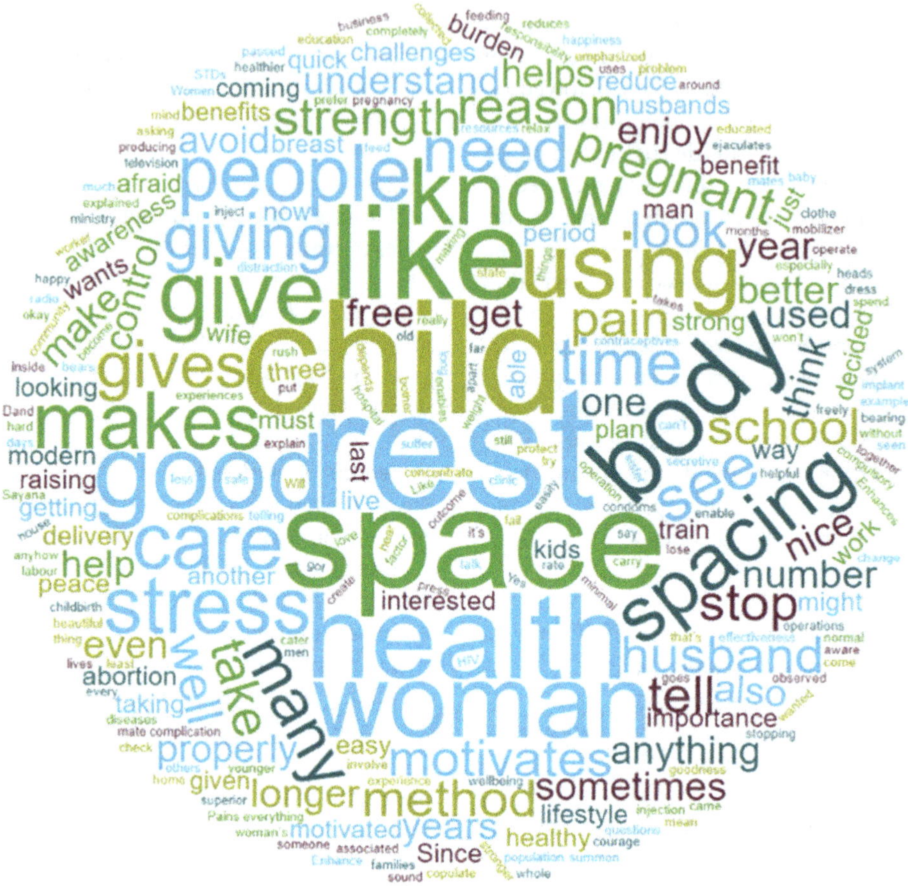

Fig. 1 What respondents describe as benefits of FP

previous history of personal negative experience of not using a method or a negative experience of someone close to them. Excerpts below describe how these women expressed these experiences in their own words:

> *"Death of a neighbor when she was giving birth to the 10th child"* **[FGD women in union aged 18-24 years, Rivers]**

> *"My girlfriend got pregnant 2 or three times and had abortions, that made me use family planning"* **[FGD Unmarried women aged 18-25 years, Rivers]**

> *"... I met a woman who was poor, even to pay the children school fees was the problem but the husband will always want her to give birth. I ask her what was the problem, she said that the man said that he is the only son of his parent. I told her the*

Table 4 Factors that encourage women to use modern FP

Encouraging factors	Number of coded segments
Affordability	21
Availability	26
Economic hardship	7
Experience of others	11
No side effects	43
Partners support	6
Sensitization/awareness	101
Others	35

Table 5 Decision makers regarding number of children

Decision makers	Number of coded segments
Both couple/partners	110
Husbands/Male partners	103
Wife/Female partners	58
Health providers	2
Mother-in-law	4
Religious leaders	2
Others	6

best thing for you now is to quietly do FP method without the husband knowing, because the husband won't even agree to it. Another example is a man who got married to a girl at her tender age and the man just want her to be giving birth and the girl was tired I told her is just to use modern FP quietly ..." **[IDI religious leader, Enugu]**

"After giving birth to my first daughter, I was using withdrawal method and the method failed me and produced this baby, now I am using the pills and I am okay with it" **[FGD, Women in union aged 18–24 using modern FP, Anambra]**

"My neighbor who is above 40years of age got pregnant after 10 years. She thought she had stopped and the pregnancy came in when she didn't expect it. That was what I saw that made me use modern FP method" **[FGD, Women in union aged 18-24 years using modern FP, Ogun]**

"I also use tablet method there was a particular month that I forgot to use it and I got pregnant, on the naming day my husband ran out from the house luckily for me I was working in the secretariat as a cleaner and I was also involve in thrift in the office that was how I use the money to do my naming ceremony when I explain to my friend she then advise that I use the implant method of 5 years which I did" **[FGD, Women in union aged 25-49 years using modern FP, Ogun]**

"The reason I decided to use FP is because of my daughter. I just gave birth to the previous pregnancy, I suffered so much I didn't even know that I was going to be alive so now I want to rest at least 2-3years" **[IDI, Women aged 18-49 years who use DMPA-SC self-inject, Niger]**

"My friend told me her mother uses Igi Ibepe (meaning fused-end of a pawpaw fruit) and after some time it failed, and she got pregnant after which she aborts the pregnancy, now she's using modern FP, so, that experience made me use modern FP" **[FGD, Women in Union aged 18-24 years using modern FP, Ogun]**

Enablers, internal and external triggers

When asked what made it easy for partners to use FP, respondents mentioned the following common factors: Partner encouragement, personal experience, Accessibility and availability, awareness of FP and its benefits; willingness to space children and costs. Excerpts below describes some of the views of respondents:

"It is my husband because he wants it, so after talking to me about it and giving me much advice on what I will gain from it, I have to obey and it favoured me also". **[FGD, women in union, 18–24 years, Enugu state].**

"Some people believe if you are on family planning in your next world you will not have a child. Some people too, they believe that if you do family planning, you will be barren for life, even when you want to have a child, you won't have a child" **[IDI, FP focal person, Rivers]**

"They don't like it, some of them because I know of a man whose wife gave birth to triplet as her first issue and she is a young girl that just got married, I spoke with the husband to let her take family planning because it is not easy for her with the 3 children at once and she doesn't have any helper, the man said no that if the wife knows about it, she will start misbehaving because she is free and if she does it, she cannot get pregnant so it will be an eye opener for the girl. She is young and still in secondary school, he said no, he doesn't want her to go that side because if she does it will be an eye opener and she will know more than she should know". **[FGD, women in union, 25–49 years, Enugu]**

Similarly, respondents were asked what would make it easy for them to continue use of FP. More mentions were made of the following: use of appointment cards, phone calls from health workers, reminders (text messages, phone alarms and reminders from partners).

"Some of these family planning last for 3 months, people like me it might even pass 6 months before I will remember that I am supposed to renew it every 3 months so it better for them to be sending alert, when you go to the nurse, she should register you and send you a reminder of the month you are to come back or else we will forget" **[FGD Women in union aged 25-49 years using modern FP, Anambra]**

"They can tell her husband to remind her about her appointment" **[IDI, Husbands of current user, Niger]**

"Where I did my own, they gave me a card and they wrote the date and the month when I will come back to renew it. It makes it easier for me to remember" **[FGD, women in union aged 18-24 years using modern FP, Rivers]**

More women from Oyo and Niger states mentioned the use of appointment cards as an enabler for continued use of FP. Among Kwara respondents, there was more mention of phone calls and reminders (text messages, partner's reminder).

The study also revealed that FP presents parents with the opportunity to properly train their children due to proper spacing (Table 6).

> *"The health centre is near to my home, so it makes it easy for me and the charges is a little amount compare to the expenses you will spend when you get pregnant"* **[FGD, women in union 25–49 years, Enugu].**

> *"Sincerely even if you have not decided to do FP, the way it is been advertised, publicized and the way its benefits are explained, you will want to do it like me it is injectable I use but the way I see people using the implants me too I will love to put it"***[FGD, women in union aged 25-49 years, Niger].**

Discussion

In this study, we explored the triggers, ideation and motivational factors of modern family planning methods including DMPA-SC across selected states in Nigeria, including; Oyo, Ogun, Rivers, Enugu, Anambra, Delta, Niger, Kwara and Lagos. Though several factors were found to influence the utilization of modern contraceptive methods, there were disparities in the motivational and enabling factors that exerted high influence over utilization. Understanding of the benefits of contraceptive utilization, sensitization/awareness creation, lack of side effects, economic hardship and accessibility to contraceptive services; be it geographical or financial accessibility was found to exert considerable influence over contraceptive utilization. Based on the findings of this study, several other factors were reported to encourage or motivate women to use modern contraceptive methods. These include; fear of unwanted/unintended pregnancy, availability and affordability of contraceptive methods, suitability and convenience, recommendation by friends or health workers, encouragement from partners, confidentiality of contraceptive methods and effectiveness of contraceptive methods. Our findings suggest that an increase in contraceptive use can be achieved by enhancing women's empowerment through spousal support, sensitization, awareness creation, financial support and positive peer influence. This brings to limelight, the effect of decision-making autonomy by women and improved knowledge level as major factors to be considered in health-related programmes to yield population control benefits to the societies in general [9].

Also, the cost of acquiring diverse contraceptive methods could determine the utilization rate. This implies that disadvantaged women will be most-at-risk of the consequences of not being able to afford contraceptives. These could include the cost to travel to a health facility or amount of time spent, or cost to purchase the service or commodities known as the indirect and direct cost respectively [20, 21]. Though family planning services in public health facilities may be with small fee for some methods, the costs of commodities could be high for some types of contraceptive methods. On the availability of contraceptive methods, though many of the health facilities and community clinics may claim to have varieties of modern contraceptives, only a limited number of key methods may actually be available. The most contraceptives methods that are usually available are condoms, injectables and pills. However, other methods like the DMPA-SC, intrauterine device (IUD), implant and other long term methods are less readily available or accessible. This finding is consistent with a previous report [11].

The fear of side effect for different contraceptive methods could hamper contraceptive use. To this effect, women may see it as a risky medical process which could lead to infertility, increase in weight gain and sometimes

Table 6 Identified Motivators, Abilities and Triggers

Motivators	Abilities	Triggers
• Fear of unwanted pregnancy • Benefits of FP • Economic situation • Accessibility and Suitability • Encouragement from partners • Negative experiences from personal and close relatives • Long lasting methods • Methods with less side effects • Awareness about methods • Cost-Affordability • Influence from friends • Availability of methods • Effectiveness of methods • Privacy of methods	• Ability to self-administer • Willingness to use • Self will • Personal experience • Personal conviction	• Appointment cards • Phone calls • Text message reminders • Partner reminder • Home visits by health worker or community volunteer

irregular bleeding. A study revealed that women who discontinued modern contraceptive methods explained that they found it difficult to give birth when they wanted to and that it took them long time to conceive, which was clearly unusual to them [22]. The perceptions of women about the side effects of modern contraceptives to a large extent also determine the level of utilization in Nigeria. Though most medicines and other medical procedures have their side effects, patients and clients continue to use them. However, with the use of modern contraceptive methods, side effects could be the major reasons why women could decline use. Common side effects which lead to non-use of contraceptive use have previously been reported to include waist and abdominal pains, high body temperature, increase in weight, irregular menstrual flow and hypertension had kept a number of clients away [23].

For the decision makers regarding the number of children to have in a family, prominently, respondents reported that both couple/partners and husband/male partner as key decision makers. Others such as wife/female partner, health workers, mother-in-law and religious leaders could also influence the family size. Some gender practices such as women's inability to make decisions concerning their reproductive health, due to early and forced marriages could greatly influence women decision-making power on the number of children they wanted for the family. These poor marriage practices, specifically in several rural communities in Nigeria has taken away self-confidence of women and also put them in a position that makes it difficult to negotiate contraceptive use with their male partners when they would actually like to stop having children.

Notably, several abilities or enablers in contraceptive utilization identified in this study include ability to self-administer the chosen method, willingness to use, self-will, personal experience and conviction. Furthermore, the triggers identified for contraceptive use include; appointment cards, phone calls, text message reminders, partner's reminder and home visits by health worker or community volunteers. The findings of this study suggest the need for interventions to promote healthy inter-pregnancy intervals to reduce adverse child health outcomes [24]. In addition, health care stakeholders would find the findings of this study interesting and a base for policy formulation and implementation.

Conclusion

Increasing utilization therefore requires a well-planned horizontal approach that considers all enabling factors influencing utilization including women's empowerment. Family planning programmes that are client centered, address socio-cultural and gender norms and ensure access to contraceptive mix methods is recommended to improve utilization rate. This study recommends improved care-seeking behaviour through community-based awareness creation to address myths and misconceptions of family planning use, establishment of contraceptive delivery teams to prevent challenges of availability and accessibility, value clarification and tasks shifting among others to deal with the issue of inadequate family planning utilization.

Abbreviations

AIDS: Acquired Immunodeficiency Syndrome; ARFH: Association for Reproductive and Family Health; CCSI: Centre for Communication and Social Impact; DMPA-SC: Depot-medroxyprogesterone acetate subcutaneous; FGDs: Focus group discussions; FP: Family planning; HIV: Human Immunodeficiency Virus; IDIs: In-depth Interviews; IUD: Intrauterine device; NDHS: Nigeria Demographic and Health Survey; NHREC: National Health Research Ethics Committee; RASUDIN: Resilient and Accelerated Scale Up of Depot-medroxyprogesterone Acetate Subcutaneous in Nigeria; SBC: Social and Behaviour Change; SDG: Sustainable Development Goal

Acknowledgements

The authors appreciate Bill and Melinda Gates Foundation for the grant.

Authors' contributions

KO, ME, OO, AH and OAL conceived and designed the study, reviewed the literature, performed data analysis and wrote the discussion of the findings. All authors critically reviewed the manuscript for its intellectual content, read and approved the final version of the manuscript. KO had the responsibility to submit the manuscript.

Author details

[1]Association for Reproductive and Family Health, 1st Floor, Block C, Millennium Builders Plaza, Abuja, Nigeria. [2]Department of Epidemiology and Medical Statistics, Faculty of Public Health, College of Medicine, University of Ibadan, Ibadan, Nigeria. [3]Family Health International (FHI360), Godab Plaza, J. S. Tarkar St, Garki, Abuja, Nigeria.

References

1. United Nations, Department of Economic and Social Affairs, Population Division. Trends in contraceptive use worldwide, 2015. 2015.
2. Adefalu AA, Ladipo OA, Akinyemi OO, Popoola OA, Latunji OO, Iyanda O. Awareness and opinions regarding contraception by women of reproductive age in North-West Nigeria. Pan Afr Med J. 2018;30 [cited 2019 Apr 2]. Available from: http://www.panafrican-med-journal.com/content/article/30/65/full/.
3. World Health Organization, UNICEF, United Nations, Department of Economic and Social Affairs, Population Division, World Bank. Trends in maternal mortality: 1990 to 2015 : estimates by WHO, UNICEF, UNFPA, World Bank Group and the United Nations Population Division. 2015. [cited 2019 Apr 2]. Available from: http://www.who.int/reproductivehealth/publications/monitoring/maternal-mortality-2015/en/.
4. World Bank. Poverty Reduction in Nigeria in the Last Decade: World Bank; 2016. [cited 2019 Apr 2]. Available from: http://elibrary.worldbank.org/doi/book/10.1596/25825.
5. Ejembi CL, Dahiru T, Aliyu AA. Contextual factors influencing modern contraceptive use in Nigeria. 2015. [cited 2019 Apr 2]; Available from: https://dhsprogram.com/publications/publication-wp120-working-papers.cfm.
6. Rosa W, editor. Transforming Our World: The 2030 Agenda for Sustainable Development. In: A New Era in Global Health. New York: Springer Publishing Company; 2017. [cited 2019 Feb 14]. Available from: http://connect.springerpub.com/lookup/doi/10.1891/9780826190123.ap02.
7. Essien EJ, Meshack AF, Peters RJ, Ogungbade GO, Osemene NI. Strategies to prevent HIV transmission among heterosexual African-American men. BMC Public Health. 2005;5(1) [cited 2019 Apr 2]. Available from: http://bmcpublichealth.biomedcentral.com/articles/10.1186/1471-2458-5-3.
8. Lotfi R, Tehrani FR, Yaghmaei F, Hajizadeh E. Barriers to condom use among women at risk of HIV/AIDS: a qualitative study from Iran. BMC Womens Health. 2012;12(1) [cited 2019 Apr 2]. Available from: http://bmcwomenshealth.biomedcentral.com/articles/10.1186/1472-6874-12-13.

9. Yaya S, Uthman OA, Ekholuenetale M, Bishwajit G. Women empowerment as an enabling factor of contraceptive use in sub-Saharan Africa: a multilevel analysis of cross-sectional surveys of 32 countries. Reprod Health. 2018;15(1) [cited 2019 Mar 22]. Available from: https://reproductive-health-journal.biomedcentral.com/articles/10.1186/s12978-018-0658-5.
10. Krenn S, Cobb L, Babalola S, Odeku M, Kusemiju B. Using behavior change communication to lead a comprehensive family planning program: the Nigerian Urban Reproductive Health Initiative. Glob Health Sci Pract. 2014;2(4):427–43.
11. Babalola S, Figueroa M-E, Krenn S. Association of Mass Media Communication with Contraceptive Use in Sub-Saharan Africa: A Meta-Analysis of Demographic and Health Surveys. J Health Commun. 2017; [cited 2019 Mar 21]. Available from: https://www.tandfonline.com/doi/abs/10.1080/10810730.2017.1373874.
12. NPC/Nigeria NPC-, International ICF. Nigeria Demographic and Health Survey 2013. 2014. [cited 2019 Apr 2]. Available from: https://dhsprogram.com/publications/publication-fr293-dhs-final-reports.cfm.
13. Ajaero CK, Odimegwu C, Ajaero ID, Nwachukwu CA. Access to mass media messages, and use of family planning in Nigeria: a spatio-demographic analysis from the 2013 DHS. BMC Public Health. 2016;16(1) [cited 2019 Mar 21]. Available from: http://bmcpublichealth.biomedcentral.com/articles/10.1186/s12889-016-2979-z.
14. Ugboaja J, Oguejiofor C, Oranu E, Igwegbe A. Assessing the influence of mass media on contraceptive use in Nigeria: a secondary analysis of 2013 Nigerian national demographic and health survey. Niger J Gen Pract. 2018;16(2):39.
15. Letamo G, Navaneetham K. Levels, trends and reasons for unmet need for family planning among married women in Botswana: a cross-sectional study. BMJ Open. 2015;5(3):–e006603.
16. Salami IC, Oladosu M. Socio-demographic factors, contraceptive use and fertility preference among married women in South- South Region of Nigeria. 2016;7.
17. Ackerson K, Zielinski R. Factors influencing use of family planning in women living in crisis affected areas of sub-Saharan Africa: a review of the literature. Midwifery. 2017;54:35–60.
18. Ahmed WAM, Shokai SB, Abduelkhair IH, Boshra AY. Factors affecting utilization of family planning services in a post-conflict setting, South Sudan: a qualitative study. AIMS Public Health. 2015;2(4):655–66.
19. Apanga PA, Adam MA. Factors influencing the uptake of family planning services in the Talensi District, Ghana. Pan Afr Med J. 2015;20 [cited 2019 Mar 18]. Available from: https://www.ncbi.nlm.nih.gov/pmc/articles/PMC4430143/.
20. Ochako R, Mbondo M, Aloo S, Kaimenyi S, Thompson R, Temmerman M, et al. Barriers to modern contraceptive methods uptake among young women in Kenya: a qualitative study. BMC Public Health. 2015;15(1) [cited 2019 Mar 18]. Available from: http://bmcpublichealth.biomedcentral.com/articles/10.1186/s12889-015-1483-1.
21. Do M, Kurimoto N. Women's empowerment and choice of contraceptive methods in selected African countries. Int Perspect Sex Reprod Health. 2012; 38(01):023–33.
22. Achana FS, Bawah AA, Jackson EF, Welaga P, Awine T, Asuo-Mante E, et al. Spatial and socio-demographic determinants of contraceptive use in the Upper East region of Ghana. Reprod Health. 2015;12(1) [cited 2019 Mar 25]. Available from: https://reproductive-health-journal.biomedcentral.com/articles/10.1186/s12978-015-0017-8.
23. Hindin MJ, McGough LJ, Adanu RM. Misperceptions, misinformation and myths about modern contraceptive use in Ghana. J Fam Plann Reprod Health Care. 2014;40(1):30–5.
24. Yaya S, Uthman OA, Ekholuenetale M, Bishwajit G, Adjiwanou V. Effects of birth spacing on adverse childhood health outcomes: evidence from 34 countries in sub-Saharan Africa. J Matern Fetal Neonatal Med. 2019;0(0):1–8.

Permissions

All chapters in this book were first published by BioMed Central; hereby published with permission under the Creative Commons Attribution License or equivalent. Every chapter published in this book has been scrutinized by our experts. Their significance has been extensively debated. The topics covered herein carry significant findings which will fuel the growth of the discipline. They may even be implemented as practical applications or may be referred to as a beginning point for another development.

The contributors of this book come from diverse backgrounds, making this book a truly international effort. This book will bring forth new frontiers with its revolutionizing research information and detailed analysis of the nascent developments around the world.

We would like to thank all the contributing authors for lending their expertise to make the book truly unique. They have played a crucial role in the development of this book. Without their invaluable contributions this book wouldn't have been possible. They have made vital efforts to compile up to date information on the varied aspects of this subject to make this book a valuable addition to the collection of many professionals and students.

This book was conceptualized with the vision of imparting up-to-date information and advanced data in this field. To ensure the same, a matchless editorial board was set up. Every individual on the board went through rigorous rounds of assessment to prove their worth. After which they invested a large part of their time researching and compiling the most relevant data for our readers.

The editorial board has been involved in producing this book since its inception. They have spent rigorous hours researching and exploring the diverse topics which have resulted in the successful publishing of this book. They have passed on their knowledge of decades through this book. To expedite this challenging task, the publisher supported the team at every step. A small team of assistant editors was also appointed to further simplify the editing procedure and attain best results for the readers.

Apart from the editorial board, the designing team has also invested a significant amount of their time in understanding the subject and creating the most relevant covers. They scrutinized every image to scout for the most suitable representation of the subject and create an appropriate cover for the book.

The publishing team has been an ardent support to the editorial, designing and production team. Their endless efforts to recruit the best for this project, has resulted in the accomplishment of this book. They are a veteran in the field of academics and their pool of knowledge is as vast as their experience in printing. Their expertise and guidance has proved useful at every step. Their uncompromising quality standards have made this book an exceptional effort. Their encouragement from time to time has been an inspiration for everyone.

The publisher and the editorial board hope that this book will prove to be a valuable piece of knowledge for researchers, students, practitioners and scholars across the globe.

List of Contributors

Tamrat Shaweno
Department of Epidemiology, Faculty of Public Health, Jimma University, Jimma, Ethiopia

Zerihun Kura
Biostatistics Unit, Department of Epidemiology, Faculty of Public Health, Jimma University, Jimma, Ethiopia

Tadesse Wuletaw Demissie
Department of Nursing, Debre Tabor Health Science College, Debra Tabor, Ethiopia

Araya Mesfin Nigatu
Department of Health Informatics, Institute of Public Health, University of Gondar, Gondar, Ethiopia

Getnet Mihretie Beyene
Department of Health Informatics, Institute of Public Health, University of Gondar, Gondar, Ethiopia
Department of Nursing, Debre Tabor University, Debra Tabor, Ethiopia

Elynn Kann Sanchez, Courtney McGuire and Lisa M. Calhoun
Carolina Population Center, University of North Carolina-Chapel Hill, Chapel Hill, USA

Gwyn Hainsworth
The Bill & Melinda Gates Foundation, Seattle, USA

Ilene S. Speizer
Carolina Population Center, University of North Carolina-Chapel Hill, Chapel Hill, USA
Gillings School of Global Public Health, Department of Maternal and Child Health, UNC, Chapel Hill, USA

Afra Nuwasiima, Agnes Watsemba, Allan Eyapu and Peter Kaddu
Living Goods, Kampala, Uganda

Justin Loiseau
Global Research & Evidence Strategy Living Goods, Nairobi, Kenya

Biruktawit Fekade Woldu and Negeso Gebeyehu Gejo
Department of Midwifery, College of Medicine and Health Sciences, Wachemo University, Hossana, Ethiopia

Tadesse Lelago Ermolo
Department of Nursing, College of Medicine and Health Sciences, Wachemo University, Hossana, Ethiopia

Lidiya Gutema Lemu
Department of Midwifery, College of Health Sciences, Mizan Tepi University, Mizan Aman, Ethiopia

Alemu Kebede, Elias Merdassa and Tariku Tesfaye Bekuma
Department of Public Health, Institute of Health Sciences, Wollega University, Nekemte, Ethiopia

Sileshi G. Abaya
Public Health, Adama Hospital Medical College, Adama, Ethiopia

Michael J. Mahande and Caroline Amour
Department of Epidemiology and Biostatistics, Institute of Public Health, Kilimanjaro Christian Medical University College, Tanzania

Ryoko Sato, Bilikisu Elewonibi and Iqbal Shah
Department of Global Health and Population, Harvard T.H. Chan School of Public Health, Boston, USA

Rachel Manongi and Amina Farah
Department of Community Health, Institute of Public Health, Kilimanjaro Christian Medical University College, Moshi, Tanzania

Sia E. Msuya
Department of Epidemiology and Biostatistics, Institute of Public Health, Kilimanjaro Christian Medical University College, Moshi, Tanzania
Department of Community Health, Institute of Public Health, Kilimanjaro Christian Medical University College, Moshi, Tanzania
Department of Community Health, KCMC Hospital, Moshi, Tanzania

Eugene Budu
Department of Population and Health, University of Cape Coast, Cape Coast, Ghana

Richard Gyan Aboagye
School of Public Health, University of Health and Allied Sciences, Ho, Ghana

Ebenezer Agbaglo
Department of English, University of Cape Coast, Cape Coast, Ghana

Francis Arthur-Holmes
Department of Sociology and Social Policy, Lingnan University, 8 Castle Peak Road, Tuen Mun, Hong Kong

Collins Adu
Department of Health Promotion, Education and Disability Studies, Kwame Nkrumah University of Science and Technology, Kumasi, Ghana

Anita Gracious Archer
School of Nursing and Midwifery, University of Health and Allied Sciences, Ho, Ghana

Yaa Boahemaa Gyasi Aderoju
Department of Adult Health Nursing, School of Nursing and Midwifery, University of Cape Coast, Cape Coast, Ghana

Abdul-Aziz Seidu
Department of Population and Health, University of Cape Coast, Cape Coast, Ghana
College of Public Health, Medical and Veterinary Services, James Cook University, Townsville, Australia

Ayaga A. Bawah, Patrick Asuming, Caesar Agula and Charles Agyei-Asabere
University of Ghana, Legon, Accra, Ghana

Elizabeth G. Henry and David Canning
TH Chan School of Public Health, Harvard University, Boston, USA

Delayehu Bekele, Feiruz Surur and Balkachew Nigatu
Department of Obstetrics and Gynecology, Saint Paul's Hospital Millennium Medical College, Addis Ababa, Ethiopia

Alula Teklu
Research Office, Saint Paul's Hospital Millennium Medical College, Addis Ababa, Ethiopia

Tewodros Getinet
Public Health Department, Saint Paul's Hospital Millennium Medical College, Addis Ababa, Ethiopia

Munir Kassa
Federal Ministry of Health, Ministry's Office, Addis Ababa, Ethiopia

Merhawi Gebremedhin and Berhe Gebremichael
School of Public Health, Haramaya University, Harar, Ethiopia

Yonas Abesha
Private Consultancy Practice, Addis Ababa, Ethiopia

James Forty, Serai Daniel Rakgoasi and Mpho Keetile
Department of Population Studies, University of Botswana, Private Bag UB, 00705 Gaborone, Botswana

Markos Desalegn
Department of Public health, College of medicine and health sciences, Jigjiga University, Jigjiga, Somali region, Ethiopia

Ayele Belachew and Muluken Gizaw
School of public health, college of health sciences, Addis Ababa University, Addis Abeba, Ethiopia

Gemechu Kejela and Robsan Gudeta
Department of public health, Institute of health sciences, Wollega University, Oromia region, Nekemte, Ethiopia

Joseph K. Wulifan and Stephen Kpinpuo
School of Business and Law, Department of Administration and Management Studies, University for Development Studies, Wa-campus, Wa, Ghana

Jacob Mazalale
Department of Economics, University of Malawi, Chancellor College, Zomba, Malawi

Christabel Kambala
Environmental Health Department, The Malawi Polytechnic, University of Malawi, Chichiri, Blantyre 3, Blantyre, Malawi

William Angko
School of Business and Law, Department of Banking and Finance, University for Development Studies, Wa-campus, Wa, Ghana

Job Asante
Faculty of Integrated Development Studies, Campus Officer, University for Development Studies, Wa-campus, Wa, Ghana

Albino Kalolo
Department of Public Health, St. Francis University College of Health and Allied Sciences, Ifakara, Tanzania

Louis Kobina Dadzie and Justice Kanor Tetteh
Department of Population and Health, University of Cape Coast, Cape Coast, Ghana

Bright Opoku Ahinkorah and Edward Kwabena Ameyaw
School of Public Health, Faculty of Health, University of Technology Sydney, Sydney, Australia

Sanni Yaya
School of International Development and Global Studies, University of Ottawa, Ottawa, Canada
The George Institute for Global Health, The University of Oxford, Oxford, UK

Biresaw Wassihun, Kidist Wosen, Asmare Getie, Kalkidan Belay, Rehal Tesfaye, Tewodros Tadesse, Yosef Alemayehu, Manaye Yihune and Addis Aklilu
College of Medicine and Health Sciences, Arba Minch University, Arba Minch, Ethiopia

Kassahun Gebayehu
Department of Nursing, College of Medicine and Health Sciences, University of Gondar, Gondar, Ethiopia

Shegaw Zeleke
Colleges of Medicine and Health Sciences, Debre Tabor University, Debre Tabor, Ethiopia

Elizabeth Corey, Stephanie Frazin, Samantha Heywood and Sadia Haider
Department of Obstetrics and Gynecology, University of Illinois at Chicago, 820 South Wood Street, Chicago, IL 60612, USA

Lemessa Assefa and Ebisa Turi
Department of Public health, Institute of Health Sciences, Wollega University, Nekemte, Ethiopia

Zemenu Shasho
Deputy of the health center, Gimbi Health Center, Western Wollega Zone, Gimbi, Ethiopia

Habtamu Kebebe Kasaye
Department of Midwifery, Institute of Health Sciences, Wollega University, Nekemte, Ethiopia

Edao Tesa
Department of Public Health, College of Medical and Health Sciences, Madda Walabu University, Goba Referral Hospital, Goba, Ethiopia

Ginenus Fekadu
Department of Pharmacy, Institute of Health Sciences, Wollega University, Nekemte, Oromia, Ethiopia
School of Pharmacy, Faculty of Medicine, The Chinese University of Hong Kong, Shatin, New territory, Hong Kong

Chris Smith
Graduate School of Tropical Medicine and Global Health, Nagasaki University, Nagasaki, Japan
Department of Population Health, London School of Hygiene & Tropical Medicine, London, UK

Rachel H. Scott and Caroline Free
Department of Population Health, London School of Hygiene & Tropical Medicine, London, UK

Tansy Edwards
MRC Tropical Epidemiology Group, London School of Hygiene & Tropical Medicine, London, UK

Kim Jonas and Catherine Mathews
Health Systems Research Unit, South African Medical Research Council, Cape Town, South Africa
Adolescent Health Research Unit, Department of Psychiatry and Mental Health, University of Cape Town, Cape Town, South Africa

Moira Kalichman and Seth Kalichman
Department of Psychology, University of Connecticut, Storrs, Mansfield, CT, USA

Chelsea Morroni
Liverpool School of Tropical Medicine, Liverpool, UK
Women's Health Research Unit, School of Public Health and Family Medicine, University of Cape Town, Cape Town, South Africa
Botswana-University of Pennsylvania Partnership, Gaborone, Botswana

Wende Safari, Mark Urassa, Baltazar Mtenga and John Changalucha
National Institute for Medical Research (NIMR), Mwanza Centre, Mwanza, Tanzania

Basia Zaba and Kathryn Church
London School of Hygiene and Tropical Medicine, London, UK

James Beard and Jim Todd
National Institute for Medical Research (NIMR), Mwanza Centre, Mwanza, Tanzania
London School of Hygiene and Tropical Medicine, London, UK

Desalegn Tsegaw Hibstu
Department of Reproductive Health, School of Public Health, College of Medicine and Health Sciences, Hawassa University, Hawassa, Ethiopia

Akalewold Alemayehu
Department of Epidemiology, School of Public Health, College of Medicine and Health Sciences, Hawassa University, Hawassa, Ethiopia

Kehinde Osinowo, Oluwaseun Ojomo and Oladapo Alabi Ladipo
Association for Reproductive and Family Health, 1st Floor, Block C, Millennium Builders Plaza, Abuja, Nigeria

Michael Ekholuenetale
Association for Reproductive and Family Health, 1st Floor, Block C, Millennium Builders Plaza, Abuja, Nigeria
Department of Epidemiology and Medical Statistics, Faculty of Public Health, College of Medicine, University of Ibadan, Ibadan, Nigeria

Abiodun Hassan
Association for Reproductive and Family Health, 1st Floor, Block C, Millennium Builders Plaza, Abuja, Nigeria
Family Health International (FHI360), Godab Plaza, J. S. Tarkar St, Garki, Abuja, Nigeria

Index

www.ingramcontent.com/pod-product-compliance
Lightning Source LLC
LaVergne TN
LVHW082127200926
848484LV00008B/2016